Recent Advances in Nutritional Psychiatry

Recent Advances in Nutritional Psychiatry

Editor

Giuseppe Grosso

MDPI • Basel • Beijing • Wuhan • Barcelona • Belgrade • Manchester • Tokyo • Cluj • Tianjin

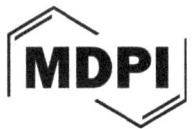

Editor
Giuseppe Grosso
Department of Biomedical and
Biotechnological Sciences
University of Catania
Catania
Italy

Editorial Office
MDPI
St. Alban-Anlage 66
4052 Basel, Switzerland

This is a reprint of articles from the Special Issue published online in the open access journal *Nutrients* (ISSN 2072-6643) (available at: www.mdpi.com/journal/nutrients/special_issues/ nutritional_psychiatry).

For citation purposes, cite each article independently as indicated on the article page online and as indicated below:

LastName, A.A.; LastName, B.B.; LastName, C.C. Article Title. *Journal Name* **Year**, *Volume Number*, Page Range.

ISBN 978-3-0365-1346-1 (Hbk)
ISBN 978-3-0365-1345-4 (PDF)

Contents

About the Editor

Giuseppe Grosso

Dr. Giuseppe Grosso's research focuses on evidence-based nutrition, a recently emerged field as the bottom line of the Health Technology Assessment applied to food and nutrition. Its main interests include the impact of dietary and lifestyle habits on common non-communicable diseases. He is interested in evidence synthesis aimed to generate policy-oriented research in the area of public health nutrition. Dr. Giuseppe Grosso is a cum laude graduated medical doctor. Dr. Grosso holds a specialization in public health and a PhD in neuropharmacology. He is currently working as a Assistant Professor of human nutrition at the Department of Biomedical and Biotechnological Sciences, University of Catania, Catania, Italy; he has been recognized as Highly Cited Researcher from Clarivate-Web of Science for the years 2019 and 2020; he is the President of the Food and Nutrition Section of the European Public Health Association (EUPHA).

Preface to "Recent Advances in Nutritional Psychiatry"

Mental health disorders represent a major public health issue due to their impact on years lived with disability, and cross-talk with other non-communicable diseases, such as cancer, cardiovascular diseases, and diabetes. Importantly, most of these conditions can be prevented by implementing healthy dietary habits. Consequently, a recently developed field of psychiatry, "nutritional psychiatry", is focused on investigating the relationships among dietary factors, eating habits, and mental disorders in order to form methods for the prevention and treatment of mental disorders.

This Special Collection from *Nutrients* will focus on both observational and molecular studies that investigate the effects of nutrients, foods, and whole dietary patterns on mental health. We invited authors to submit reviews and studies providing evidence of the effects of nutritional factors on cognitive function, depression, sleep patterns, stress, and quality of life.

Giuseppe Grosso
Editor

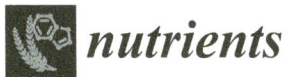 *nutrients*

Editorial

Nutritional Psychiatry: How Diet Affects Brain through Gut Microbiota

Giuseppe Grosso

Department of Biomedical and Biotechnological Sciences, University of Catania, 95123 Catania, Italy; giuseppe.grosso@unict.it; Tel.: +39-0954-781-187

Abstract: Nutritional sciences have been recognized as being of paramount importance for the prevention of non-communicable diseases. Among others, mental health disorders have been hypothesized to be influenced by dietary risk through a variety of molecular mechanisms. The improvements in the technology and implementation of-omics sciences in terms of nutrition have created the possibility of studying the relation between diet, gut microbiota and mental health. The gut–brain–axis represents the core rationale setting the stage for a relatively new discipline of study defined as "nutritional psychiatry". Research on this matter will help to better understand the relation between food and mood, sleep quality, cognition, and mental health in general.

Keywords: diet; dietary factors; lifestyle; gut microbiota; nutritional psychiatry; mental health; sleep; cognitive; mood; anxiety

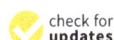 check for updates

Citation: Grosso, G. Nutritional Psychiatry: How Diet Affects Brain through Gut Microbiota. *Nutrients* **2021**, *13*, 1282. https://doi.org/10.3390/nu13041282

Received: 7 April 2021
Accepted: 12 April 2021
Published: 14 April 2021

Publisher's Note: MDPI stays neutral with regard to jurisdictional claims in published maps and institutional affiliations.

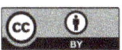
Mental health disorders have risen as common morbidities of this century [1]. They are characterized by a number of clinical conditions, among which, stress, anxiety, and depression are the most common, which could evolve and mutate into far more dangerous illnesses, including psychosis and schizophrenia [2]. In 2017, it was estimated that mental disorders accounted for about 14% of worldwide years lived with disability (depression alone accounted for over 50 million and anxiety disorders about half of that) [3]. The reasons for such a rise in the incidence of mental health disorders is unknown: from an epidemiological point of view, a better knowledge of these conditions allowed a more timely recognition and consequently, a higher rate of diagnosis. However, an increased incidence of such illnesses has been recognized, and a common hypothesis relies on the modern lifestyle and the "stressogenic" environment we live in [4,5]. In fact, lifestyles have greatly changed over the last 50 years: urbanization and the technological improvements up to the so-called "information revolution", the modern lifestyle characterized by longer days (due to night lights), the long screen-hours, accompanied by the pressure from a competitive society may finally result in a mismatch with the human genetic heritage, largely unchanged from our ancestors [6]. The resulting trends over the future projections of incidence of mental diseases are thus alarming, being anticipated that by 2030 mental health diseases will be the leading cause of disease burden globally [7].

While pharmacological therapies have been of primary use and utility to cure mental disorders, behavioral interventions have caught on in recent decades as support for conventional therapy. However, nearly no progress has been made regarding the prevention of such conditions, as no univocal risk factor has been identified. With the discovery of inflammation playing a role in several central nervous system diseases [8], an intriguing hypothesis has been postulated not long ago, suggesting that dietary factors may play a role in mental health diseases [9]. From a mechanistic point of view, a potential direct anti-inflammatory effect (i.e., omega-3 polyunsaturated fatty acids), antioxidant action (i.e., polyphenols able to pass the blood–barrier membrane, such as anthocyanins, etc.), or functional modulation (i.e., group B vitamins, glycine, L-ornithine, tryptophan amino acids, etc.), may provide the rationale for the potential effects of diet on mental health [10].

Nutrients **2021**, *13*, 1282. https://doi.org/10.3390/nu13041282

https://www.mdpi.com/journal/nutrients

This evidence has set the stage for a new discipline of study defined as "nutritional psychiatry" [11].

Today, nutritional support as supplements or dietary interventions characterize adjuvant therapy against depression, anxiety, stress, and cognitive decline [12–16]. Moreover, a great deal of studies have been conducted relating dietary variables and the prevention of mental health disorders [17–19]. Together with the aforementioned mechanisms, current evidence suggests that the rich innervation of the gastrointestinal system might deliver impulses and signals to the brain in addition to receiving them [20]. In this context, the gut microbiota may play an important role in the integrity and proper functionality of the human gut: certain dietary factors may affect the intestinal microbiome, resulting in the alteration of nutrient absorption, weakening of the intestinal barrier against toxins and bacteria per se, the determination of chronic inflammation, and subsequently, the activation of neural pathways that directly affect the functionality of the central nervous system [21]. Alterations of gut microbiota have been demonstrated in association with changes in food intake or adherence to an entire dietary pattern (in an healthy or unhealthy direction) [22]. Recent evidence also suggests that circadian rhythms and feeding time (i.e., intermittent fasting or time-restricted feeding) may also play a role in the gut microbiota profile, with consequent potential effects on systemic inflammation and mental health outcomes.

The Special Issue "Recent Advances in Nutritional Psychiatry" provided new and interesting insights on this matter including cognitive status, depression, and sleep quality. The study of Fisicaro et al. [23] showed that mocha (stove) coffee consumption may be associated with improved cognitive and mood status. Currenti et al. [24] also provided the first evidence that not only diet quality features, but also time of eating may play a role on cognitive status: specifically, individuals having their eating time restricted to 10 h were less likely to have cognitive impairment in a cohort of southern Italian older adults. A laboratory study explored the hypothesis that the content in anthocyanins of isogenic wheat lines may be determinant to exert positive effects on neurodegenerative disorders [25]. Concerning sleep quality, two studies have shown an association of higher adherence to the Mediterranean diet during pregnancy [26] and food security with sleep quality [27], respectively; a third study from our group provided the first evidence of a potential role played by dietary polyphenol content in sleep quality [28]. Diet quality has also been related to depression in two studies: Cebrino et al. [29] reported that non-depressive individuals had a higher diet quality than depressive ones in a nationwide cross-sectional study conducted in Spain; in the study of Marozoff et al. [30], the authors showed that increasing Healthy Eating Index-Canada scores were associated with fewer physician visits for depression in a prospective investigation of adults living in Alberta (Canada).

The review of Janda et al. [31] summarized the evidence from clinical trials of the therapeutic effects of Passiflora incarnata in neuropsychiatric disorders showing potential for its use against anxiety symptoms with no adverse effects to mention. Finally, the review of Wlodarczyk et al. [32] points out that the ketogenic diet might be used as an add on to common psychotherapy and pharmacology for anxiety disorders.

The growing number of studies related to nutritional psychiatry corroborates the need for a better understanding of the relation between dietary factors and mental health disorders. Future studies should fill the gap between the epidemiological and clinical evidence of the prevention of mental health disorders through dietary factors by investigating mechanistic features related to gut microbiota and its interaction with the central nervous system.

Funding: This study was a part of the ADICOS (Association between Dietary Factors and Cognitive Status) project funded by the "Piano di Incentivi per la Ricerca di Ateneo 2020/2022–Starting Grant" of the University of Catania, Italy (G.G.).

Institutional Review Board Statement: Not applicable.

Informed Consent Statement: Not applicable.

Data Availability Statement: Not applicable.

Conflicts of Interest: The author declares no conflict of interest. The funders had no role in the design of the study, in the collection, analyses, or interpretation of data, in the writing of the manuscript, or in the decision to publish the results.

References

1. Whiteford, A.H.; Degenhardt, L.; Rehm, J.; Baxter, A.J.; Ferrari, A.J.; Erskine, E.H.; Charlson, F.J.; Norman, E.R.; Flaxman, A.D.; Johns, N.; et al. Global burden of disease attributable to mental and substance use disorders: Findings from the Global Burden of Disease Study 2010. *Lancet* **2013**, *382*, 1575–1586. [CrossRef]
2. Rehm, J.; Shield, K.D. Global Burden of Disease and the Impact of Mental and Addictive Disorders. *Curr. Psychiatry Rep.* **2019**, *21*, 10. [CrossRef] [PubMed]
3. GBD 2017 Disease and Injury Incidence and Prevalence Collaborators. Global, regional, and national incidence, prevalence, and years lived with disability for 354 diseases and injuries for 195 countries and territories, 1990–2017: A systematic analy-sis for the Global Burden of Disease Study 2017. *Lancet* **2018**, *392*, 1789–1858. [CrossRef]
4. Hoare, E.; Jacka, F.; Berk, M. The impact of urbanization on mood disorders. *Curr. Opin. Psychiatry* **2019**, *32*, 198–203. [CrossRef]
5. Lewis-Fernández, R.; Hinton, D.E.; Laria, A.J.; Patterson, E.H.; Hofmann, S.G.; Craske, M.G.; Stein, D.J.; Asnaani, A.; Liao, B. Culture and the anxiety disorders: Recommendations for DSM-V. *Depress. Anxiety* **2010**, *27*, 212–229. [CrossRef]
6. Grinde, B. An approach to the prevention of anxiety-related disorders based on evolutionary medicine. *Prev. Med.* **2005**, *40*, 904–909. [CrossRef] [PubMed]
7. Patel, V.; Saxena, S.; Lund, C.; Thornicroft, G.; Baingana, F.; Bolton, P.; Chisholm, D.; Collins, P.Y.; Cooper, J.L.; Eaton, J.; et al. The Lancet Commission on global mental health and sustainable development. *Lancet* **2018**, *392*, 1553–1598. [CrossRef]
8. Caruso, G.; Fresta, C.G.; Grasso, M.; Santangelo, R.; Lazzarino, G.; Lunte, S.M.; Caraci, F. Inflammation as the Common Biological Link Between Depression and Cardiovascular Diseases: Can Carnosine Exert a Protective Role? *Curr. Med. Chem.* **2020**, *27*, 1782–1800. [CrossRef]
9. Grosso, G. Nutrition and aging: Is there a link to cognitive health? *Int. J. Food Sci. Nutr.* **2020**, *71*, 265–266. [CrossRef] [PubMed]
10. Godos, J.; Currenti, W.; Angelino, D.; Mena, P.; Castellano, S.; Caraci, F.; Galvano, F.; Del Rio, D.; Ferri, R.; Grosso, G. Diet and Mental Health: Review of the Recent Updates on Molecular Mechanisms. *Antioxidants* **2020**, *9*, 346. [CrossRef] [PubMed]
11. Logan, A.C.; Jacka, F.N. Nutritional psychiatry research: An emerging discipline and its intersection with global urbanization, environmental challenges and the evolutionary mismatch. *J. Physiol. Anthr.* **2014**, *33*, 22. [CrossRef] [PubMed]
12. Grosso, G.; Pajak, A.; Marventano, S.; Castellano, S.; Galvano, F.; Bucolo, C.; Drago, F.; Caraci, F. Role of Omega-3 Fatty Acids in the Treatment of Depressive Disorders: A Comprehensive Meta-Analysis of Randomized Clinical Trials. *PLoS ONE* **2014**, *9*, e96905. [CrossRef]
13. Caruso, G.; Godos, J.; Castellano, S.; Micek, A.; Murabito, P.; Galvano, F.; Ferri, R.; Grosso, G.; Caraci, F. The Therapeutic Potential of Carnosine/Anserine Supplementation against Cognitive Decline: A Systematic Review with Meta-Analysis. *Biomedicines* **2021**, *9*, 253. [CrossRef]
14. Young, L.M.; Pipingas, A.; White, D.J.; Gauci, S.; Scholey, A. A Systematic Review and Meta-Analysis of B Vitamin Supple-mentation on Depressive Symptoms, Anxiety, and Stress: Effects on Healthy and 'At-Risk'Individuals. *Nutrients* **2019**, *11*, 2232. [CrossRef]
15. Cheng, Y.; Huang, Y.; Huang, W. The effect of vitamin D supplement on negative emotions: A systematic review and meta-analysis. *Depress. Anxiety* **2020**, *37*, 549–564. [CrossRef]
16. Marx, W.; Lane, M.; Rocks, T.; Ruusunen, A.; Loughman, A.; Lopresti, A.; Marshall, S.; Berk, M.; Jacka, F.; Dean, O.M. Effect of saffron supplementation on symptoms of depression and anxiety: A systematic review and meta-analysis. *Nutr. Rev.* **2019**, *77*, 557–571. [CrossRef]
17. Wu, P.-Y.; Chen, K.-M.; Belcastro, F. Dietary patterns and depression risk in older adults: Systematic review and meta-analysis. *Nutr. Rev.* **2020**. [CrossRef]
18. McCabe, D.; Lisy, K.; Lockwood, C.; Colbeck, M. The impact of essential fatty acid, B vitamins, vitamin C, magnesium and zinc supplementation on stress levels in women. *JBI Database Syst. Rev. Implement. Rep.* **2017**, *15*, 402–453. [CrossRef]
19. Godos, J.; Grosso, G.; Castellano, S.; Galvano, F.; Caraci, F.; Ferri, R. Association between diet and sleep quality: A systematic review. *Sleep Med. Rev.* **2021**, *57*, 101430. [CrossRef] [PubMed]
20. Salvucci, E. The human-microbiome superorganism and its modulation to restore health. *Int. J. Food Sci. Nutr.* **2019**, *70*, 781–795. [CrossRef] [PubMed]
21. Ceppa, F.; Mancini, A.; Tuohy, K. Current evidence linking diet to gut microbiota and brain development and function. *Int. J. Food Sci. Nutr.* **2018**, *70*, 1–19. [CrossRef]
22. Marx, W.; Moseley, G.; Berk, M.; Jacka, F. Nutritional psychiatry: The present state of the evidence. *Proc. Nutr. Soc.* **2017**, *76*, 427–436. [CrossRef]
23. Fisicaro, F.; Lanza, G.; Pennisi, M.; Vagli, C.; Cantone, M.; Pennisi, G.; Ferri, R.; Bella, R. Moderate Mocha Coffee Consumption Is Associated with Higher Cognitive and Mood Status in a Non-Demented Elderly Population with Subcortical Ischemic Vascular Disease. *Nutrients* **2021**, *13*, 536. [CrossRef]

24. Currenti, W.; Godos, J.; Castellano, S.; Caruso, G.; Ferri, R.; Caraci, F.; Grosso, G.; Galvano, F. Association between Time Restricted Feeding and Cognitive Status in Older Italian Adults. *Nutrients* **2021**, *13*, 191. [CrossRef] [PubMed]
25. Tikhonova, M.A.; Shoeva, O.Y.; Tenditnik, M.V.; Ovsyukova, M.V.; Akopyan, A.A.; Dubrovina, N.I.; Amstislavskaya, T.G.; Khlestkina, E.K. Evaluating the Effects of Grain of Isogenic Wheat Lines Differing in the Content of Anthocyanins in Mouse Models of Neurodegenerative Disorders. *Nutrients* **2020**, *12*, 3877. [CrossRef]
26. Flor-Alemany, M.; Nestares, T.; Alemany-Arrebola, I.; Marín-Jiménez, N.; Borges-Cosic, M.; Aparicio, V.A. Influence of Dietary Habits and Mediterranean Diet Adherence on Sleep Quality during Pregnancy. The GESTAFIT Project. *Nutrients* **2020**, *12*, 3569. [CrossRef]
27. Isaura, E.R.; Chen, Y.-C.; Su, H.-Y.; Yang, S.-H. The Relationship between Food Security Status and Sleep Disturbance among Adults: A Cross-Sectional Study in an Indonesian Population. *Nutrients* **2020**, *12*, 3411. [CrossRef] [PubMed]
28. Godos, J.; Ferri, R.; Castellano, S.; Angelino, D.; Mena, P.; Del Rio, D.; Caraci, F.; Galvano, F.; Grosso, G. Specific Dietary (Poly)phenols Are Associated with Sleep Quality in a Cohort of Italian Adults. *Nutrients* **2020**, *12*, 1226. [CrossRef]
29. Cebrino, J.; De La Cruz, S.P. Diet Quality and Sociodemographic, Lifestyle, and Health-Related Determinants among People with Depression in Spain: New Evidence from a Cross-Sectional Population-Based Study (2011–2017). *Nutrients* **2020**, *13*, 106. [CrossRef] [PubMed]
30. Marozoff, S.; Veugelers, P.J.; Dabravolskaj, J.; Eurich, D.T.; Ye, M.; Maximova, K. Diet Quality and Health Service Utilization for Depression: A Prospective Investigation of Adults in Alberta's Tomorrow Project. *Nutrients* **2020**, *12*, 2437. [CrossRef] [PubMed]
31. Janda, K.; Wojtkowska, K.; Jakubczyk, K.; Antoniewicz, J.; Skonieczna-Żydecka, K. *Passiflora incarnata* in Neuropsychiatric Disorders—A Systematic Review. *Nutrients* **2020**, *12*, 3894. [CrossRef] [PubMed]
32. Włodarczyk, A.; Cubała, W.J.; Wielewicka, A. Ketogenic Diet: A Dietary Modification as an Anxiolytic Approach? *Nutrients* **2020**, *12*, 3822. [CrossRef] [PubMed]

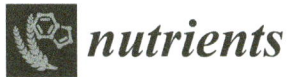

nutrients

MDPI

Article

Association between Time Restricted Feeding and Cognitive Status in Older Italian Adults

Walter Currenti [1], Justyna Godos [2], Sabrina Castellano [3], Giuseppe Caruso [4], Raffaele Ferri [2], Filippo Caraci [2,4], Giuseppe Grosso [1,*] and Fabio Galvano [1]

1. Department of Biomedical and Biotechnological Sciences, University of Catania, 95123 Catania, Italy; currentiw@gmail.com (W.C.); fgalvano@unict.it (F.G.)
2. Oasi Research Institute—IRCCS, 94018 Troina, Italy; justyna.godos@gmail.com (J.G.); rferri@oasi.en.it (R.F.); fcaraci@unict.it (F.C.)
3. Department of Educational Sciences, University of Catania, 95124 Catania, Italy; sabrina.castellano@unict.it
4. Department of Drug Sciences, University of Catania, 95125 Catania, Italy; forgiuseppecaruso@gmail.com
* Correspondence: giuseppe.grosso@unict.it; Tel.: +39-0954-781-187

Abstract: Background: Due to the increased life expectancy, the prevalence of aging-related health conditions, such as cognitive impairment, dementia and Alzheimer's disease is increasing. Among the modifiable risk factors, dietary factors have proved to be of primary importance in preserving and improving mental health and cognitive status in older adults, possibly through the modulation of adult neurogenesis, neuronal plasticity and brain signaling. Feeding/fasting timing manipulation has emerged as an innovative strategy to counteract and treat cognitive decline. The aim of this study was to investigate the association between the timing of the feeding period and cognitive status in a cross-sectional cohort of adults living in the Mediterranean area. Methods: Demographic and dietary characteristics of 883 adults living in Southern Italy (Sicily) were analyzed. Food frequency questionnaires were used to calculate the time window between the first and the last meal of an average day. Participants with an eating time window duration of more than 10 h were then identified, as well as those with eating time restricted to less than 10 h (TRF). Results: After adjusting for potential confounding factors, individuals adherent to TRF were less likely to have cognitive impairment, compared to those with no eating time restrictions [odds ratio (OR) = 0.28; 95% confidence intervals (CI): 0.07–0.90]; a similar association was found for individuals having breakfast (OR = 0.37, 95% CI: 0.16–0.89), but not for those having dinner. Conclusions: The results of this study reveal that time restricted eating may be positively associated with cognitive status, and thus exert plausible effects on brain health.

Keywords: time restricted feeding; intermittent fasting; chrononutrition; cognitive; brain diseases; brain; aging; risk factor; cohort; Mediterranean diet

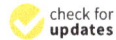
check for updates

Citation: Currenti, W.; Godos, J.; Castellano, S.; Caruso, G.; Ferri, R.; Caraci, F.; Grosso, G.; Galvano, F. Association between Time Restricted Feeding and Cognitive Status in Older Italian Adults. *Nutrients* 2021, 13, 191. https://doi.org/10.3390/nu13010191

Received: 31 December 2020
Accepted: 7 January 2021
Published: 9 January 2021

Publisher's Note: MDPI stays neutral with regard to jurisdictional claims in published maps and institutional affiliations.

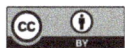
1. Introduction

Due to the increased life expectancy, aging-related health conditions are becoming a relevant socio-economic burden for all populations worldwide [1]. In fact, in recent years a significant rise in the prevalence of neurodegenerative diseases, including a progressive global deterioration of cognitive abilities in multiple domains, such as learning, memory, orientation, language, comprehension and judgment has been observed in older adults [2]. To date, there is no effective pharmacological treatment capable of curing dementia [3]; thus, it is important to prevent or delay the onset of cognitive deterioration.

Despite the fact that the causes of neurological diseases are multifactorial, there is a growing body of evidence showing that modifiable risk factors, such as nutrition and lifestyle, play an important role in the prevention of neurodegenerative diseases [4]. Among modifiable risk factors, dietary factors have been identified as playing a potential role in preserving and possibly improving mental health and cognitive status in older adults [5]. Recent scientific evidence demonstrated the beneficial effect of plant-based foods and beverages, rich in polyphenols [6], toward cognitive health, including fruits and vegetables [7]), nuts, whole grains and legumes [8–10], and coffee [11]. However, not only plant-based foods and/or manipulation of macronutrient intake have an effect; in fact nutritional interventions that consist of reducing global calories or increasing the fasting window between two meals have often been reported to improve healthspan and lifespan in a variety of organisms in laboratory settings, with increasing evidence that they are effective in humans [12]. However, only recently some studies have been published on intermittent fasting (IF) and outcomes related to cognitive status, although results are unequivocal [13,14].

Time-restricted feeding (TRF) is a form of IF in which all nutrient intake occurs within a few hours (usually ≤12 h) everyday, without any attempt to alter nutrient quality or calories. The concept of TRF arose within the context of circadian rhythms, which are daily circa 24-h rhythms in physiology, metabolism and behavior sustained under constant light or dark conditions [15]. TRF has been hypothesized to modify brain neurochemistry and neuronal network activity in ways that optimize brain function and peripheral energy metabolism [16,17]. Indeed, favorable effects of IF toward insulin metabolism, regulation of autophagy and neuro-inflammation, modulation of the expression of brain derived neurotrophic factor (BDNF) and regulation of behavior have been previously demonstrated; and importantly, all of the foregoing may affect neurogenesis and neuroplasticity [18]. However, most of the studies have been conducted in laboratory settings and studies on humans, even though observational, are lacking [19]. The aim of this study was to investigate the association between time feeding period and cognitive status in a cohort of adults living in the Mediterranean area.

2. Materials and Methods

2.1. Study Population

The MEAL study is an observational study aiming to investigate the association between nutritional and lifestyle habits characterizing the classical Mediterranean area and non-communicable diseases. The baseline data comprised a sample of 2044 men and women aged 18 or more years old randomly selected and enrolled between 2014 and 2015 in the main districts of the city of Catania, southern Italy. Details of the study protocol are published elsewhere [20]. Briefly, data collection was performed through the registered records of local general practitioners stratified by sex and 10-year age groups. The theoretical sample size was set at 1500 individuals to provide a specific relative precision of 5% (Type I error, 0.05; Type II error, 0.10), taking into account an anticipated 70% participation rate. Out of 2405 individuals invited, the final sample size was 2044 participants (response rate of 85%). Given the outcome investigated has a major impact at older ages, the analysis for the present study was restricted to individuals of age of 50 years old or older ($n = 916$). Aims of the study were introduced to all participants and informed written consent was obtained. The study protocol has been reviewed and approved by the concerning ethical committee and all the study procedures were carried out in accordance with the Declaration of Helsinki (1989) of the World Medical Association.

2.2. Data Collection

Face-to-face assisted personal interviews were conducted and electronic data collection was performed using tablet computers. All participants were provided with a paper copy of the questionnaire to visualize the response options. Nonetheless, final answers were registered directly by the interviewer. The demographic data including gender, age at recruitment, highest educational degree achieved, occupation (specifies the character of the most important employment during the year before the investigation) or last occupation before retirement, and marital status were collected. Occupational status was categorized as (i) unemployed, (ii) low (unskilled workers), (iii) medium (partially skilled workers), and (iv) high (skilled workers). Educational status was categorized as (i) low (primary/secondary), (ii) medium (high school), and (iii) high (university). The International Physical Activity Questionnaire (IPAQ) was used to assess physical activity [21], it included a set of questionnaires (five domains) investigating the time spent being physically active in the last 7 days. According to the IPAQ guidelines, physical activity level was categorized as (i) low, (ii) moderate, and (iii) high. Smoking status was categorized as (i) non-smoker, (ii) ex-smoker, and (iii) current smoker, while alcohol consumption was categorized as (i) none, (ii) moderate drinker (0.1–12 g/d) and (iii) regular drinker (>12 g/d). Data regarding health status including information about anthropometric measurements assessed through standard methods and previous or current cardiometabolic diseases and cancer were also collected [22].

2.3. Dietary Assessment

In order to assess the dietary intake, two food frequency questionnaires (FFQ, a long and a short version) previously tested for validity and reliability for the Sicilian population were administered [23,24]. The determination of the food intake, the energy content as well as the macro- and micro-nutrients intake were obtained through comparison with food composition tables of the Italian Research Center for Foods and Nutrition (Available online: https://www.crea.gov.it/-/tabella-di-composizione-degli-alimenti accessed on 17 July 2020). Intake of seasonal foods referred to consumption during the period in which the food was available and then adjusted by its proportional intake in one year. FFQs with unreliable intakes (<1000 or >6000 kcal/d) were excluded from the analyses (n = 22) leaving a total of 883 individuals included in the analysis.

2.4. Time Feeding

Participants were asked whether and what time, on average, they consumed their daily meals over the last 6 months (including breakfast, snacks, lunch and dinner). Consequently, the window of time between the first and the last meal of an average day was calculated; participants were finally categorized in those having an eating time window duration of more than 10 h and those with time restricted feeding less than 10 h (TRF).

2.5. Cognitive Evaluation

Cognitive status was evaluated using the Short Portable Mental Status Questionnaire (SPMSQ) [25], designed to measure cognitive impairment in both general and hospital population [26] also applied to the Italian population [27]. This 10-item tool was administered by the clinician in the office or in a hospital. The pre-defined categories for interpretation of the screening tool were (i) intact, less than 3 errors; (ii) mild, 3 to 4 errors; (iii) moderate, 5 to 7 errors, and (iv) severe, 8 or more errors. For this study, we considered more than 2 errors as a cut off point for impaired cognitive status.

2.6. Statistical Analysis

We analyzed the baseline cross-sectional data from this cohort. Exposure variables were eating time window (TRF vs. no eating time restriction), having breakfast and having dinner (vs. skipping). Categorical variables are presented as frequencies of occurrence and percentages; differences between groups were tested with Chi-squared test. Continuous variables are presented as means and standard deviations (SDs); differences between groups were tested with Student's t-test or Mann-Whitney U-test for normally and not-normally distributed variables, respectively. The relation between exposure variables and cognitive status was tested through multivariate logistic regression analysis adjusted for baseline characteristics (age, sex, marital, educational and occupational status, smoking and alcohol drinking habits, and physical activity level). All reported p values were based on two-sided tests and compared to a significance level of 5%. SPSS 17 (SPSS Inc., Chicago, IL, USA) software was used for all the statistical calculations.

3. Results

Background characteristics of the study population according to feeding time window duration and meal habits are presented in Table 1. Among those having TRF there were less individuals with low educational and occupational status, more former smokers, less overweight, obesity, type-2 diabetes, hypertension, dyslipidemia and CVD (Table 1). Also regarding breakfast and dinner there were some differences among groups: for instance, among those having breakfast there were more older women, lower educational and occupational status, more never smokers, hypertensive, dyslipidemic and previous CVD; regarding dinner, there was a significant different distribution of occupational status categories despite with no clear trends (Table 1).

Table 1. Background characteristics of the study population according to eating time window duration (TRF vs. no restriction), breakfast (yes vs. no), and dinner (yes vs. no).

	TRF			Breakfast			Dinner		
	Yes (*n* = 98)	No (*n* = 785)	*p*-Value	Yes (*n* = 702)	No (*n* = 181)	*p*-Value	Yes (*n* = 859)	No (*n* = 24)	*p*-Value
Sex, *n* (%)			0.226			<0.001			0.499
Men	48 (49)	334 (42.5)		281 (40)	101 (55.8)		370 (43.1)	12 (50)	
Women	50 (51)	451 (57.5)		421 (60)	80 (44.2)		489 (56.9)	12 (50)	
Age, mean (SD)	65.2 (9.4)	65.1 (9.6)	0.057	65.5 (9)	62.8 (9.6)	0.001	65 (9.6)	61.5 (7.9)	0.080
Educational status, *n* (%)			0.008			0.001			0.480
Low	38 (38.8)	413 (52.6)		380 (54.1)	71 (39.2)		441 (51.3)	10 (41.7)	
Medium	45 (45.9)	240 (30.6)		210 (29.9)	75 (41.4)		277 (32.2)	8 (33.3)	
High	15 (15.3)	132 (16.8)		112 (16)	35 (19.3)		141 (16.4)	6 (25)	
Occupational status, *n* (%)			0.001			<0.001			0.022
Unemployed	9 (9.9)	194 (28.4)		184 (29.8)	19 (12.3)		199 (26.6)	4 (16.7)	
Low	25 (27.5)	110 (16.1)		93 (15)	42 (27.1)		126 (16.8)	9 (37.5)	
Medium	30 (33)	204 (29.9)		187 (30.3)	47 (30.3)		231 (30.8)	3 (12.5)	
High	27 (29.7)	174 (25.5)		154 (24.9)	47 (30.3)		193 (25.8)	8 (33.3)	
Smoking status, *n* (%)			<0.001			<0.001			0.815
Never smoker	37 (37.8)	460 (58.6)		419 (59.7)	78 (43.1)		485 (56.5)	12 (50)	
Former smoker	43 (43.9)	144 (18.3)		126 (17.9)	61 (33.7)		181 (21.1)	6 (25)	
Current smoker	18 (18.4)	181 (23.1)		157 (22.4)	42 (23.2)		193 (22.5)	6 (25)	
Physical activity level, *n* (%)			0.659			0.142			0.183
Low	23 (25)	173 (26.3)		161 (27.5)	35 (21.5)		193 (26.6)	3 (12.5)	
Moderate	43 (46.7)	327 (49.8)		290 (49.5)	80 (49.1)		354 (48.8)	16 (66.7)	
High	26 (28.3)	157 (23.9)		135 (23)	48 (29.4)		178 (24.6)	5 (20.8)	
BMI categories, *n* (%)			<0.001			0.286			0.203
Normal	44 (62)	256 (33.7)		253 (37.3)	47 (30.7)		292 (35.9)	8 (44.4)	
Overweight	27 (38)	312 (41.1)		273 (40.3)	66 (43.1)		330 (40.6)	9 (50)	
Obese	0 (0)	192 (25.3)		152 (22.4)	40 (26.1)		191 (23.5)	1 (5.6)	
Health status, *n* (%)									
Type-2 diabetes	9 (9.2)	135 (17.2)	0.043	120 (17.1)	24 (13.3)	0.213	143 (16.6)	1 (4.2)	0.103
Hypertension	61 (62.2)	599 (76.3)	0.003	536 (76.4)	124 (68.5)	0.030	646 (75.2)	14 (58.3)	0.061
Dyslipidemias	13 (13.3)	289 (36.8)	<0.001	273 (38.9)	29 (16)	<0.001	297 (34.6)	5 (20.8)	0.162
CVD	8 (8.3)	128 (16.9)	0.031	128 (18.9)	8 (4.6)	<0.001	135 (16.3)	1 (4.2)	0.110
Cancer	8 (8.2)	66 (8.4)	0.934	62 (8.8)	12 (6.6)	0.340	70 (8.1)	4 (16.7)	0.137

Nutrients and food group consumption across TRF, breakfast and dinner eaters are shown in Table 2. Individuals having TRF consumed more fibre, vitamin C, vitamin E, fruit, legumes, less potassium, less meat (total and red), and dairy products (Table 2); those having breakfast had lower intake of vitamin C and vitamin E while consumed more total meat, nuts and dairy products and less legumes; finally, those having dinner had lower energy intake, carbohydrate intake, fibre, PUFA, vitamin C, vitamin E, sodium, and higher intake of vitamin D and fish (Table 2).

Table 2. Mean (and standard deviation) of micro-, macro-nutrients and major food groups intake according to feeding time window duration (time feeding restricted to 10 vs. no restriction), breakfast (yes vs. no), and dinner (yes vs. no).

	TRF			Breakfast			Dinner		
	Yes (*n* = 98)	No (*n* = 785)	*p*-Value	Yes (*n* = 702)	No (*n* = 181)	*p*-Value	Yes (*n* = 859)	No (*n* = 24)	*p*-Value
	Mean (SD)			Mean (SD)			Mean (SD)		
Energy intake (kcal/d)	2110.8 (759.6)	2039.8 (637.1)	0.310	2034.4 (631.6)	2099.5 (724.4)	0.231	2040 (639.9)	2320 (967.3)	0.038
Energy intake (kJ/d)	8606.97 (3161.637)	8257.8 (2614.5)	0.224	8230.6 (2585.3)	8552.3 (3017.9)	0.150	8262.1 (2626.6)	9530 (4078.4)	0.022
Macronutrients									
Carbohydrates (g/d)	299 (108.9)	314.6 (117)	0.186	297.8 (107.2)	312.2 (119.2)	0.116	299.4 (108.5)	348 (146.5)	0.032
Fiber (g/d)	35.6 (14.5)	32.3 (13.7)	0.027	32.3 (13.9)	34.2 (13.5)	0.098	32.6 (13.8)	38.2 (14.3)	0.049
Protein (g/d)	84.4 (29.5)	84.8 (28.6)	0.900	84.8 (29)	84.7 (27.9)	0.981	84.6 (28.6)	89.4 (32.7)	0.422
Fat (g/d)	60.5 (30.9)	59.2 (20.6)	0.595	59.3 (20.3)	59.8 (27.4)	0.791	59.3 (21.3)	65.6 (40)	0.165
Cholesterol (mg/d)	174.3 (91.8)	190.1 (85.9)	0.089	190.4 (87.2)	180.7 (84.8)	0.179	188.7 (86.8)	177.2 (86.9)	0.522
SFA	22.9 (12.1)	23.6 (9.1)	0.541	23.7 (8.9)	23.1 (11.5)	0.520	23.5 (9.2)	26 (17.7)	0.207
MUFA	26 (13.1)	25.2 (8)	0.358	25.2 (8)	25.7 (11.3)	0.485	25.2 (8.6)	27.8 (15.3)	0.169
PUFA g	11.4 (5.7)	10.9 (4.2)	0.345	11 (4.3)	11.2 (5)	0.209	7.3 (6.5)	10.7 (14.1)	0.015
Total Omega-3	1.69 (0.83)	1.76 (0.85)	0.480	1.8 (0.9)	1.7 (0.8)	0.325	1.76 (0.85)	1.48 (0.44)	0.107
Micronutrients									
Vitamin A (Retinol)	897.92 (379)	867.3 (428.8)	0.500	872.5 (427.2)	863.8 (410.2)	0.806	869 (425)	929 (368.7)	0.494
Vitamin C (mg/d)	203.4 (118.6)	153,9 (92.4)	<0.001	154 (94.2)	180.5 (104.2)	0.001	158.4 (96.9)	198.3 (88.9)	0.047
Vitamin E (mg/d)	9.8 (4.4)	8.5 (3)	<0.001	8.5 (3)	9.2 (3.9)	0.013	8.6 (3.2)	10 (4.5)	0.039
Vitamin B12	5.6 (4.2)	6.2 (4.3)	0.206	6.3 (4.5)	5.8 (3.5)	0.157	6.2 (4.4)	5 (2.1)	0.211
Vitamin D	5.6 (6.3)	5.6 (5.4)	0.963	5.7 (5.6)	5.5 (5.1)	0.677	5.7 (5.6)	3.5 (1)	0.050
Sodium (mg/d)	2699.9 (1248.6)	2767.8 (1065.3)	0.560	2744.5 (1016.9)	2821.9 (1324.9)	0.393	2743.7 (1070.5)	3354 (1468.8)	0.007
Potassium (mg/d)	3649.8 (1331.8)	3987.3 (1456.4)	0.020	3651.4 (1345.9)	3826.7 (1358.3)	0.119	3673.6 (1344.3)	4212.6 (1458.5)	0.053
Food groups									
Cereals (total, g/d)	222 (129.5)	228,2 (132.1)	0.662	226.2 (129.5)	232.7 (140.4)	0.556	226.4 (131)	268.2 (151.4)	0.125
Vegetables (g/d)	264.7 (118.5)	261 (148)	0.526	258.1 (140.4)	274 (161.2)	0.190	260.6 (145.9)	288.5 (105.9)	0.353
Fruit (g/d)	482.2 (337.1)	398.52 (313)	0.014	401.77 (322.4)	431.2 (293.1)	0.265	405.3 (316.7)	497.6 (310.3)	0.159
Legumes (g/d)	46.1 (40.6)	36.5 (35.3)	0.013	36.4 (36)	42.3 (35.7)	0.047	37.5 (36.1)	40.6 (34.2)	0.677
Nuts (total, g/d)	14.8 (19.2)	21.3 (33.1)	0.057	22 (34.6)	15.3 (17.7)	0.011	20.8 (32.1)	17 (23.2)	0.564
Fish (g/d)	66.5 (70.2)	65.3 (61.5)	0.861	65.6 (63.7)	65 (58.1)	0.909	66.2 (63.2)	39.5 (14.9)	0.039
Meat (total, g/d)	57.4 (31.6)	70.5 (39.9)	0.002	70.7 (41.1)	63 (30.9)	0.018	69.2 (39.6)	66 (30.4)	0.698
Red meat (g/d)	27.4 (19.6)	33.84 (24.7)	0.023	33.7 (27.3)	31.1 (21.1)	0.248	33.1 (26.3)	33 (20.8)	0.974
Processed Meat (g/d)	13.8 (22.4)	13.4 (16)	0.85	13.5 (16.5)	13.7 (18.3)	0.878	13.3 (16.8)	20.1 (19.4)	0.052
Dairy products (g/d)	157.9 (176.3)	194.8 (171.4)	0.046	202.1 (175.4)	146.7 (152.2)	<0.001	191 (171.2)	196.8 (212.3)	0.862
Alcohol (total, g/d)	8.79 (11.3)	8.23 (12.8)	0.681	8 (12.6)	9.4 (13.1)	0.187	8.2 (12.6)	11.2 (16.2)	0.253
Coffee (mL/d)	57.1 (38.8)	60.4 (44.1)	0.484	59.1 (44.1)	63.7 (41.6)	0.207	60 (43.8)	61.5 (36)	0.870
Tea (mL/d)	70.3 (128.19)	57.6 (122.2)	0.337	60 (127.5)	54.9 (102.9)	0.615	59.2 (123.3)	52.1 (107.2)	0.785
Olive oil (mL/d)	7.6 (3.1)	7.2 (3.1)	0.267	7.2 (3.2)	7.5 (3.1)	0.313	7.3 (3.2)	6.8 (3.2)	0.435

A total of 82 individuals had impaired cognitive status: most of them resulted having mild impairment, while four participants reported moderate impairment. Cognitive impaired individuals were older, with higher proportion less physically active, and had higher rates of hypertension (Supplementary Table S1). Table 3 reports the associations between the exposure variables and cognitive status. The multivariate model shows that individuals having TRF were less likely to have cognitive impairment compared to those with no eating time restrictions [odds ratio (OR) = 0.28; 95% confidence intervals (CI): 0.07–0.90)]; a similar association was found for those individuals having breakfast (OR = 0.37, 95% CI: 0.16–0.89), but no for dinner (Table 3).

Table 3. Association between feeding time window duration (time feeding restricted to 10 vs. no restriction), breakfast (yes vs. no), dinner (yes vs. no), and cognitive status in the study sample.

	Cognitive Impairment, OR (95% CI)					
	TRF	*p*-Value	**Breakfast**	*p*-Value	**Dinner**	*p*-Value
Model 1	0.39 (0.14–1.10)	0.077	0.45 (0.22–0.94)	0.034	0.59 (0.17–2.1)	0.238
Model 2	0.42 (0.15–1.20)	0.105	0.51 (0.25–1.10)	0.078	0.46 (0.13–1.66)	0.418
Model 3	0.28 (0.07–0.90)	0.049	0.37 (0.16–0.89)	0.025	0.48 (0.13–1.85)	0.289

Model 1 is unadjusted. Model 2 includes adjustment for age and sex. Model 3 includes adjustment for variables as model 2 + educational and occupational level, smoking status, physical activity level, BMI categories, and type-2 diabetes, hypertension, dyslipidemia, previous history of CVD and cancer.

4. Discussion

In the present cross-sectional study, the relation between TRF and cognitive status was investigated in a cohort of Italian adults. Individuals who practiced TRF were less likely to screen positive for impaired cognitive status, and among those practicing TRF only those who did not skip breakfast were less likely to screen positive for impaired cognitive status. Interestingly, the results of TRF in humans seem to depend on the time of day of the eating window and not only related to fasting duration per se [28–32]. In fact, studies showed that restricting food intake starting from the middle of the day (skipping dinner) reduced body fat, fasting glucose, insulin resistance, hyperlipidemia and inflammation [29,30]. Conversely, restricting the entire food daily intake to the late afternoon (skipping breakfast) either produced mostly null results or worsened cardiometabolic health [28,31,32]. The circadian system may explain these dichotomous time-of-day effects. Circadian rhythms are self-sustained ~24 h oscillations in physiology, metabolism and behavior induced by coordinated transcriptional–translational feedback loops involving clock genes such as CLOCK, BMAL1 CRY1/2 and PER1/2 which in turn cause oscillations in a numerous of downstream targets. Jamshed and colleagues [33] investigated the effects of early TRF (skipping dinner) on gene expression, circulating hormones and cardiometabolic risk on eleven overweight adults. After only 4 days of early TRF they found changes in the expression of 6 circadian clock genes and upregulation of both SIRT1 and LC3A that have a role in autophagy. Autophagy has been shown to play a determinant role in protecting against multiple chronic disorders such as diabetes, heart disease, cancer, and neurodegenerative diseases, by recycling used and damaged proteins and organelles.

To our knowledge, our study is the first to focus on the relation between TRF and cognitive status in humans. Unfortunately, our current understanding regarding IF on cognitive status and neurodegenerative diseases is mainly inferred from in vitro or animal studies because human studies are lacking. There are very few interventional studies exploring the effects of TRF on humans and they mainly concern metabolic aspects such as weight reduction and/or insulin resistance. Sutton and colleagues [34] found that a 5-week of 8-h early time restricted feeding improved insulin levels, insulin sensitivity, b cell responsiveness, blood pressure, and oxidative stress levels in men with prediabetes even though food intake was matched to the control arm and no weight loss occurred. Similarly, another study conducted during orthodox religious fasting reported that time restricted eating might be associated with better metabolic and glycemic profile [35,36]. Maintaining adequate blood pressure prevents cerebral microhemorrhages which contribute to cognitive impairment, geriatric psychiatric syndromes, and gait disorders [37]. These findings are also relevant because metabolic syndrome is another major risk factor for a variety of neurological diseases [38].

Fasting per se may counteract aging which is the most recognized risk factor for cognitive impairment, dementia and neurological disease [16]. In fact, aging is associated with many morpho-functional changes that can affect behaviour, cognition and susceptibility to neurodegenerative disorders such as Alzheimer's disease (AD) and Parkinson's disease (PD) [39]. Over the years the most relevant changes occur in the hippocampus and in the prefrontal cortex which are crucial for spatial and working memory [40,41]. It has been demonstrated that the deterioration of these two structures is widely responsible for the decline seen in cognitive functions during aging [42]. Aging is characterized by a deterioration in the extent of dendritic branching both in apical and basilar dendrites in the hippocampus and in the superficial cortical layer of the prefrontal cortex [43] leading to reduction in cognitive function [44]. Moreover, aged neurons show an increased density of calcium channels that leads to an alteration of after-hyperpolarization (AHP) potential. In fact after depolarization, neurons utilize potassium channels to repolarize but when AHP is increased, neurons need to reset longer to resting potential [45]. This coincides with a reduction in levels of BDNF which correlates with age-related cognitive deficits [46]. Many studies have shown that Intermittent fasting may enhance synaptic plasticity, neurogenesis and neuroprotection especially by an increase in BDNF [47,48]. BDNF has an effect also in neural precursor cells (NPC) which reside in the dentate gyrus of the hippocampus in which they are relevant for the formation of new neurons that integrate into the hippocampal circuitry and play roles in spatial pattern separation, a fundamental domain of learning and memory [49–51].

Another physiological mechanism during aging is the progressive loss of synapses in some regions of the human brain that leads to worsened communication between neurons and is associated with increased inflammation and oxidative stress [52]. Findings in rodents suggest that IF enhances neuronal resilience to excitotoxic stress, preventing learning deficit [53] due to hippocampal cell death and stimulating neurogenesis [49,54]. The consequent increased expression of synaptic proteins regulating calcium homeostasis [55] attenuates the typical decline in motor coordination and spatial learning typically observed in old rats.

IF may exert also neuroprotective effects by an improved mitochondrial respiratory activity [56] due to an upregulation of PGC1α which contributes to mitochondrial biogenesis and detoxification [57]. The upregulation of PGC1α modulates also the expression of nitric oxide (NO) which has antioxidant and protective properties in the endothelium and may preserve the brain microvasculature [58,59]. Interestingly a TRF protocol was also reported to diminish ROS production, improve endothelial function [60] and reduce levels of pro-inflammatory cytokines as TNFα, IL-1β and IL-6 [54]. In neurodegenerative diseases, these changes related to aging occur at a much faster rate and it has been hypothesized that intermittent fasting could also have a beneficial effect on their treatment. Compared to ad libitum-fed controls, mice and rats on an IF diet exhibit less neuronal dysfunction, degeneration and fewer clinical symptoms in models of AD, PD and Huntington's disease (HD) [16]. In a different in vivo study carried out by Chaix et al. [61], there were 17 serum metabolites that were higher in TRF than ad libitum feeding group, including anserine and carnosine, which have shown therapeutic potential against the oxidative stress observed in pathologies characterized by cognitive dysfunctions [62,63]. Differently from caloric restriction, IF could prevent cognitive decline in a triple transgenic AD mouse model by acting on mitochondrial dysfunction and oxidative imbalance without reductions in β-amyloid protein and phospho-tau levels [64]. Moreover, it has recently been demonstrated that TRF protocol improves sleep, motor coordination and autonomic nervous system function in mouse models of Huntington's disease [65,66].

Current evidence, even though limited and conflicting [67,68] has associated TRF with changes in human gut microbiota. In particular, Zeb et al. demonstrated that TRF may modulate microbial composition and increase its relative abundance, thereby influencing the host metabolism and nutritional status [68]. Consequently, gut microbiome imbalance has been associated with numerous inflammatory, immune and nervous system-related diseases through a communication pathway called microbiome-brain axis [69], also influencing brain development and function [70].

This study has a major strength to be the first reporting an association between TRF and cognitive status, suggesting this hypothesis to be further tested in future studies. However, albeit among the first reported in the scientific literature, the findings of this study should be considered in light of some limitations. First, the cross-sectional nature of the study cannot allow us to draft conclusions on the association between TRF and cognitive status. However, this type of study is important to be performed in order to provide preliminary results of potential interest in spite of clinical intervention trials; in fact, it is crucial to have preliminary data before setting up intervention trials strongly affecting the eating habits of older individuals at risk of cognitive impairment and altered cognitive function (lack of compliance). Another limitation of our study includes the possibility of residual confounding due to the characteristics of individuals having TRF, as they demonstrated to be potentially more health conscious with higher socio-educational level and, thus, at lower risk of age-related disorders. Despite the fact that we adjusted for all these potential confounding factors, we cannot rule out the possibility of existence of related unmeasured confounders. Finally, despite statistically significant, we found wide CIs for the association between TRF and cognitive status: although the direction of the association is significant, the strength of these findings should be confirmed in future studies with larger sample, more cases and more individuals exposed to the variable of interest.

5. Conclusions

In conclusion, restricting the daily time feeding window is associated with reduced odds of impaired cognitive status especially when it is obtained through restricting food intake starting from the middle of the day in alignment with circadian rhythms. Therefore, large sample interventional human studies in which cognitive status, regional brain volumes, neural network activity, and biochemical analyses of cerebrospinal fluid are needed to clarify the impact of TRF on mental health.

Supplementary Materials: The following are available online at https://www.mdpi.com/2072-664 3/13/1/191/s1, Table S1: Background characteristics by cognitive status.

Author Contributions: Conceptualization, W.C., J.G., G.G., F.G.; methodology W.C., J.G., G.G., F.G.; formal analysis, W.C., J.G., G.G., F.G.; writing—original draft preparation, W.C., J.G., S.C., G.C., R.F., F.C., G.G., F.G.; writing—review and editing, W.C., J.G., S.C., G.C., R.F., F.C., G.G., F.G.; supervision, R.F., F.C., G.G., F.G. All authors have read and agreed to the published version of the manuscript.

Funding: This research received no external funding.

Institutional Review Board Statement: The study was conducted according to the guidelines of the Declaration of Helsinki, and approved by the Institutional Review Board (or Ethics Committee) of University of Catania (protocol code 802/23 December 2014).

Informed Consent Statement: Informed consent was obtained from all subjects involved in the study.

Data Availability Statement: The data presented in this study are available on request from the corresponding author.

Acknowledgments: W.C. is a PhD student in the International PhD Program in Neuroscience at the University of Catania.

Conflicts of Interest: The authors declare no conflict of interest. The funders had no role in the design of the study; in the collection, analyses, or interpretation of data; in the writing of the manuscript, or in the decision to publish the results.

References

1. Fernandes, L.; Paúl, C. Editorial: Aging and mental health. *Front. Aging Neurosci.* **2017**, *9*, 25. [CrossRef]
2. GBD 2017 Disease and Injury Incidence and Prevalence Collaborators. Global, regional, and national incidence, prevalence, and years lived with disability for 354 diseases and injuries for 195 countries and territories, 1990–2017: A systematic analysis for the Global Burden of Disease Study 2017. *Lancet* **2018**, *392*, 1789–1858. [CrossRef]
3. Tricco, A.C.; Soobiah, C.; Berliner, S.; Ho, J.M.; Ng, C.H.; Ashoor, H.M.; Chen, M.H.; Hemmelgarn, B.; Straus, S.E. Efficacy and safety of cognitive enhancers for patients with mild cognitive impairment: A systematic review and meta-analysis. *CMAJ* **2013**, *185*, 1393–1401. [CrossRef] [PubMed]
4. Adan, R.A.H.; van der Beek, E.M.; Buitelaar, J.K.; Cryan, J.F.; Hebebrand, J.; Higgs, S.; Schellekens, H.; Dickson, S.L. Nutritional psychiatry: Towards improving mental health by what you eat. *Eur. Neuropsychopharmacol.* **2019**, *29*, 1321–1332. [CrossRef] [PubMed]
5. Grosso, G. Nutrition and aging: Is there a link to cognitive health? *Int. J. Food Sci. Nutr.* **2020**, *71*, 265–266. [CrossRef] [PubMed]
6. Godos, J.; Caraci, F.; Castellano, S.; Currenti, W.; Galvano, F.; Ferri, R.; Grosso, G. Association between dietary flavonoids intake and cognitive function in an italian cohort. *Biomolecules* **2020**, *10*, 1300. [CrossRef]
7. Angelino, D.; Godos, J.; Ghelfi, F.; Tieri, M.; Titta, L.; Lafranconi, A.; Marventano, S.; Alonzo, E.; Gambera, A.; Sciacca, S.; et al. Fruit and vegetable consumption and health outcomes: An umbrella review of observational studies. *Int. J. Food Sci. Nutr.* **2019**, *70*, 652–667. [CrossRef]
8. Akbaraly, T.N.; Brunner, E.J.; Ferrie, J.E.; Marmot, M.G.; Kivimaki, M.; Singh-Manoux, A. Dietary pattern and depressive symptoms in middle age. *Br. J. Psychiatry* **2009**, *195*, 408–413. [CrossRef]
9. Godos, J.; Currenti, W.; Angelino, D.; Mena, P.; Castellano, S.; Caraci, F.; Galvano, F.; Del Rio, D.; Ferri, R.; Grosso, G. Diet and mental health: Review of the recent updates on molecular mechanisms. *Antioxidants* **2020**, *9*, 346. [CrossRef]
10. Broughton, P.M.; Bullock, D.G.; Cramb, R. Improving the quality of plasma cholesterol measurements in primary care. *Scand. J. Clin. Lab. Investig. Suppl.* **1990**, *198*, 43–48. [CrossRef]
11. Grosso, G.; Godos, J.; Galvano, F.; Giovannucci, E.L. Coffee, caffeine, and health outcomes: An umbrella review. *Annu. Rev. Nutr.* **2017**, *37*, 131–156. [CrossRef] [PubMed]
12. Wahl, D.; Coogan, S.C.; Solon-Biet, S.M.; de Cabo, R.; Haran, J.B.; Raubenheimer, D.; Cogger, V.C.; Mattson, M.P.; Simpson, S.J.; Le Couteur, D.G. Cognitive and behavioral evaluation of nutritional interventions in rodent models of brain aging and dementia. *Clin. Interv. Aging* **2017**, *12*, 1419–1428. [CrossRef] [PubMed]
13. Ooi, T.C.; Meramat, A.; Rajab, N.F.; Shahar, S.; Ismail, I.S.; Azam, A.A.; Sharif, R. Intermittent Fasting Enhanced the Cognitive Function in Older Adults with Mild Cognitive Impairment by Inducing Biochemical and Metabolic changes: A 3-Year Progressive Study. *Nutrients* **2020**, *12*, 2644. [CrossRef] [PubMed]
14. Harder-Lauridsen, N.M.; Rosenberg, A.; Benatti, F.B.; Damm, J.A.; Thomsen, C.; Mortensen, E.L.; Pedersen, B.K.; Krogh-Madsen, R. Ramadan model of intermittent fasting for 28 d had no major effect on body composition, glucose metabolism, or cognitive functions in healthy lean men. *Nutrition* **2017**, *37*, 92–103. [CrossRef]
15. Xie, Y.; Tang, Q.; Chen, G.; Xie, M.; Yu, S.; Zhao, J.; Chen, L. New insights into the circadian rhythm and its related diseases. *Front. Physiol.* **2019**, *10*, 682. [CrossRef]
16. Longo, V.D.; Mattson, M.P. Fasting: Molecular mechanisms and clinical applications. *Cell Metab.* **2014**, *19*, 181–192. [CrossRef]
17. Currenti, W.; Godos, J.; Castellano, S.; Mogavero, M.P.; Ferri, R.; Caraci, F.; Grosso, G.; Galvano, F. Time restricted feeding and mental health: A review of possible mechanisms on affective and cognitive disorders. *Int. J. Food Sci. Nutr.* **2020**, 1–11. [CrossRef]
18. Francis, N. Intermittent fasting and brain health: Efficacy and potential mechanisms of action. *OBM Geriat.* **2020**, *4*, 1–19. [CrossRef]
19. Sofi, F. FASTING-MIMICKING DIET a clarion call for human nutrition research or an additional swan song for a commercial diet? *Int. J. Food Sci. Nutr.* **2020**, *71*, 921–928. [CrossRef]
20. Grosso, G.; Marventano, S.; D'Urso, M.; Mistretta, A.; Galvano, F. The Mediterranean healthy eating, ageing, and lifestyle (MEAL) study: Rationale and study design. *Int. J. Food Sci. Nutr.* **2017**, *68*, 577–586. [CrossRef]
21. Craig, C.L.; Marshall, A.L.; Sjöström, M.; Bauman, A.E.; Booth, M.L.; Ainsworth, B.E.; Pratt, M.; Ekelund, U.; Yngve, A.; Sallis, J.F.; et al. International physical activity questionnaire: 12-country reliability and validity. *Med. Sci. Sports Exerc.* **2003**, *35*, 1381–1395. [CrossRef] [PubMed]
22. Mistretta, A.; Marventano, S.; Platania, A.; Godos, J.; Galvano, F.; Grosso, G. Metabolic profile of the Mediterranean healthy Eating, Lifestyle and Aging (MEAL) study cohort. *Med. J. Nutr. Metab.* **2017**, *10*, 131–140. [CrossRef]
23. Buscemi, S.; Rosafio, G.; Vasto, S.; Massenti, F.M.; Grosso, G.; Galvano, F.; Rini, N.; Barile, A.M.; Maniaci, V.; Cosentino, L.; et al. Validation of a food frequency questionnaire for use in Italian adults living in Sicily. *Int. J. Food Sci. Nutr.* **2015**, *66*, 426–438. [CrossRef] [PubMed]
24. Marventano, S.; Mistretta, A.; Platania, A.; Galvano, F.; Grosso, G. Reliability and relative validity of a food frequency questionnaire for Italian adults living in Sicily, Southern Italy. *Int. J. Food Sci. Nutr.* **2016**, *67*, 857–864. [CrossRef]
25. Pfeiffer, E. A short portable mental status questionnaire for the assessment of organic brain deficit in elderly patients. *J. Am. Geriatr. Soc.* **1975**, *23*, 433–441. [CrossRef]
26. Erkinjuntti, T.; Sulkava, R.; Wikström, J.; Autio, L. Short Portable Mental Status Questionnaire as a screening test for dementia and delirium among the elderly. *J. Am. Geriatr. Soc.* **1987**, *35*, 412–416. [CrossRef]

27. Pilotto, A.; Ferrucci, L. Verso una definizione clinica della fragilità: Utilità dell'approccio multidimensionale. *G Gerontol.* **2011**, *59*, 125–129.
28. Carlson, O.; Martin, B.; Stote, K.S.; Golden, E.; Maudsley, S.; Najjar, S.S.; Ferrucci, L.; Ingram, D.K.; Longo, D.L.; Rumpler, W.V.; et al. Impact of reduced meal frequency without caloric restriction on glucose regulation in healthy, normal-weight middle-aged men and women. *Metab. Clin. Exp.* **2007**, *56*, 1729–1734. [CrossRef]
29. Gill, S.; Panda, S. A Smartphone App Reveals Erratic Diurnal Eating Patterns in Humans that Can Be Modulated for Health Benefits. *Cell Metab.* **2015**, *22*, 789–798. [CrossRef]
30. Moro, T.; Tinsley, G.; Bianco, A.; Marcolin, G.; Pacelli, Q.F.; Battaglia, G.; Palma, A.; Gentil, P.; Neri, M.; Paoli, A. Effects of eight weeks of time-restricted feeding (16/8) on basal metabolism, maximal strength, body composition, inflammation, and cardiovascular risk factors in resistance-trained males. *J. Transl. Med.* **2016**, *14*, 290. [CrossRef]
31. Stote, K.S.; Baer, D.J.; Spears, K.; Paul, D.R.; Harris, G.K.; Rumpler, W.V.; Strycula, P.; Najjar, S.S.; Ferrucci, L.; Ingram, D.K.; et al. A controlled trial of reduced meal frequency without caloric restriction in healthy, normal-weight, middle-aged adults. *Am. J. Clin. Nutr.* **2007**, *85*, 981–988. [CrossRef] [PubMed]
32. Tinsley, G.M.; Forsse, J.S.; Butler, N.K.; Paoli, A.; Bane, A.A.; La Bounty, P.M.; Morgan, G.B.; Grandjean, P.W. Time-restricted feeding in young men performing resistance training: A randomized controlled trial. *Eur. J. Sport Sci.* **2017**, *17*, 200–207. [CrossRef] [PubMed]
33. Jamshed, H.; Beyl, R.A.; Della Manna, D.L.; Yang, E.S.; Ravussin, E.; Peterson, C.M. Early Time-Restricted Feeding Improves 24-Hour Glucose Levels and Affects Markers of the Circadian Clock, Aging, and Autophagy in Humans. *Nutrients* **2019**, *11*, 1234. [CrossRef] [PubMed]
34. Sutton, E.F.; Beyl, R.; Early, K.S.; Cefalu, W.T.; Ravussin, E.; Peterson, C.M. Early Time-Restricted Feeding Improves Insulin Sensitivity, Blood Pressure, and Oxidative Stress Even without Weight Loss in Men with Prediabetes. *Cell Metab.* **2018**, *27*, 1212–1221. [CrossRef] [PubMed]
35. Karras, S.N.; Koufakis, T.; Adamidou, L.; Antonopoulou, V.; Karalazou, P.; Thisiadou, K.; Mitrofanova, E.; Mulrooney, H.; Petróczi, A.; Zebekakis, P.; et al. Effects of orthodox religious fasting versus combined energy and time restricted eating on body weight, lipid concentrations and glycaemic profile. *Int. J. Food Sci. Nutr.* **2020**, 1–11. [CrossRef]
36. Karras, S.N.; Koufakis, T.; Adamidou, L.; Polyzos, S.A.; Karalazou, P.; Thisiadou, K.; Zebekakis, P.; Makedou, K.; Kotsa, K. Similar late effects of a 7-week orthodox religious fasting and a time restricted eating pattern on anthropometric and metabolic profiles of overweight adults. *Int. J. Food Sci. Nutr.* **2020**, 1–11. [CrossRef] [PubMed]
37. Ungvari, Z.; Tarantini, S.; Hertelendy, P.; Valcarcel-Ares, M.N.; Fülöp, G.A.; Logan, S.; Kiss, T.; Farkas, E.; Csiszar, A.; Yabluchanskiy, A. Cerebromicrovascular dysfunction predicts cognitive decline and gait abnormalities in a mouse model of whole brain irradiation-induced accelerated brain senescence. *Geroscience* **2017**, *39*, 33–42. [CrossRef]
38. Farooqui, A.A.; Farooqui, T.; Panza, F.; Frisardi, V. Metabolic syndrome as a risk factor for neurological disorders. *Cell. Mol. Life Sci.* **2012**, *69*, 741–762. [CrossRef]
39. Anderton, B.H. Ageing of the brain. *Mech. Ageing Dev.* **2002**, *123*, 811–817. [CrossRef]
40. Weber, M.; Wu, T.; Hanson, J.E.; Alam, N.M.; Solanoy, H.; Ngu, H.; Lauffer, B.E.; Lin, H.H.; Dominguez, S.L.; Reeder, J.; et al. Cognitive deficits, changes in synaptic function, and brain pathology in a mouse model of normal aging(1,2,3). *ENeuro* **2015**, *2*. [CrossRef]
41. Chersi, F.; Burgess, N. The cognitive architecture of spatial navigation: Hippocampal and striatal contributions. *Neuron* **2015**, *88*, 64–77. [CrossRef] [PubMed]
42. West, R.L. An application of prefrontal cortex function theory to cognitive aging. *Psychol. Bull.* **1996**, *120*, 272–292. [CrossRef] [PubMed]
43. Grill, J.D.; Riddle, D.R. Age-related and laminar-specific dendritic changes in the medial frontal cortex of the rat. *Brain Res.* **2002**, *937*, 8–21. [CrossRef]
44. Cubelos, B.; Nieto, M. Intrinsic programs regulating dendrites and synapses in the upper layer neurons of the cortex. *Commun. Integr. Biol.* **2010**, *3*, 483–486. [CrossRef] [PubMed]
45. Matthews, E.A.; Linardakis, J.M.; Disterhoft, J.F. The fast and slow afterhyperpolarizations are differentially modulated in hippocampal neurons by aging and learning. *J. Neurosci.* **2009**, *29*, 4750–4755. [CrossRef] [PubMed]
46. Navarro-Martínez, R.; Fernández-Garrido, J.; Buigues, C.; Torralba-Martínez, E.; Martinez-Martinez, M.; Verdejo, Y.; Mascarós, M.C.; Cauli, O. Brain-derived neurotrophic factor correlates with functional and cognitive impairment in non-disabled older individuals. *Exp. Gerontol.* **2015**, *72*, 129–137. [CrossRef]
47. Fusco, S.; Pani, G. Brain response to calorie restriction. *Cell. Mol. Life Sci.* **2013**, *70*, 3157–3170. [CrossRef]
48. Kaptan, Z.; Akgün-Dar, K.; Kapucu, A.; Dedeakayoğulları, H.; Batu, Ş.; Üzüm, G. Long term consequences on spatial learning-memory of low-calorie diet during adolescence in female rats; hippocampal and prefrontal cortex BDNF level, expression of NeuN and cell proliferation in dentate gyrus. *Brain Res.* **2015**, *1618*, 194–204. [CrossRef]
49. Marosi, K.; Mattson, M.P. BDNF mediates adaptive brain and body responses to energetic challenges. *Trends Endocrinol. Metab.* **2014**, *25*, 89–98. [CrossRef]
50. Vivar, C.; van Praag, H. Functional circuits of new neurons in the dentate gyrus. *Front. Neural Circuits* **2013**, *7*, 15. [CrossRef]
51. Mattson, M.P.; Duan, W.; Lee, J.; Guo, Z. Suppression of brain aging and neurodegenerative disorders by dietary restriction and environmental enrichment: Molecular mechanisms. *Mech. Ageing Dev.* **2001**, *122*, 757–778. [CrossRef]

52. Johnson, D.A.; Johnson, J.A. Nrf2—A therapeutic target for the treatment of neurodegenerative diseases. *Free Radic. Biol. Med.* **2015**, *88*, 253–267. [CrossRef] [PubMed]

53. Qiu, G.; Spangler, E.L.; Wan, R.; Miller, M.; Mattson, M.P.; So, K.-F.; de Cabo, R.; Zou, S.; Ingram, D.K. Neuroprotection provided by dietary restriction in rats is further enhanced by reducing glucocortocoids. *Neurobiol. Aging* **2012**, *33*, 2398–2410. [CrossRef] [PubMed]

54. Arumugam, T.V.; Phillips, T.M.; Cheng, A.; Morrell, C.H.; Mattson, M.P.; Wan, R. Age and energy intake interact to modify cell stress pathways and stroke outcome. *Ann. Neurol.* **2010**, *67*, 41–52. [CrossRef] [PubMed]

55. Singh, R.; Lakhanpal, D.; Kumar, S.; Sharma, S.; Kataria, H.; Kaur, M.; Kaur, G. Late-onset intermittent fasting dietary restriction as a potential intervention to retard age-associated brain function impairments in male rats. *Age* **2012**, *34*, 917–933. [CrossRef] [PubMed]

56. Cerqueira, F.M.; Cunha, F.M.; Laurindo, F.R.M.; Kowaltowski, A.J. Calorie restriction increases cerebral mitochondrial respiratory capacity in a NO•-mediated mechanism: Impact on neuronal survival. *Free Radic. Biol. Med.* **2012**, *52*, 1236–1241. [CrossRef]

57. Liang, H.; Ward, W.F. PGC-1alpha: A key regulator of energy metabolism. *Adv. Physiol. Educ.* **2006**, *30*, 145–151. [CrossRef]

58. Borniquel, S.; Valle, I.; Cadenas, S.; Lamas, S.; Monsalve, M. Nitric oxide regulates mitochondrial oxidative stress protection via the transcriptional coactivator PGC-1alpha. *FASEB J.* **2006**, *20*, 1889–1891. [CrossRef]

59. Bernier, M.; Wahl, D.; Ali, A.; Allard, J.; Faulkner, S.; Wnorowski, A.; Sanghvi, M.; Moaddel, R.; Alfaras, I.; Mattison, J.A.; et al. Resveratrol supplementation confers neuroprotection in cortical brain tissue of nonhuman primates fed a high-fat/sucrose diet. *Aging* **2016**, *8*, 899–916. [CrossRef]

60. Headland, M.L.; Clifton, P.M.; Keogh, J.B. Effect of intermittent energy restriction on flow mediated dilatation, a measure of endothelial function: A short report. *Int. J. Environ. Res. Public Health* **2018**, *15*, 1166. [CrossRef]

61. Chaix, A.; Zarrinpar, A.; Miu, P.; Panda, S. Time-restricted feeding is a preventative and therapeutic intervention against diverse nutritional challenges. *Cell Metab.* **2014**, *20*, 991–1005. [CrossRef] [PubMed]

62. Caruso, G.; Caraci, F.; Jolivet, R.B. Pivotal role of carnosine in the modulation of brain cells activity: Multimodal mechanism of action and therapeutic potential in neurodegenerative disorders. *Prog. Neurobiol.* **2019**, *175*, 35–53. [CrossRef] [PubMed]

63. Caruso, G.; Benatti, C.; Blom, J.M.C.; Caraci, F.; Tascedda, F. The many faces of mitochondrial dysfunction in depression: From pathology to treatment. *Front. Pharmacol.* **2019**, *10*, 995. [CrossRef] [PubMed]

64. Halagappa, V.K.M.; Guo, Z.; Pearson, M.; Matsuoka, Y.; Cutler, R.G.; Laferla, F.M.; Mattson, M.P. Intermittent fasting and caloric restriction ameliorate age-related behavioral deficits in the triple-transgenic mouse model of Alzheimer's disease. *Neurobiol. Dis.* **2007**, *26*, 212–220. [CrossRef] [PubMed]

65. Wang, H.-B.; Loh, D.H.; Whittaker, D.S.; Cutler, T.; Howland, D.; Colwell, C.S. Time-Restricted Feeding Improves Circadian Dysfunction as well as Motor Symptoms in the Q175 Mouse Model of Huntington's Disease. *ENeuro* **2018**, *5*. [CrossRef] [PubMed]

66. Whittaker, D.S.; Loh, D.H.; Wang, H.-B.; Tahara, Y.; Kuljis, D.; Cutler, T.; Ghiani, C.A.; Shibata, S.; Block, G.D.; Colwell, C.S. Circadian-based Treatment Strategy Effective in the BACHD Mouse Model of Huntington's Disease. *J. Biol. Rhythm.* **2018**, *33*, 535–554. [CrossRef]

67. Gabel, K.; Marcell, J.; Cares, K.; Kalam, F.; Cienfuegos, S.; Ezpeleta, M.; Varady, K.A. Effect of time restricted feeding on the gut microbiome in adults with obesity: A pilot study. *Nutr. Health* **2020**, *26*, 79–85. [CrossRef]

68. Zeb, F.; Wu, X.; Chen, L.; Fatima, S.; Ijaz-Ul-Haq; Chen, A.; Xu, C.; Jianglei, R.; Feng, Q.; Li, M. Time-restricted feeding is associated with changes in human gut microbiota related to nutrient intake. *Nutrition* **2020**, *78*, 110797. [CrossRef]

69. Salvucci, E. The human-microbiome superorganism and its modulation to restore health. *Int. J. Food Sci. Nutr.* **2019**, *70*, 781–795. [CrossRef]

70. Ceppa, F.; Mancini, A.; Tuohy, K. Current evidence linking diet to gut microbiota and brain development and function. *Int. J. Food Sci. Nutr.* **2019**, *70*, 1–19. [CrossRef]

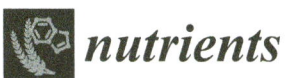

Article

Moderate Mocha Coffee Consumption Is Associated with Higher Cognitive and Mood Status in a Non-Demented Elderly Population with Subcortical Ischemic Vascular Disease

Francesco Fisicaro [1,†] , **Giuseppe Lanza** [2,3,*,†] , **Manuela Pennisi** [1] , **Carla Vagli** [4] , **Mariagiovanna Cantone** [5] , **Giovanni Pennisi** [2] , **Raffaele Ferri** [3] and **Rita Bella** [4]

1 Department of Biomedical and Biotechnological Sciences, University of Catania, Via Santa Sofia 97, 95123 Catania, Italy; drfrancescofisicaro@gmail.com (F.F.); manuela.pennisi@unict.it (M.P.)
2 Department of Surgery and Medical-Surgery Specialties, University of Catania, Via Santa Sofia 78, 95123 Catania, Italy; pennigi@unict.it
3 Department of Neurology IC, Oasi Research Institute-IRCCS, Via Conte Ruggero 78, 94018 Troina, Italy; rferri@oasi.en.it
4 Department of Medical and Surgical Sciences and Advanced Technologies, University of Catania, Via Santa Sofia 87, 95123 Catania, Italy; carlavagli@gmail.com (C.V.); rbella@unict.it (R.B.)
5 Department of Neurology, Sant'Elia Hospital, ASP Caltanissetta, Via Luigi Russo 6, 93100 Caltanissetta, Italy; m.cantone@asp.cl.it
* Correspondence: glanza@oasi.en.it; Tel.: +39-095-3782448
† These authors contributed equally to this work.

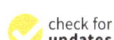
check for
updates

Citation: Fisicaro, F.; Lanza, G.; Pennisi, M.; Vagli, C.; Cantone, M.; Pennisi, G.; Ferri, R.; Bella, R. Moderate Mocha Coffee Consumption Is Associated with Higher Cognitive and Mood Status in a Non-Demented Elderly Population with Subcortical Ischemic Vascular Disease. *Nutrients* **2021**, *13*, 536. https://doi.org/10.3390/nu13020536

Academic Editor: Marilyn C Cornelis
Received: 22 December 2020
Accepted: 3 February 2021
Published: 6 February 2021

Publisher's Note: MDPI stays neutral with regard to jurisdictional claims in published maps and institutional affiliations.

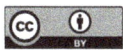

Abstract: To date, interest in the role of coffee intake in the occurrence and course of age-related neurological and neuropsychiatric disorders has provided an inconclusive effect. Moreover, no study has evaluated mocha coffee consumption in subjects with mild vascular cognitive impairment and late-onset depression. We assessed the association between different quantities of mocha coffee intake over the last year and cognitive and mood performance in a homogeneous sample of 300 non-demented elderly Italian subjects with subcortical ischemic vascular disease. Mini Mental State Examination (MMSE), Stroop Colour-Word Interference Test (Stroop T), 17-items Hamilton Depression Rating Scalfe (HDRS), Activities of Daily Living (ADL), and Instrumental ADL were the outcome measures. MMSE, HDRS, and Stroop T were independently and significantly associated with coffee consumption, i.e., better scores with increasing intake. At the post-hoc analyses, it was found that the group with a moderate intake (two cups/day) had similar values compared to the heavy drinkers (≥three cups/day), with the exception of MMSE. Daily mocha coffee intake was associated with higher cognitive and mood status, with a significant dose-response association even with moderate consumption. This might have translational implications for the identification of modifiable factors for vascular dementia and geriatric depression.

Keywords: coffee consumption; caffeine; cerebrovascular disease; executive dysfunction; geriatric depression; dose-response association

1. Introduction

The progressive aging of the population has led to an increased rate of some age-related diseases, such as cognitive impairment and dementia, including Alzheimer's disease (AD) and vascular dementia (VaD), as well as some late-onset neuropsychiatric disorders (i.e., geriatric depression). As an "umbrella term", vascular cognitive impairment (VCI) encompasses a wide range of cognitive deficits due to neurovascular disorders, such as those resulting in subcortical ischemic vascular disease (SIVD), secondary to lacunar infarcts and vascular white matter lesions (WMLs) [1,2]. As such, VCI includes all types of vascular-related cognitive disorders, from the involvement of a single cognitive domain without dementia (called mild VCI) to a clear VaD [3].

Nutrients **2021**, *13*, 536. https://doi.org/10.3390/nu13020536 https://www.mdpi.com/journal/nutrients

In addition to cognitive impairment, behaviour and mood abnormalities are frequently found in association with ischemic lesions of the prefrontal-subcortical loops underlying mood and affecting control [1,2]. Indeed, SIVD is commonly associated with late-life depression, referred to as "vascular depression" [3], a clinical-radiological condition which has been found to be different from early-onset major depression [4,5]. Namely, the "vascular depression" hypothesis posits that cerebrovascular disease may predispose, precipitate, or perpetuate geriatric depression, thus shedding light on the complex relationships between late-life depression, WMLs, and cognition. Over time, the progression of WMLs and cognitive deficit also predicts a poor course of depression and drug-resistant response, both related to a worsening of the underlying SIVD [6]. Although still debated, a "disconnection hypothesis", wherein focal vascular damage and WML location seem to play a crucial factor, contributes to the disease onset and course, as well as to clinical symptomatology and its severity. More recently, neuroinflammation and chronic hypoperfusion have also been linked to the vascular processes underlying cognitive dysfunction and late-life depression, eventually influencing their development and course [7–10].

Overall, both cognitive impairment and geriatric depression cause a significant impact on the social and healthcare-related burden worldwide [11–13]. Epidemiological evidence also supports the concept that modifiable vascular and lifestyle-related factors are related with the onset of cognitive impairment and movement disorders [14–20]. To date, an early identification and prompt management of cardio- and cerebrovascular risk factors are the only effective measures to prevent dementia and other types of cognitive disorders, such as Mild Cognitive Impairment (MCI) and VCI [21,22]. Therefore, a comprehensive description and quantification of these factors is the preliminary step towards the elucidation of the causes and mechanisms underlying the onset and progression of dementia, as well as the design of new disease-modifying strategies [23–31].

Some dietary components of the Mediterranean diet have been traditionally considered as preventing factors of cardiovascular diseases (including stroke), and some age-related cognitive disorders (such as AD and VaD) [32–36]. Recently, there has been increasing interest in the exploration of the role of coffee intake in some neurological and neuropsychiatric disorders, although large epidemiological investigations are still inconclusive in terms of a protective role of caffeine in the risk of cognitive disorders. Indeed, while many studies have found a protective role of coffee in cognitive impairment [37], an extensive neuropsychological evaluation was not always performed, and the association was not found, or at least not for all, cognitive domains [37]. Similarly, there is still no consensus regarding a dose-response effect on cognition or mood [37–41].

Regarding the risk of depression, a systematic review and dose-response meta-analysis of observational studies on coffee, tea, and caffeine [42], including 23 datasets accounting for a total of 8146 individuals with depression, found that, compared to those with lower coffee consumption, the higher intakes had a pooled relative risk of depression of 0.76 (95% confidence interval 0.64, 0.91). The dose-response effect suggested a nonlinear "J-shaped" relation between coffee consumption and risk of depression, with a peak of effect for 400 mL/day, suggesting a protective role of coffee in the risk of depression [42]. Another meta-analysis of observational studies confirmed that coffee and caffeine consumption were significantly associated with a decreased risk of depression [43].

The roasted seeds of *Coffea* sp. are used for coffee extraction. The composition of a coffee beverage basically depends on species, roast, and preparation methods [44–46], which vary according to geographic and cultural factors, all affecting the chemical profile. For instance, in Italian coffee shops, the espresso method, in which hot water at high pressure is passed through about 8 g of finely-ground coffee powder producing a serving of 30 mL, is basically the rule. Another common preparation of coffee in Italy, particularly at home and in the Southern regions, is through a mocha, i.e., an aluminium or stainless-steel machine, in which hot water (approx. 70 °C) is forced up through the coffee in the pot top [47].

Methods of preparation influence diterpenes and caffeine concentration. Cafestol and kahweol content per cup is approximately 7.2 mg in boiled coffee, 2.3 mg in mocha coffee, 1.0 mg in espresso coffee, but only 0.02 mg in filtered coffee [48]. In Italian-made coffee, the contact time of water with the solid coffee is very short, thus accounting for the lower concentration of lipids than boiled coffee, although it is substantially higher than paper-filtered coffee [48]. However, albeit the concentration of diterpene in Italian-made coffee is considerable [48], the size of the cup is much smaller than in other European countries. On these bases, differences in the effects of mocha coffee are expected.

As drank daily by millions of persons worldwide and due to the caffeine content, coffee is the most common psychophysical stimulating agent, whose consumption is known to result in heightened alertness and arousal, as well as in better mental performance [49]. Studies in male rats also indicate that long-lasting caffeine intake might prevent cognitive deficits [50]. The main proposed mechanisms, among others, are based on the finding that caffeine, as an antioxidant compound, can limit oxidative stress [51] and exert neuronal protection against the disruption of the blood–brain barrier (BBB) [52].

In addition to its short-term effects, a systematic review of human studies has assessed the chronically assumed impact of coffee on cerebral functions, providing hints on the protective role in cognitive disorders till dementia, with a higher effect in females than in males [53]. However, the association was not observed for every cognitive domain and a clear dose-response association is still lacking [37]. It has also been shown that the risk of depression decreased with increasing caffeinated coffee consumption in women [40].

Similarly, the effects of coffee on VCI and geriatric depression remain basically unexplored, with previous studies frequently producing contradictory results. In a previous study [41], the association of coffee intake in midlife with the risk of dementia, its neuropathological correlates, and cognitive impairment was examined among 3494 men, including 418 decedents who underwent brain autopsy. Although dementia was diagnosed in 226 men (including 118 AD and 80 VaD) and cognitive impairment in 347, there was no association between coffee intake and the risk of cognitive impairment, overall dementia, AD, VaD, or moderate/high levels of neuropathologic lesions. However, men in the highest quartile of caffeine intake were less likely to have any lesion type at autopsy than men in the lowest quartile [41]. A few years later, the association between coffee intake and silent brain infarcts in magnetic resonance imaging (MRI) in 242 middle-age healthy individuals demonstrated that brain lesions were observed less frequently in those consuming three cups or more of coffee per day [54].

Lastly, a recent umbrella review evaluating current evidence of the relation between coffee consumption and human health suggested that there might be a possible association between coffee intake and decreased risk of AD [55]. However, the evidence was concluded from studies investigating the consumption of regular coffee, while data on mocha are lacking.

Based on these considerations, in the present study we aimed to estimate the association between mocha coffee consumption and cognitive and mood status in a homogeneous population of non-demented elderly Italian subjects with SIVD. We hypothesized that daily coffee intake would positively influence cognitive performance and mood status, with a dose-response association.

2. Materials and Methods

2.1. Participants

In this cross-sectional study, a population of 300 individuals was consecutively enrolled from the Cerebrovascular Diseases Centre of the "Azienda Ospedaliera Universitaria Policlinico Gaspare Rodolico-San Marco" of Catania, Italy. All subjects were referred to an expert neurologist (R.B.) because of non-specific cognitive deficits, with or without concomitant mood complaints.

An age ≥ 65 years, a Mini Mental State Examination score (MMSE) ≥ 24, and brain MRI-based evidence of lacunar state or ischemic WMLs were the inclusion criteria. Coffee consumption over the last year was focused to mocha, as it represents the most common preparation of coffee consumed by elderly people in Southern Italy. Exclusion criteria were: overt dementia, consumption of other coffee preparations different from mocha, any medical condition or drug affecting cognitive functions and/or mood status, alcohol or drug abuse, and any contraindication to MRI. Namely, 46 subjects mainly drinking espresso coffee or with a mixed coffee consumption (i.e., espresso and mocha) were excluded.

Signed informed consent was provided by all individuals before participation in the study, which was approved by the Ethics Committee of the "Azienda Ospedaliera Universitaria Policlinico Gaspare Rodolico-San Marco" of Catania, Italy (approval code 292/prot. n. 871) and performed according to the 1964 Declaration of Helsinki and its subsequent amendments.

2.2. Assessment

All participants underwent a detailed clinical and demographic history and a full neurological examination. In particular, information about past medical history, coffee consumption, smoking habit, and drugs taken was collected and confirmed by the subjects and their relatives/caregivers.

High blood pressure was considered as drug therapy intake or a measured systolic blood pressure ≥ 140 mmHg and/or diastolic blood pressure ≥ 90 mmHg. Hyperlipidemia and diabetes were assessed by a recent laboratory test or self-reported diagnosis and drug treatment. Given the lack of a validated food-frequency questionnaire on mocha coffee consumption, information on coffee data was collected via a diet record. The intake of coffee was classified as: <1 cup/day (non-drinkers or occasional consumers), 1 cup/day (light consumers), 2 cups/day (moderate consumers), and ≥ 3 cups/day (heavy consumers), as adapted from a recently published study [56].

Neuropsychological evaluation, performed by a trained neurologist (F.F.), who was blind with respect to coffee consumption, included: a screening test of cognitive functions, i.e., the Mini Mental State Examination (MMSE) [57]; a test evaluating executive functions and other frontal lobe abilities, i.e., the Stroop Colour-Word Interference Test (Stroop T) [58]; an assessment of depressive symptoms through a standardized questionnaire, i.e., the 17-item Hamilton Depression Rating Scale (HDRS) [59]; a scoring of the functional status according to the Activities of Daily Living (ADL) and the Instrumental ADL (IADL) [60].

As known, frontal lobe abilities are typically involved in this population, who may manifest attention deficit and executive dysfunction early, which causes impairment in complex information use, strategy formulation, and emotional-behavioural control [61]. Compared with AD, subjects with VCI also show a less pronounced impairment of episodic memory, but more depressive symptoms and greater variability in the disease course [6]. Moreover, SIVD due to small vessel disease contributes to the deterioration of psychomotor speed, global cognitive function, impaired executive control, and loss of activities of daily living, eventually leading to a considerable risk of dementia [62]. Cognitive impairment is also common in vascular depression, particularly executive dysfunction, a finding which is also predictive of poor antidepressant response [63].

All subjects underwent brain MRI, which was carried out with a 1.5 Tesla General Electric machine (General Electric Healthcare, Milwaukee, WI, USA). The neuroimaging exam included T1-, T2-, fluid-attenuated inversion recovery (FLAIR), and proton density-weighted scans (slice thickness 5 mm, slice gap 0.5 mm). The Fazekas visual scale was used for grading WMLs in all participants: 0 = lack of foci; 1 = punctuate foci; 2 = initially confluent foci; 3 = large confluent foci [64]. Lacunar lesions had to be of 3–20 mm, multiple (>5) cavitated lesions, with T2-weighted or FLAIR hyperintensity in the deep grey matter, corona radiata, and internal capsule. Foci less than 2 mm were considered perivascular spaces, with the exception of the anterior commissure, where larger perivascular spaces can be present. Another author (G.L.), blind to the clinical features and coffee intake, independently reviewed all the scans.

2.3. Statistical Analysis

Subjects' characteristics at baseline, based on the subgroups of coffee consumption, were handled as means and standard deviations (continuous variables) or frequencies (categorical variables). Comparison of continuous variables obtained from the four groups of subjects was first carried out by means of the one-way ANOVA, while the comparison of categorical variables obtained from the same groups of subjects was performed by means of the chi-square test.

Then, based on results obtained from the above analyses, we checked for any simultaneous association of coffee consumption, as well as age, sex, education, and smoking (independent factors/predictors), on the scores obtained at the MMSE, HDRS, and Stroop T, separately (dependent variables) by means of the General Regression Models of the software STATISTICA v.6 StatSoft Inc., Tulsa, OK, USA (employed for all the statistical tests in this study). This module allows us to build models for design with categorical predictor variables, as well as with continuous predictor variables. For each dependent variable, the statistical significance of the association of coffee consumption was obtained by taking into account the effect of the other independent factors. Post-hoc comparisons between the different pairs of groups were then carried-out, for significant comparisons at the previous analysis, with both the Fisher Least Significant Difference (LSD) and the Tukey Honestly Significant Difference (HSD) tests.

Lastly, we analysed the association between MMSE, HDRS, or Stroop T and coffee consumption by calculating the Pearson's correlation coefficient and, following Cohen's [65] indications, we considered a correlation coefficient 0.10, 0.30, and 0.50 as corresponding to small, medium, and large sizes, respectively.

3. Results

The comparison between the different parameters in the four groups of subjects, established on the basis of their daily coffee consumption, is reported in Tables 1 and 2. In Table 1, showing the comparison of continuous variables, a significant difference was found not only in most of the outcome measures (i.e., MMSE, HDRS, and Stroop T), but also in age and education, which might be viewed as factors potentially affecting the results. This was also observed for the comparison of some of the categorical variables (Table 2), such as sex and smoking.

In order to disentangle the association of coffee intake from that of other parameters that were found to be significantly different in the subject groups, we built an analysis design by using the above-mentioned General Regression Models module, using age, sex, education, smoking and coffee consumption as independent predictors, and MMSE, HDRS, Stroop T, ADL, and IADL as dependent variables. Accordingly, we were able to assess that MMSE, HDRS, and Stroop T scores were significantly and independently different in the three coffee consumption subgroups, with a generally lower severity of HDRS with increasing coffee intake ($F = 22.669$, $p < 0.000001$), as well as with better MMSE ($F = 4.105$, $p < 0.0071$) and Stroop T ($F = 4.806$, $p < 0.0028$). The results of MMSE, HDRS, and Stroop T are graphically displayed in Figure 1 as bar graphs of continuous outcome variables obtained from the four groups of subjects (i.e., non-drinkers and drinkers of different cups of mocha coffee per day).

Post-hoc analyses of the differences between the various pairs of groups showed that, for MMSE, the group with highest coffee daily consumption ($\geq$three cups/day) had significantly higher values than the other groups (with both the Fisher LSD and the Tukey HSD tests). Additionally, regarding HDRS, the coffee $\geq$three group had the smallest scores which were, however, not significantly different from those of the coffee two group, and both groups (i.e., coffee $\geq$three and coffee two) had significantly lower scores than the other groups. Similarly, for the Stroop T, in which a significant decrease was observed with increasing coffee consumption, the post-hoc comparisons revealed no difference between coffee two and $\geq$three groups.

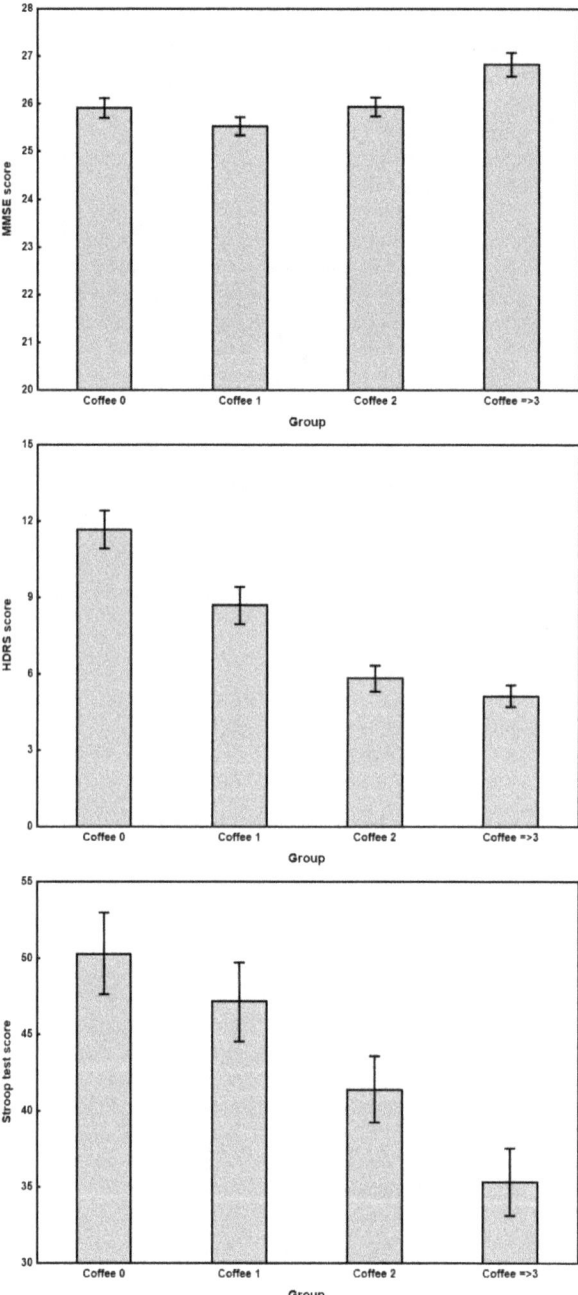

Figure 1. Bar graphs of continuous outcome variables obtained from the four groups of subjects and showing significant differences in Table 1. Data are shown as means (columns) and standard error (wishers). Coffee 0 = non-coffee drinkers; Coffee 1 = consumers of 1 cup daily; Coffee 2 = consumers of 2 cups daily; Coffee $\geq$ 3 = consumers of 3 or more cups daily; MMSE = Mini Mental State Examination; HDRS = 17-item Hamilton Depression Rating Scale; Stroop T = Stroop Colour-Word Interference Test.

Table 1. Comparison of continuous variables obtained from the four groups of subjects.

	Coffee 0 cup/day (n = 73)		Coffee 1 cup/day (n = 69)		Coffee 2 cups/day (n = 87)		Coffee ≥ 3 cups/day (n = 71)		ANOVA	
	Mean	SD	Mean	SD	Mean	SD	Mean	SD	$F_{3,296}$	$p<$
Age, years	73.9	6.2	72.9	5.7	73.5	6.4	70.9	5.6	3.623	0.014
Education, years	6.5	3.7	6.9	4.0	7.5	4.0	8.2	3.9	2.635	0.05
MMSE	25.9	1.8	25.5	1.6	25.9	1.9	26.8	2.1	6.212	0.00042
ADL	5.6	0.7	5.5	0.7	5.6	0.6	5.8	0.6	2.112	NS
IADL	7.2	1.3	6.8	1.5	7.1	1.2	7.3	1.2	1.814	NS
HDRS	11.7	6.4	8.7	6.0	5.8	4.8	5.1	3.6	23.790	0.000001
Stroop T	50.3	22.9	47.1	21.6	41.4	20.4	35.3	18.6	7.182	0.00011

Legend: SD = standard deviation; MMSE = Mini Mental State Examination; ADL = Activities of Daily Living; IADL = Instrumental Activities of Daily Living; HDRS = 17-item Hamilton Depression Rating Scale; Stroop T = Stroop Colour-Word Interference Test; NS = not significant.

Table 2. Comparison of categorical variables obtained from the four groups of subjects.

	Coffee 0 cup/day (n = 73)	Coffee 1 cup/day (n = 69)	Coffee 2 cups/day (n = 87)	Coffee ≥ 3 cups/day (n = 71)	Chi-Square	$p<$
Sex, male/female	28/45	32/37	48/39	48/23	13.60	0.004
Hypertension, yes/no	60/13	50/19	70/17	59/12	3.05	NS
Diabetes, yes/no	15/58	20/49	24/63	26/45	4.62	NS
Hypercholesterolemia, yes/no	22/51	19/50	29/58	28/43	2.54	NS
Coronary artery disease, yes/no	10/63	13/56	9/78	14/57	3.52	NS
Tobacco smoking, yes/no/ex	7/54/12	13/47/9	15/57/15	26/37/8	17.90	0.006
Atrial fibrillation, yes/no	11/62	7/62	8/79	9/62	1.56	NS
Neurologic signs, yes/no	29/44	30/39	36/51	32/39	0.49	NS
Family history, yes/no	8/65	13/56	8/79	8/63	3.70	NS
History of depression, yes/no	15/58	17/52	29/67	16/55	2.40	NS
MRI, lacunar/Fazekas 1/2/3	13/15/29/16	8/22/24/15	15/21/32/19	12/21/24/14	3.81	NS

Legend: ex = former smokers; MRI = magnetic resonance imaging; Fazekas 1/2/3 = white matter lesion severity based on the Fazekas visual scale: 0 = lack of foci; 1 = punctuate foci; 2 = initially confluent foci; 3 = large confluent foci; NS = not significant.

The simple (not adjusted) regression analysis between HDRS and individual daily coffee consumption in the whole group of subjects showed a correlation coefficient that can be considered to be medium-to-large, according to Cohen [65] (-0.386; $p < 0.000001$). The same analysis yielded a correlation coefficient of 0.193 ($p < 0.0008$, small-to-medium size) between coffee consumption and MMSE, and of 0.256 ($p < 0.000001$, close to medium size) between daily coffee consumption and Stroop T.

4. Discussion

4.1. Main Findings

This is the first study focused on the association between a specific coffee preparation method (i.e., mocha) and cognitive impairment and late-life depression in a homogeneous population of non-demented elderly subjects with SIVD. Most of the previous studies, indeed, explored the effects of boiled or filtered coffee, which are very popular in other European countries and in the USA [66]. An association between coffee consumption and cognitive and mood performance in VCI subjects, along with a dose-response association already observed with a moderate intake (two cups/day), without difference for heavier drinkers (with the exception of the MMSE results), are the main findings of this study.

A number of longitudinal and cross-sectional population-based studies hypothesized a protective role of coffee in cognitive impairment [37], although not all performed an extensive neuropsychological evaluation and, among them, the association was not found in all cognitive domains. In general, with increasing quantity of coffee, a positive dose-response effect was observed in cognitive batteries evaluating verbal memory, reaction time, and visuo-spatial skills [38], with higher lifetime coffee intake associated with higher scores [39]. On the other hand, in a cohort of elderly subjects, a significant association between coffee intake and overall cognitive and mnesic performance was found, although, after adjustment for age, intelligence quotient, and social status, this association became not significant [67]. In our population, we found a significant difference in age and education among the four groups, but the General Regression Model showed that the associations between mocha coffee intake and both cognition and mood were independent from the socio-demographic variables.

Other longitudinal studies found a negative association between coffee intake and cognitive disorder in a sample of healthy elderly men from different European countries [68], especially in women [69–71]. In particular, higher coffee consumption was associated with a moderately better maintenance of cognitive status over five years in older females with vascular diseases [72]. Such gender-related association was not evident in the present population of VCI subjects, as well as the association with vascular burden. Even for these aspects, previous evidence in this type of population is scarce and not tailored to the coffee preparation method. Regarding the gender-related effect, an earlier prospective study [73] on 455 participants (314 men) found that the incidence of small vessel disease was lower in male drinkers than male non-drinkers and occasional drinkers, whereas the incidence of WMLs was lower in female drinkers than female non-drinkers or occasional drinkers. In the multivariate analyses including age, sex, smoking status, body-mass index, and coffee consumption, the incidence of microbleeds was significantly lower in male drinkers compared to non-drinkers [73]. Regarding the vascular burden, a recent study [74] assessing the impact of some dietary intake (including coffee) on cognitive outcome and MRI parameters in old age demonstrated an inverse association between coffee consumption and cognitive performance. Moreover, moderate-to-heavy coffee drinking was associated with better white matter preservation and cerebral blood flow in cognitively stable elders [74].

It should be reported that some prospective reports did not observe any association between coffee intake and cognitive disorders [41,75–77]. Among 418 subjects who underwent brain autopsy, there was no association between coffee consumption and the risk of cognitive impairment, VaD, AD, or moderate/severe neuropathological lesions [41]. In 2015, a meta-analysis reached the conclusion that coffee or tea consumption was not associated with a risk of cognitive decline [78]. Nonetheless, the majority of systematic reviews and meta-analyses seem to converge on a positive effect of caffeine on cognitive decline [79–81], with a greater impact in females than in males [53], along with the minimum risk at a daily intake of one–two cups of coffee [82]. Similarly, two meta-analyses showed that coffee intake was significantly associated with a reduced risk of depression [42,43]. Accordingly, we found that subjects with the highest daily coffee consumption had significantly better MMSE compared to the other groups.

Finally, little is known about coffee and depression in older adults, as well as a dose-response association. According to our data, the positive association with HDRS and Stroop T seems to be dose-dependent, with a significant association reached with a moderate intake (two cups/day) and not further increasing with higher intake. In this context, it has been previously demonstrated that drinking coffee or tea was associated with lower risk for depression in older adults [83], whereas in another study on middle-age participants, those who drank at least four cups of coffee per day showed a significantly lower risk of depression than participants drinking ≤one cup, although an inverse linear dose-response association was not observed [84]. Finally, a very recent multicentre cross-sectional study on 1992 elderly Japanese women [85] found that coffee intake was associated with a lower prevalence of depressive symptoms in a fully adjusted model. Caffeine intake was also associated with depressive symptoms, although the association was not statistically significant, suggesting that the association might also be related to other substances in coffee or other factors related to coffee intake [85].

A recent study in Italy has evaluated the association between modification or constant habits in coffee intake and the occurrence of MCI in a sample of elderly subjects followed-up for 3.5 years [86]. This study found that individuals who usually drink a moderate daily quantity of coffee (one–two cups) exhibited a lower rate of MCI compared to non-drinkers or occasional consumers. Those who increased coffee consumption (>one cup) shower a higher incidence rate of MCI than subjects with constant habits (up to +/− one cup) or those without consumption. Additionally, no significant association between higher quantity of coffee intake (>two cups) and the incidence of MCI compared with non-drinkers or occasional consumers was observed [86]. Conversely, heavy and prolonged coffee consumption is associated with the risk of WMLs in later life, likely through an increase in arterial stiffness, vascular resistance, and cerebral vasoconstriction. This may result in reduced cerebral blood flow and eventually lead to an increased rate and severity of vascular lesions [87].

Lastly, tobacco smoking reduces the half-life of caffeine [88], a finding that might contribute to a weaker protective effect of coffee in smokers. Therefore, given that smokers are often coffee consumers, a weaker protective role is likely to take place in males, with the rate of smokers being higher in males than in females [89–91]. Although in our sample we found a significant difference in smoking habits among the groups, there was no significant smoking-related independent association with the outcome measures.

4.2. Limitations

These findings need to be considered in light of some limitations. Firstly, due to its cross-sectional design, this study is prone to several biases, including that of drinking habit as an effect of cognitive status rather than causally related [53]. Additionally, population-based studies may suffer from item response bias in the measures of cognition. Therefore, we cannot establish a causal association between these factors. Similarly, although a dose-response association is likely to occur, a causal relationship cannot be established. Future investigations, along with multidimensional follow-up, will verify the possibility of a protective role of mocha coffee consumption in the measures of interest, as well as a dose-response effect.

Secondly, not all cognitive domains were explored in this study, although we focused on those domains typically and early affected in subjects with VCI.

The self-reported coffee drinking habits may represent an additional limitation, although measurement errors are often inevitable for dietary exposures, especially in older individuals or in some with cognitive impairment, who may hardly have a reliable record of their usual consumption.

Fourthly, although the results were adjusted for possible confounding factors, we cannot entirely exclude the potential association with unmeasured confounders. For instance, coffee consumption may be related to other lifestyle and social factors that may account for part of the associations observed. This also holds true for medications assumed for the control of co-morbid conditions.

Lastly, although we hypothesized that caffeine would have contributed to the results, the potential contribution of other compounds contained in coffee (for instance, flavonoids) cannot be excluded and deserves further investigation.

5. Conclusions

Moderate mocha coffee consumption was associated with higher cognition and mood status in non-demented elderly subjects with VCI. If confirmed in larger populations, these findings may be implicated in the delay or even prevention of some age-related cognitive disorders and late-life mood disturbances. Prospective studies will elucidate the potential protective effect of different methods of coffee preparation both in aged healthy individuals and in patients with cognitive decline and geriatric depression, thus contributing to disentangling the exciting relationships between coffee intake and the aging brain.

Author Contributions: Conceptualization, F.F. and R.B.; methodology, M.P. and C.V.; validation, G.P. and R.F.; formal analysis, R.F.; data curation, M.C.; writing—original draft preparation, F.F. and G.L.; writing—review and editing, M.P. and C.V.; visualization, G.L. and M.C.; supervision, G.P.; project administration, R.B. All authors have read and agreed to the published version of the manuscript.

Funding: This research received no external funding.

Institutional Review Board Statement: The study was conducted according to the guidelines of the Declaration of Helsinki, and approved by the Ethics Committee of the "Azienda Ospedaliera Universitaria Policlinico Gaspare Rodolico-San Marco" of Catania, Italy (approval code 292/prot. n. 871).

Informed Consent Statement: Informed consent was obtained from all subjects involved in the study.

Data Availability Statement: The data that support the findings of this study are openly available in "Mendeley Data" at https://data.mendeley.com/datasets/vnzpzcw224/1.

Conflicts of Interest: The authors declare no conflict of interest.

References

1. Cummings, J.L. Frontal-Subcortical Circuits and Human Behavior. *Arch. Neurol.* **1993**, *50*, 873–880. [CrossRef]
2. Lanza, G.; Bella, R.; Giuffrida, S.; Cantone, M.; Pennisi, G.; Spampinato, C.; Giordano, D.; Malaguarnera, G.; Raggi, A.; Pennisi, M. Preserved Transcallosal Inhibition to Transcranial Magnetic Stimulation in Nondemented Elderly Patients with Leukoaraiosis. *BioMed Res. Int.* **2013**, *2013*, 351680. [CrossRef]
3. Aizenstein, H.J.; Baskys, A.; Boldrini, M.; Butters, M.A.; Diniz, B.S.; Jaiswal, M.K.; Jellinger, K.A.; Kruglov, L.S.; Meshandin, I.A.; Mijajlovic, M.D.; et al. Vascular Depression Consensus Report—A Critical Update. *BMC Med.* **2016**, *14*, 161. [CrossRef]
4. Bella, R.; Ferri, R.; Cantone, M.; Pennisi, M.; Lanza, G.; Malaguarnera, G.; Spampinato, C.; Giordano, D.; Raggi, A.; Pennisi, G. Motor Cortex Excitability in Vascular Depression. *Int. J. Psychophysiol.* **2011**, *82*, 248–253. [CrossRef]
5. Concerto, C.; Lanza, G.; Cantone, M.; Pennisi, M.; Giordano, D.; Spampinato, C.; Ricceri, R.; Pennisi, G.; Aguglia, E.; Bella, R. Different Patterns of Cortical Excitability in Major Depression and Vascular Depression: A Transcranial Magnetic Stimulation Study. *BMC Psychiatry* **2013**, *13*, 300. [CrossRef]
6. Taylor, W.D.; Aizenstein, H.J.; Alexopoulos, G.S. The Vascular Depression Hypothesis: Mechanisms Linking Vascular Disease with Depression. *Mol. Psychiatry* **2013**, *18*, 963–974. [CrossRef] [PubMed]
7. Alexopoulos, G.S. Mechanisms and Treatment of Late-Life Depression. *Transl. Psychiatry* **2019**, *9*. [CrossRef] [PubMed]
8. Vagli, C.; Fisicaro, F.; Vinciguerra, L.; Puglisi, V.; Rodolico, M.S.; Giordano, A.; Ferri, R.; Lanza, G.; Bella, R. Cerebral Hemodynamic Changes to Transcranial Doppler in Asymptomatic Patients with Fabry's Disease. *Brain Sci.* **2020**, *10*, 546. [CrossRef] [PubMed]
9. Vinciguerra, L.; Lanza, G.; Puglisi, V.; Pennisi, M.; Cantone, M.; Bramanti, A.; Pennisi, G.; Bella, R. Transcranial Doppler Ultrasound in Vascular Cognitive Impairment-No Dementia. *PLoS ONE* **2019**, *14*, e0216162. [CrossRef] [PubMed]
10. Puglisi, V.; Bramanti, A.; Lanza, G.; Cantone, M.; Vinciguerra, L.; Pennisi, M.; Bonanno, L.; Pennisi, G.; Bella, R. Impaired Cerebral Haemodynamics in Vascular Depression: Insights From Transcranial Doppler Ultrasonography. *Front. Psychiatry* **2018**, *9*, 316. [CrossRef]
11. Naylor, M.D.; Karlawish, J.H.; Arnold, S.E.; Khachaturian, A.S.; Khachaturian, Z.S.; Lee, V.M.-Y.; Baumgart, M.; Banerjee, S.; Beck, C.; Blennow, K.; et al. Advancing Alzheimer's Disease Diagnosis, Treatment, and Care: Recommendations from the Ware Invitational Summit. *Alzheimers Dement.* **2012**, *8*, 445–452. [CrossRef]
12. Cantone, M.; Catalano, M.A.; Lanza, G.; La Delfa, G.; Ferri, R.; Pennisi, M.; Bella, R.; Pennisi, G.; Bramanti, A. Motor and Perceptual Recovery in Adult Patients with Mild Intellectual Disability. *Neural Plast.* **2018**. [CrossRef]
13. Lanza, G.; Bella, R.; Cantone, M.; Pennisi, G.; Ferri, R.; Pennisi, M. Cognitive Impairment and Celiac Disease: Is Transcranial Magnetic Stimulation a Trait d'Union between Gut and Brain? *Int. J. Mol. Sci.* **2018**, *19*, 2243. [CrossRef]
14. Solfrizzi, V.; Capurso, C.; D'Introno, A.; Colacicco, A.M.; Santamato, A.; Ranieri, M.; Fiore, P.; Capurso, A.; Panza, F. Lifestyle-Related Factors in Predementia and Dementia Syndromes. *Expert Rev. Neurother.* **2008**, *8*, 133–158. [CrossRef]
15. Solfrizzi, V.; Panza, F.; Frisardi, V.; Seripa, D.; Logroscino, G.; Imbimbo, B.P.; Pilotto, A. Diet and Alzheimer's Disease Risk Factors or Prevention: The Current Evidence. *Expert Rev. Neurother.* **2011**, *11*, 677–708. [CrossRef]
16. Panza, F.; Solfrizzi, V.; Logroscino, G.; Maggi, S.; Santamato, A.; Seripa, D.; Pilotto, A. Current Epidemiological Approaches to the Metabolic-Cognitive Syndrome. *J. Alzheimers Dis.* **2012**, *30* (Suppl. 2), S31–S75. [CrossRef]
17. Richard, E.; Moll van Charante, E.P.; van Gool, W.A. Vascular Risk Factors as Treatment Target to Prevent Cognitive Decline. *J. Alzheimers Dis.* **2012**, *32*, 733–740. [CrossRef] [PubMed]
18. Lanza, G.; Pino, M.; Fisicaro, F.; Vagli, C.; Cantone, M.; Pennisi, M.; Bella, R.; Bellomo, M. Motor Activity and Becker's Muscular Dystrophy: Lights and Shadows. *Phys. Sportsmed.* **2019**, 1–10. [CrossRef] [PubMed]
19. Lanza, G.; Casabona, J.A.; Bellomo, M.; Cantone, M.; Fisicaro, F.; Bella, R.; Pennisi, G.; Bramanti, P.; Pennisi, M.; Bramanti, A. Update on Intensive Motor Training in Spinocerebellar Ataxia: Time to Move a Step Forward? *J. Int. Med. Res.* **2019**. [CrossRef]
20. Lanza, G.; Ferri, R. The Neurophysiology of Hyperarousal in Restless Legs Syndrome: Hints for a Role of Glutamate/GABA. *Adv. Pharmacol.* **2019**, *84*, 101–119. [CrossRef] [PubMed]
21. Vinciguerra, L.; Lanza, G.; Puglisi, V.; Fisicaro, F.; Pennisi, M.; Bella, R.; Cantone, M. Update on the Neurobiology of Vascular Cognitive Impairment: From Lab to Clinic. *Int. J. Mol. Sci.* **2020**, *21*, 2977. [CrossRef]
22. Fisicaro, F.; Lanza, G.; Cantone, M.; Ferri, R.; Pennisi, G.; Nicoletti, A.; Zappia, M.; Bella, R.; Pennisi, M. Clinical and Electrophysiological Hints to TMS in de Novo Patients with Parkinson's Disease and Progressive Supranuclear Palsy. *J. Pers. Med.* **2020**, *10*, 274. [CrossRef] [PubMed]

23. Di Marco, L.Y.; Marzo, A.; Muñoz-Ruiz, M.; Ikram, M.A.; Kivipelto, M.; Ruefenacht, D.; Venneri, A.; Soininen, H.; Wanke, I.; Ventikos, Y.A.; et al. Modifiable Lifestyle Factors in Dementia: A Systematic Review of Longitudinal Observational Cohort Studies. *J. Alzheimers Dis.* **2014**, *42*, 119–135. [CrossRef] [PubMed]

24. Bordet, R.; Ihl, R.; Korczyn, A.D.; Lanza, G.; Jansa, J.; Hoerr, R.; Guekht, A. Towards the Concept of Disease-Modifier in Post-Stroke or Vascular Cognitive Impairment: A Consensus Report. *BMC Med.* **2017**, *15*. [CrossRef]

25. Pennisi, M.; Lanza, G.; Cantone, M.; D'Amico, E.; Fisicaro, F.; Puglisi, V.; Vinciguerra, L.; Bella, R.; Vicari, E.; Malaguarnera, G. Acetyl-L-Carnitine in Dementia and Other Cognitive Disorders: A Critical Update. *Nutrients* **2020**, *12*, 1389. [CrossRef]

26. Cantone, M.; Lanza, G.; Fisicaro, F.; Pennisi, M.; Bella, R.; Di Lazzaro, V.; Di Pino, G. Evaluation and Treatment of Vascular Cognitive Impairment by Transcranial Magnetic Stimulation. *Neural Plast.* **2020**, *2020*. [CrossRef]

27. Lanza, G.; Calì, F.; Vinci, M.; Cosentino, F.I.I.; Tripodi, M.; Spada, R.S.; Cantone, M.; Bella, R.; Mattina, T.; Ferri, R. A Customized Next-Generation Sequencing-Based Panel to Identify Novel Genetic Variants in Dementing Disorders: A Pilot Study. *Neural Plast.* **2020**, *2020*, e8078103. [CrossRef]

28. Lanza, G.; Cantone, M.; Musso, S.; Borgione, E.; Scuderi, C.; Ferri, R. Early-Onset Subcortical Ischemic Vascular Dementia in an Adult with MtDNA Mutation 3316G>A. *J. Neurol.* **2018**, *265*, 968–969. [CrossRef] [PubMed]

29. Fisicaro, F.; Lanza, G.; Bella, R.; Pennisi, M. "Self-Neuroenhancement": The Last Frontier of Noninvasive Brain Stimulation? *J. Clin. Neurol.* **2020**, *16*, 158–159. [CrossRef]

30. Lanza, G.; Centonze, S.S.; Destro, G.; Vella, V.; Bellomo, M.; Pennisi, M.; Bella, R.; Ciavardelli, D. Shiatsu as an Adjuvant Therapy for Depression in Patients with Alzheimer's Disease: A Pilot Study. *Complement. Ther. Med.* **2018**, *38*, 74–78. [CrossRef]

31. Fisicaro, F.; Lanza, G.; Grasso, A.A.; Pennisi, G.; Bella, R.; Paulus, W.; Pennisi, M. Repetitive Transcranial Magnetic Stimulation in Stroke Rehabilitation: Review of the Current Evidence and Pitfalls. *Ther. Adv. Neurol. Disord.* **2019**, *12*. [CrossRef] [PubMed]

32. Godos, J.; Caraci, F.; Castellano, S.; Currenti, W.; Galvano, F.; Ferri, R.; Grosso, G. Association Between Dietary Flavonoids Intake and Cognitive Function in an Italian Cohort. *Biomolecules* **2020**, *10*, 1300. [CrossRef]

33. Godos, J.; Currenti, W.; Angelino, D.; Mena, P.; Castellano, S.; Caraci, F.; Galvano, F.; Del Rio, D.; Ferri, R.; Grosso, G. Diet and Mental Health: Review of the Recent Updates on Molecular Mechanisms. *Antioxidants* **2020**, *9*, 346. [CrossRef]

34. Pennisi, M.; Malaguarnera, G.; Di Bartolo, G.; Lanza, G.; Bella, R.; Chisari, E.M.; Cauli, O.; Vicari, E.; Malaguarnera, M. Decrease in Serum Vitamin D Level of Older Patients with Fatigue. *Nutrients* **2019**, *11*, 2531. [CrossRef]

35. Pennisi, M.; Di Bartolo, G.; Malaguarnera, G.; Bella, R.; Lanza, G.; Malaguarnera, M. Vitamin D Serum Levels in Patients with Statin-Induced Musculoskeletal Pain. *Dis. Markers* **2019**, *2019*, 3549402. [CrossRef]

36. Pennisi, M.; Lanza, G.; Cantone, M.; Ricceri, R.; Ferri, R.; D'Agate, C.C.; Pennisi, G.; Di Lazzaro, V.; Bella, R. Cortical Involvement in Celiac Disease before and after Long-Term Gluten-Free Diet: A Transcranial Magnetic Stimulation Study. *PLoS ONE* **2017**, *12*, e0177560. [CrossRef] [PubMed]

37. Panza, F.; Solfrizzi, V.; Barulli, M.R.; Bonfiglio, C.; Guerra, V.; Osella, A.; Seripa, D.; Sabbà, C.; Pilotto, A.; Logroscino, G. Coffee, Tea, and Caffeine Consumption and Prevention of Late-Life Cognitive Decline and Dementia: A Systematic Review. *J. Nutr. Health Aging* **2015**, *19*, 313–328. [CrossRef] [PubMed]

38. Jarvis, M.J. Does Caffeine Intake Enhance Absolute Levels of Cognitive Performance? *Psychopharmacology* **1993**, *110*, 45–52. [CrossRef] [PubMed]

39. Johnson-Kozlow, M.; Kritz-Silverstein, D.; Barrett-Connor, E.; Morton, D. Coffee Consumption and Cognitive Function among Older Adults. *Am. J. Epidemiol.* **2002**, *156*, 842–850. [CrossRef] [PubMed]

40. Lucas, D.M.; Mirzaei, D.F.; Pan, D.A.; Okereke, D.O.I.; Willett, D.W.C.; O'Reilly, D.É.J.; Koenen, D.K.; Ascherio, D.A. Coffee, Caffeine, and Risk of Depression Among Women. *Arch. Intern. Med.* **2011**, *171*, 1571. [CrossRef]

41. Gelber, R.P.; Petrovitch, H.; Masaki, K.H.; Ross, G.W.; White, L.R. Coffee Intake in Midlife and Risk of Dementia and Its Neuropathologic Correlates. *J. Alzheimers Dis.* **2011**, *23*, 607–615. [CrossRef]

42. Grosso, G.; Micek, A.; Castellano, S.; Pajak, A.; Galvano, F. Coffee, Tea, Caffeine and Risk of Depression: A Systematic Review and Dose-Response Meta-Analysis of Observational Studies. *Mol. Nutr. Food Res.* **2016**, *60*, 223–234. [CrossRef] [PubMed]

43. Wang, L.; Shen, X.; Wu, Y.; Zhang, D. Coffee and Caffeine Consumption and Depression: A Meta-Analysis of Observational Studies. *Aust. N. Z. J. Psychiatry* **2016**, *50*, 228–242. [CrossRef] [PubMed]

44. Lane, J.D.; Pieper, C.F.; Phillips-Bute, B.G.; Bryant, J.E.; Kuhn, C.M. Caffeine Affects Cardiovascular and Neuroendocrine Activation at Work and Home. *Psychosom. Med.* **2002**, *64*, 595–603. [CrossRef] [PubMed]

45. Nurminen, M.L.; Niittynen, L.; Korpela, R.; Vapaatalo, H. Coffee, Caffeine and Blood Pressure: A Critical Review. *Eur. J. Clin. Nutr.* **1999**, *53*, 831–839. [CrossRef]

46. Urgert, R.; Katan, M.B. The Cholesterol-Raising Factor from Coffee Beans. *J. R. Soc. Med.* **1996**, *89*, 618–623. [CrossRef]

47. D'Amicis, A.; Scaccini, C.; Tomassi, G.; Anaclerio, M.; Stornelli, R.; Bernini, A. Italian Style Brewed Coffee: Effect on Serum Cholesterol in Young Men. *Int. J. Epidemiol.* **1996**, *25*, 513–520. [CrossRef]

48. Casiglia, E.; Bongiovì, S.; Paleari, C.D.; Petucco, S.; Boni, M.; Colangeli, G.; Penzo, M.; Pessina, A.C. Haemodynamic Effects of Coffee and Caffeine in Normal Volunteers: A Placebo-Controlled Clinical Study. *J. Intern. Med.* **1991**, *229*, 501–504. [CrossRef]

49. Yoshimura, H. The Potential of Caffeine for Functional Modification from Cortical Synapses to Neuron Networks in the Brain. *Curr. Neuropharmacol.* **2005**, *3*, 309–316. [CrossRef] [PubMed]

50. Vila-Luna, S.; Cabrera-Isidoro, S.; Vila-Luna, L.; Juárez-Díaz, I.; Bata-García, J.L.; Alvarez-Cervera, F.J.; Zapata-Vázquez, R.E.; Arankowsky-Sandoval, G.; Heredia-López, F.; Flores, G.; et al. Chronic Caffeine Consumption Prevents Cognitive Decline from Young to Middle Age in Rats, and Is Associated with Increased Length, Branching, and Spine Density of Basal Dendrites in CA1 Hippocampal Neurons. *Neuroscience* **2012**, *202*, 384–395. [CrossRef]
51. Prasanthi, J.R.P.; Dasari, B.; Marwarha, G.; Larson, T.; Chen, X.; Geiger, J.D.; Ghribi, O. Caffeine Protects against Oxidative Stress and Alzheimer's Disease-like Pathology in Rabbit Hippocampus Induced by Cholesterol-Enriched Diet. *Free Radic. Biol. Med.* **2010**, *49*, 1212–1220. [CrossRef]
52. Chen, X.; Ghribi, O.; Geiger, J.D. Caffeine Protects against Disruptions of the Blood-Brain Barrier in Animal Models of Alzheimer's and Parkinson's Diseases. *J. Alzheimers Dis.* **2010**, *20* (Suppl. 1), S127–S141. [CrossRef] [PubMed]
53. Arab, L.; Khan, F.; Lam, H. Epidemiologic Evidence of a Relationship between Tea, Coffee, or Caffeine Consumption and Cognitive Decline. *Adv. Nutr.* **2013**, *4*, 115–122. [CrossRef] [PubMed]
54. Nakaguchi, H.; Matsuno, A.; Okubo, T.; Hoya, K. Relationship between Silent Brain Infarction and Amount of Daily Coffee Consumption in Middle Age. *J. Stroke Cerebrovasc. Dis.* **2016**, *25*, 1678–1682. [CrossRef]
55. Grosso, G.; Godos, J.; Galvano, F.; Giovannucci, E.L. Coffee, Caffeine, and Health Outcomes: An Umbrella Review. *Annu. Rev. Nutr.* **2017**, *37*, 131–156. [CrossRef]
56. Grioni, S.; Agnoli, C.; Sieri, S.; Pala, V.; Ricceri, F.; Masala, G.; Saieva, C.; Panico, S.; Mattiello, A.; Chiodini, P.; et al. Espresso Coffee Consumption and Risk of Coronary Heart Disease in a Large Italian Cohort. *PLoS ONE* **2015**, *10*, e0126550. [CrossRef]
57. Folstein, M.F.; Folstein, S.E.; McHugh, P.R. "Mini-Mental State". A Practical Method for Grading the Cognitive State of Patients for the Clinician. *J. Psychiatr. Res.* **1975**, *12*, 189–198. [CrossRef]
58. Scarpina, F.; Tagini, S. The Stroop Color and Word Test. *Front. Psychol.* **2017**, *8*. [CrossRef] [PubMed]
59. Hamilton, M. A Rating Scale for Depression. *J. Neurol. Neurosurg. Psychiatry* **1960**, *23*, 56–62. [CrossRef] [PubMed]
60. Katz, S. Assessing self-maintenance: Activities of daily living, mobility, and instrumental activities of daily living. *J. Am. Geriatr. Soc.* **1983**, *31*, 721–727. [CrossRef]
61. Wallin, A.; Román, G.C.; Esiri, M.; Kettunen, P.; Svensson, J.; Paraskevas, G.P.; Kapaki, E. Update on Vascular Cognitive Impairment Associated with Subcortical Small-Vessel Disease2. *J. Alzheimers Dis.* **2018**, *62*, 1417–1441. [CrossRef] [PubMed]
62. Jokinen, H.; Kalska, H.; Ylikoski, R.; Madureira, S.; Verdelho, A.; van der Flier, W.M.; Scheltens, P.; Barkhof, F.; Visser, M.C.; Fazekas, F.; et al. Longitudinal Cognitive Decline in Subcortical Ischemic Vascular Disease–the LADIS Study. *Cerebrovasc. Dis.* **2009**, *27*, 384–391. [CrossRef] [PubMed]
63. Bella, R.; Pennisi, G.; Cantone, M.; Palermo, F.; Pennisi, M.; Lanza, G.; Zappia, M.; Paolucci, S. Clinical Presentation and Outcome of Geriatric Depression in Subcortical Ischemic Vascular Disease. *Gerontology* **2010**, *56*, 298–302. [CrossRef] [PubMed]
64. Fazekas, F.; Chawluk, J.B.; Alavi, A.; Hurtig, H.I.; Zimmerman, R.A. MR Signal Abnormalities at 1.5 T in Alzheimer's Dementia and Normal Aging. *Am. J. Roentgenol.* **1987**, *149*, 351–356. [CrossRef]
65. Cohen, J. *Statistical Power Analysis for the Behavioral Sciences*, 2nd ed.; L. Erlbaum Associates: Hillsdale, NJ, USA, 1988; ISBN 978-0-8058-0283-2.
66. McCusker, R.R.; Goldberger, B.A.; Cone, E.J. Caffeine Content of Specialty Coffees. *J. Anal. Toxicol.* **2003**, *27*, 520–522. [CrossRef]
67. Corley, J.; Jia, X.; Kyle, J.A.M.; Gow, A.J.; Brett, C.E.; Starr, J.M.; McNeill, G.; Deary, I.J. Caffeine Consumption and Cognitive Function at Age 70: The Lothian Birth Cohort 1936 Study. *Psychosom. Med.* **2010**, *72*, 206–214. [CrossRef]
68. van Gelder, B.M.; Buijsse, B.; Tijhuis, M.; Kalmijn, S.; Giampaoli, S.; Nissinen, A.; Kromhout, D. Coffee Consumption Is Inversely Associated with Cognitive Decline in Elderly European Men: The FINE Study. *Eur. J. Clin. Nutr.* **2007**, *61*, 226–232. [CrossRef]
69. Ritchie, K.; Carrière, I.; de Mendonca, A.; Portet, F.; Dartigues, J.F.; Rouaud, O.; Barberger-Gateau, P.; Ancelin, M.L. The Neuroprotective Effects of Caffeine: A Prospective Population Study (the Three City Study). *Neurology* **2007**, *69*, 536–545. [CrossRef] [PubMed]
70. Santos, C.; Lunet, N.; Azevedo, A.; de Mendonça, A.; Ritchie, K.; Barros, H. Caffeine Intake Is Associated with a Lower Risk of Cognitive Decline: A Cohort Study from Portugal. *J. Alzheimers Dis.* **2010**, *20* (Suppl. 1), S175–S185. [CrossRef]
71. Arab, L.; Biggs, M.L.; O'Meara, E.S.; Longstreth, W.T.; Crane, P.K.; Fitzpatrick, A.L. Gender Differences in Tea, Coffee, and Cognitive Decline in the Elderly: The Cardiovascular Health Study. *J. Alzheimers Dis.* **2011**, *27*, 553–566. [CrossRef]
72. Vercambre, M.-N.; Berr, C.; Ritchie, K.; Kang, J.H. Caffeine and Cognitive Decline in Elderly Women at High Vascular Risk. *J. Alzheimers Dis.* **2013**, *35*. [CrossRef] [PubMed]
73. Shinoda, M.; Fujii, M.; Takahashi, O.; Kawatsu, A.; Uemura, A.; Niimi, Y. Inverse Relationship between Coffee Consumption and Cerebral Microbleeds in Men, but Not Women. *J. Stroke Cerebrovasc. Dis.* **2015**, *24*, 2196–2199. [CrossRef]
74. Haller, S.; Montandon, M.-L.; Rodriguez, C.; Herrmann, F.R.; Giannakopoulos, P. Impact of Coffee, Wine, and Chocolate Consumption on Cognitive Outcome and MRI Parameters in Old Age. *Nutrients* **2018**, *10*, 1391. [CrossRef]
75. Van Boxtel, M.P.J.; Schmitt, J.A.J.; Bosma, H.; Jolles, J. The Effects of Habitual Caffeine Use on Cognitive Change: A Longitudinal Perspective. *Pharmacol. Biochem. Behav.* **2003**, *75*, 921–927. [CrossRef]
76. Laitala, V.S.; Kaprio, J.; Koskenvuo, M.; Räihä, I.; Rinne, J.O.; Silventoinen, K. Coffee Drinking in Middle Age Is Not Associated with Cognitive Performance in Old Age. *Am. J. Clin. Nutr.* **2009**, *90*, 640–646. [CrossRef]
77. Fredholm, B.B.; Bättig, K.; Holmén, J.; Nehlig, A.; Zvartau, E.E. Actions of Caffeine in the Brain with Special Reference to Factors That Contribute to Its Widespread Use. *Pharmacol. Rev.* **1999**, *51*, 83–133.

78. Kim, Y.-S.; Kwak, S.M.; Myung, S.-K. Caffeine Intake from Coffee or Tea and Cognitive Disorders: A Meta-Analysis of Observational Studies. *Neuroepidemiology* **2015**, *44*, 51–63. [CrossRef] [PubMed]
79. Santos, C.; Costa, J.; Santos, J.; Vaz-Carneiro, A.; Lunet, N. Caffeine Intake and Dementia: Systematic Review and Meta-Analysis. *J. Alzheimers Dis.* **2010**, *20* (Suppl. 1), S187–S204. [CrossRef]
80. Chen, J.Q.A.; Scheltens, P.; Groot, C.; Ossenkoppele, R. Associations Between Caffeine Consumption, Cognitive Decline, and Dementia: A Systematic Review. *J. Alzheimers Dis.* **2020**. [CrossRef] [PubMed]
81. Liu, Q.-P.; Wu, Y.-F.; Cheng, H.-Y.; Xia, T.; Ding, H.; Wang, H.; Wang, Z.-M.; Xu, Y. Habitual Coffee Consumption and Risk of Cognitive Decline/Dementia: A Systematic Review and Meta-Analysis of Prospective Cohort Studies. *Nutrition* **2016**, *32*, 628–636. [CrossRef] [PubMed]
82. Wu, L.; Sun, D.; He, Y. Coffee Intake and the Incident Risk of Cognitive Disorders: A Dose-Response Meta-Analysis of Nine Prospective Cohort Studies. *Clin. Nutr.* **2017**, *36*, 730–736. [CrossRef]
83. Guo, X.; Park, Y.; Freedman, N.D.; Sinha, R.; Hollenbeck, A.R.; Blair, A.; Chen, H. Sweetened Beverages, Coffee, and Tea and Depression Risk among Older US Adults. *PLoS ONE* **2014**, *9*, e94715. [CrossRef]
84. Navarro, A.M.; Abasheva, D.; Martínez-González, M.Á.; Ruiz-Estigarribia, L.; Martín-Calvo, N.; Sánchez-Villegas, A.; Toledo, E. Coffee Consumption and the Risk of Depression in a Middle-Aged Cohort: The SUN Project. *Nutrients* **2018**, *10*, 1333. [CrossRef]
85. Kimura, Y.; Suga, H.; Kobayashi, S.; Sasaki, S. Three-Generation Study of Women on Diets and Health Study Group Intake of Coffee Associated with Decreased Depressive Symptoms among Elderly Japanese Women: A Multi-Center Cross-Sectional Study. *J. Epidemiol.* **2020**, *30*, 338–344. [CrossRef]
86. Solfrizzi, V.; Panza, F.; Imbimbo, B.P.; D'Introno, A.; Galluzzo, L.; Gandin, C.; Misciagna, G.; Guerra, V.; Osella, A.; Baldereschi, M.; et al. Coffee Consumption Habits and the Risk of Mild Cognitive Impairment: The Italian Longitudinal Study on Aging. *J. Alzheimers Dis.* **2015**, *47*, 889–899. [CrossRef]
87. Park, J.; Han, J.W.; Lee, J.R.; Byun, S.; Suh, S.W.; Kim, J.H.; Kim, K.W. Association between Lifetime Coffee Consumption and Late Life Cerebral White Matter Hyperintensities in Cognitively Normal Elderly Individuals. *Sci. Rep.* **2020**, *10*, 421. [CrossRef] [PubMed]
88. Benowitz, N.L.; Hall, S.M.; Modin, G. Persistent Increase in Caffeine Concentrations in People Who Stop Smoking. *BMJ* **1989**, *298*, 1075–1076. [CrossRef]
89. Santos, A.-C.; Barros, H. Smoking Patterns in a Community Sample of Portuguese Adults, 1999–2000. *Prev. Med.* **2004**, *38*, 114–119. [CrossRef] [PubMed]
90. Emma, R.; Caponnetto, P.; Cibella, F.; Caruso, M.; Conte, G.; Benfatto, F.; Ferlito, S.; Gulino, A.; Polosa, R. Short and Long Term Repeatability of Saccharin Transit Time in Current, Former, and Never Smokers. *Front. Physiol.* **2020**, *11*, 1109. [CrossRef] [PubMed]
91. Maniaci, A.; Iannella, G.; Cocuzza, S.; Vicini, C.; Magliulo, G.; Ferlito, S.; Cammaroto, G.; Meccariello, G.; De Vito, A.; Nicolai, A.; et al. Oxidative Stress and Inflammation Biomarker Expression in Obstructive Sleep Apnea Patients. *J. Clin. Med.* **2021**, *10*, 277. [CrossRef] [PubMed]

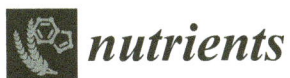

MDPI

Article

Diet Quality and Sociodemographic, Lifestyle, and Health-Related Determinants among People with Depression in Spain: New Evidence from a Cross-Sectional Population-Based Study (2011–2017)

Jesús Cebrino [1] and Silvia Portero de la Cruz [2,*]

[1] Department of Preventive Medicine and Public Health, Faculty of Medicine, University of Seville, Avda. Doctor Fedriani S/N, 41009 Seville, Spain; jcebrino@us.es

[2] Department of Nursing, Pharmacology and Physiotherapy, Faculty of Medicine and Nursing, University of Córdoba, Avda. Menéndez Pidal S/N, 14071 Córdoba, Spain

* Correspondence: n92pocrs@uco.es; Tel.: +34-957-218-093

Abstract: The role of diet quality in depression is an emerging research area and it appears that diet quality could be an important modifying factor. The aims of this study were to report the prevalence of diet quality among individuals with and without a self-reported diagnosis of depression aged from 16 to 64 years old in Spain, to analyze the time trends of the frequency of food consumption and diet quality from 2011 to 2017 in individuals with a self-reported diagnosis of depression, and to explore the associations between poor/improvable diet quality and sociodemographic, lifestyle, and health-related factors. A nationwide cross-sectional study was conducted in 42,280 participants with and without a self-reported diagnosis of depression who had participated in the 2011/2012 and 2017 Spanish National Health Surveys and the 2014 European Health Survey in Spain. A logistic regression analysis was performed to identify the variables associated with diet quality. The overall prevalence of diet quality among depressive and non-depressive individuals revealed 65.71% and 70.27% were in need of improvement, respectively. Moreover, having a poor or improvable diet quality is associated with male gender, people aged 16–24 years old and 25–44 years old, separated or divorced, and also in smokers.

Keywords: depressive disorder; diet; mental disorders; nutrition surveys; population; trends

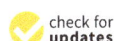
Citation: Cebrino, J.; Portero de la Cruz, S. Diet Quality and Sociodemographic, Lifestyle, and Health-Related Determinants among People with Depression in Spain: New Evidence from a Cross-Sectional Population-Based Study (2011–2017). *Nutrients* **2021**, *13*, 106. https://doi.org/10.3390/nu13010106

Received: 6 December 2020
Accepted: 27 December 2020
Published: 30 December 2020

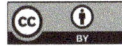
1. Introduction

Depression ranks globally among the top 10 disability causes [1,2], affecting approximately 5% to 6% of people each year worldwide and 11% to 15% of people in their lifetime [3]. Moreover, depression is often recurrent or chronic and has a negative impact on people's functioning and somatic health [4]. Additionally, it has been associated with a poor quality of life, physical decline, higher risk of premature death, and a greater economic burden [5]. Thus, depression is an important public health concern, for which there is an urgent need to identify modifiable factors to reduce its prevalence [6].

The role of diet quality in mental health illnesses and, in particular, depression is an emerging research area, and it appears that diet quality could be a major modifying factor [7–10]. Although some authors have found no associations [8], others show a link between a healthy dietary pattern and a reduced likelihood of depressive symptoms [7,11]. However, direct evidence is not readily available [12–14].

Some studies have found that depressive symptoms were associated with higher intakes of sugar, sodium, and saturated fat [15,16] or frequent consumption of meat and eggs [9,17] and lower intakes of low-calorie foods [18] and antioxidants, fruit and vegetables [19], fish [9], or legumes [20]. However, further studies are needed to assess the influence of types of diet on depression [21]. For example, the impact of soft drinks on mental health has drawn considerable interest from researchers in recent years due to the fact that numerous studies have suggested a consistent association between soft drink consumption and depressive symptoms [22–24].

It seems clear that the factors associating depression with diet quality include sociodemographic and economic conditions. For example, depression is more prevalent in people with low socioeconomic status [25,26], probably due to the fact that higher diet quality or "healthy foods" often have limited uptake because they are more costly [27,28]. In addition, any observed association between depression and diet quality might be accounted for by lifestyle habits, given that people with depression engage in less leisure-time physical activity than those without depression [29], due to a lack of energy and greater fatigue, which are common symptoms of depression [30]. Moreover, the lack of interest in various activities, for example, the motivation to cook or enjoy meals, may be explained by depressive symptoms [31].

Nowadays, drugs and psychological interventions are used to reduce symptoms of depression. Nevertheless, psychological interventions only reduce the incidence rate of depression by 20–25% [32] and medications show minimal benefits in the sub-threshold of depression [33]. Considering the rise in the number of people with depression worldwide [34], preventive strategies are needed in order to reduce its prevalence. For this reason, it is important to reflect on numerous factors affecting the development of depression [35], with particular attention given to modifiable behavior such as a diet that can potentially prevent this disorder [36]. In recent years, there has been a shift of focus from studying single nutrients toward dietary patterns [37]. This particular study uses diet quality scores to evaluate dietary patterns, based on the dietary guidelines of the Spanish Society of Community Nutrition (SSCN) [38]. Moreover, this study is the first to show the relationship between numerous different sociodemographic, lifestyle, and health-related characteristics and diet quality independently and simultaneously in a large, representative sample of the population with a self-reported diagnosis of depression in Spain, aged between 16–64 years old, conducted from 2011 to 2017. Therefore, the main objectives of the present study were to report the prevalence of diet quality among individuals with and without a self-reported diagnosis of depression aged from 16 to 64 years old in Spain, to analyze the time trends of the frequency of food consumption and diet quality from 2011 to 2017 in individuals with a self-reported diagnosis of depression, and to explore the associations between poor/improvable diet quality and sociodemographic, lifestyle, and health-related factors.

2. Materials and Methods

2.1. Study Design

A quantitative, observational, nationwide, cross-sectional study.

2.2. Data Source and Study Population

The data were obtained from the personalized interviews in the Spanish National Health Survey (SNHS) 2011/2012 (from July 2011 to July 2012) [39], the European Health Survey in Spain (EHSS) 2014 (from January 2014 to January 2015) [40], and the SNHS 2017 (from October 2016 to October 2017) [41]. The SNHS and EHSS had a cross-sectional and population-based design and were conducted at the national level, focusing on the non-institutionalized population (representativeness is ensured by assigning a weighting coefficient to each participant), through an interview. These surveys were carried out by the National Institute of Statistics and the Ministry of Health, Consumer Affairs, and Social Welfare in Spain. These personal interviews were multistage probabilistic, stratified sampling by census areas (first stage), sections (second stage), and individuals (third stage). The selected households were initially contacted through a letter from the Ministry of Health, Consumer Affairs, and Social Welfare in Spain requesting their collaboration, in which they were informed that they had been selected for the survey and that this survey was confidential and they were notified of the upcoming visit of a duly authorized interviewer. A detailed description of SNHS and EHSS methodologies can be found elsewhere [39–41].

For the data analyzed, the inclusion criteria were: people aged from 16 to 64 years old, who were resident in Spain during the years of the surveys. Figure 1 shows the flowchart of the study population. From the initial 47,962 participants (SNHS 2011/2012: n = 14,988; EHSS 2014: n = 16,136; SNHS 2017: n = 16,838), we excluded 5682 individuals who did not respond or refused to answer the interview questions (SNHS 2011/2012: n = 1534; EHSS 2014: n = 1458; SNHS 2017: n = 2690). For the cross-sectional analysis, we included 3217 participants with a self-reported diagnosis of depression (SNHS 2011/2012: n = 930; EHSS 2014: n = 1168; SNHS 2017: n = 1119) and 39,063 without a self-reported diagnosis of depression (SNHS 2011/2012: n = 12,524; EHSS 2014: n = 13,510; SNHS 2017: n = 13,029).

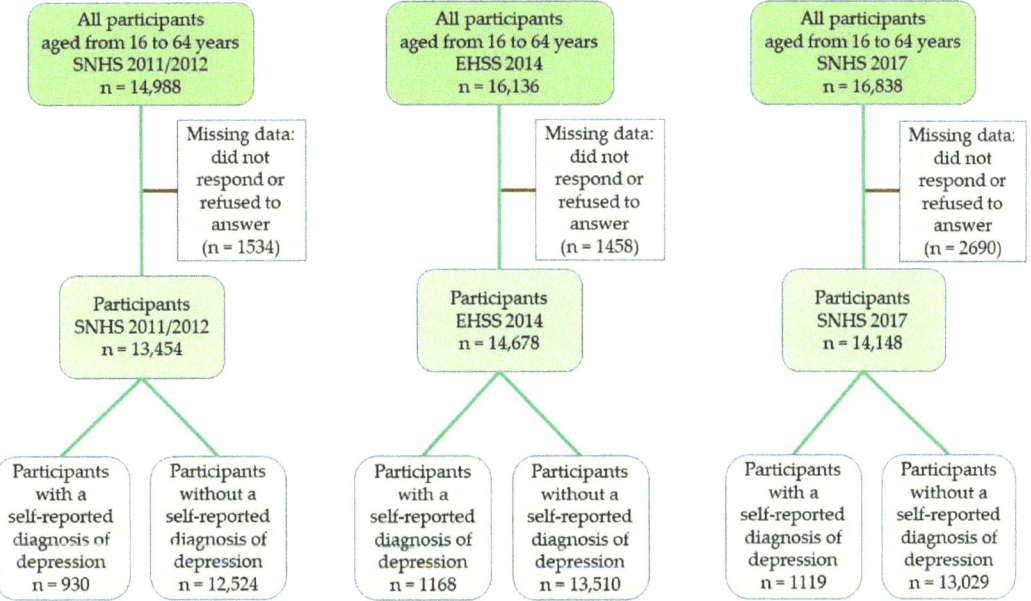

Figure 1. Flowchart of the study population. SNHS: Spanish National Health Survey 2011/2012 and 2017; EHSS: European Health Survey in Spain 2014.

For the purpose of the current study, we assessed the presence of depression through the health status module of an adult questionnaire from SNHS 2011/2012 [39] and 2017 [41] and EHSS 2014 [40]. The adult questionnaire collects individual information on a person aged 15 and over (for SNHS 2011/2012 and SNHS 2017) and 16 and over (for EHSS 2014). This information covers all the survey's health variables and is structured into three modules: (i) health status module, (ii) healthcare module, and (iii) health determinants module. The health status module collects information on perceived health status, chronic disease and limitation, diseases and health problems, accidents, restriction of activity, physical, sensory, and cognitive limitations, limitations on daily activities, mental health, stress, and job satisfaction. We identified individuals suffering from depression as those that answered "yes" to the question "Have you ever been diagnosed depression by a physician?".

2.3. Variables

2.3.1. Diet Quality

The dependent variable was diet quality. This variable was measured using the Spanish Health Eating Index (SHEI) [42]. This instrument was developed to measure how well diets meet the food-based dietary guidelines of the Spanish Society of Community Nutrition (SSCN) [38] and contain 10 items that represent food groups from the dietary guidelines. Each variable represents: (i) bread or grains, (ii) leafy greens, salads, and vegetables, (iii) fresh fruit (excluding juices), (iv) dairy products (milk, cheese, yoghurt), (v) meat (chicken, beef, pork, lamb, etc.), (vi) legumes, (vii) cold meats and cuts, (viii) sweets (biscuits, pastries, jams, cereals with sugar, sweets, etc.), (ix) soft drinks with sugar, and (x) variety of the diet, built on the recommendations of SSCN. These items were identically worded in the questionnaires and identical in the SNHS 2011/2012 and 2017, and EHSS 2014. Each of the items is divided into 5 categories, which refer to the frequency of food consumption: never or hardly ever, less than once a week, once or twice a week, three or more times a week, but not daily, and daily. The food groups were categorized as follows: bread or grains, leafy greens, salads and vegetables, fresh fruit (excluding juices), dairy products (milk, cheese, yogurt), which represent the food groups for daily consumption; meat (chicken, beef, pork, lamb, etc.) and legumes correspond to the weekly consumption food groups; cold meats and cuts, sweets (biscuits, pastries, jams, cereals with sugar, sweets, etc.) and soft drinks with sugar correspond to the occasional food groups; and the last represents the variety of the diet, a fundamental objective in a healthy diet. Each food group received a score, which ranged from 0 to 10 according to the criteria established in the Supplementary Table S1, where 10 points in a food group means that it complies with the recommendations proposed by the Spanish Society of Community Nutrition [38]. Total (overall) SHEI scores range from 0 to 100 and are the sum of the frequency of consumption of 10 food groups. The SHEI result contains three categories: poor diet, diet in need of improvement, and good diet, using the cut-off points previously established in the questionnaire validation [42]: poor diet quality (SHEI score <51), diet in need of improvement (SHEI score between 51 and 80), and good diet quality (SHEI score >80).

2.3.2. Sociodemographic Variables

The independent variables were: year of the surveys (2011/2012, 2014, 2017), gender (female, male), age group (16–24 years, 25–44 years, 45–64 years), marital status (single, married, widowed, separated/divorced), level of education (without studies, primary, secondary or professional training, university), nationality (Spanish, foreign), and size of the town of residence (<10,000 inhabitants, ≥10,000 inhabitants).

Social class, as an independent variable, was assigned according to the categories proposed by the Spanish Society of Epidemiology [43]. This variable was classified into: Class I (directors and managers of companies with 10 or more employees and professionals normally qualified with university degrees), Class II (directors and managers of companies with less than 10 salaried employees and professionals normally qualified with university degrees and other technical support professionals. Athletes and artists), Class III (intermediate professions and self-employed workers), Class IV (supervisors and workers in skilled technical work), Class V (skilled workers in the primary sector and other semi-skilled workers), Class VI (unskilled workers). For the purposes of this study, these six original classes were rearranged into three groups (Classes I and II, Classes III and IV, Classes V and VI).

2.3.3. Health-Related Variables

Body mass index (BMI), which was calculated from the self-reported values of body weight and height, was classified according to the World Health Organization [44]. Thus, the following categories were used: underweight (BMI <18.50 kg/m^2), normal-weight (BMI ranged between 18.50 and 24.99 kg/m^2), overweight (BMI ranged between 25.00 and 29.99 kg/m^2), and obesity (BMI ≥30 kg/m^2).

Other health-related variables in the study were: current smoking habit (yes, no), consumption of alcoholic beverages in the past 12 months prior to the survey (yes, no), and self-perceived health status (very good, good, fair, poor, very poor).

2.3.4. Lifestyle Behavior

Lifestyle behavior included: physical activity in main activity (physically active in the main activity, not physically active in main activity), physical activity during leisure time (yes, no), and the number of days in the last 7 days when the respondent walked for at least 10 min at a time (maximum 7 days).

2.4. Ethical Aspects

The data obtained from these surveys are available on the Ministry of Health, Consumer Affairs, and Social Welfare of Spain and the National Institute of Statistics websites [39–41] in the form of anonymized microdata: no special authorization is, therefore, required for their use. According to the SNHS and EHSS methodology, the microdata files are stored anonymously and are available to the public. In accordance with Spanish law, when secondary data are used, there is no need for approval from an Ethics Committee. The research data is available here as a Supplementary File.

2.5. Statistical Analysis

A descriptive analysis was performed by calculating the counts and percentages for the qualitative variables and the continuous variables by calculating the arithmetic mean and standard deviation (SD). Sociodemographic, lifestyle, health-related characteristics, and the diet quality of people with and without a self-reported diagnosis of depression were compared using the Chi-square test for contingency tables or Fisher's exact test if the number of expected frequencies was greater than 5. For the bivariate analysis, Student's t-test for means in normal distribution variables was used. Linear regression models were used to identify statistically significant trends in the frequency of food consumption in the period of 2011–2017. The regression coefficient and the coefficient of determination (R^2) were calculated to assess the direction, average magnitude of the change, and performance of the models. In addition, logistic regression was performed to identify the variables associated with the diet quality of people with a self-reported diagnosis of depression. It should be noted that the variable for diet quality of people with a self-reported diagnosis of depression was classified as "good diet" (a score over 80 on the SHEI) and "poor/improvable diet" (a score less than or equal to 80) for the bivariate and multivariate analysis. All the variables with a significant association in the bivariate analysis were included in the multivariate analysis. Crude and adjusted Odds Ratios (OR) were calculated with 95% confidence intervals. The Wald statistic was used to exclude one by one from the model any variables with a $p \geq 0.15$ (backward methodical selection procedure). The goodness of fit was verified with the Hosmer–Lemeshow test. All the hypothesis contrasts were bilateral and in all the statistical tests with a 95% confidence level ($p < 0.05$) were considered significant values. The statistical power for all the analyses conducted was 80%. The variables that were part of the final multivariate-adjusted model were gender, age group, marital status, current smoking habit, consumption of alcoholic beverages in the past 12 months prior to the survey, and number of days in the last 7 days when the respondent had walked for at least 10 min at a time. The statistical analysis was carried out using IBM SPSS Statistics version 25 (IBM Corp, Armonk, NY, USA), licensed to the University of Seville (Spain).

3. Results

3.1. Sociodemographic, Lifestyle Habits and Health-Related Variables

The total number of individuals with a self-reported diagnosis of depression included in the study was 3217. Participants with a self-reported diagnosis of depression were more often females (68.67% vs. 48.97%, $p < 0.001$), 45–64 years old (72.09% vs. 45.57%, $p < 0.001$), Spanish (95.37% vs. 91.62%, $p < 0.001$), current smokers (37.24% vs. 31.09%, $p < 0.001$), and not physically active (86.23% vs. 80.42%, $p < 0.001$) compared to people without a self-reported diagnosis of depression (Table 1).

Table 1. Sociodemographic, lifestyle, and health-related variables according to depressive status in people aged from 16 to 64 years (N = 42,280) (2011–2017).

Variables	Participants with a Self-Reported Diagnosis of Depression n = 3217 (%)	Participants without a Self-Reported Diagnosis of Depression n = 39,063 (%)	*p*-Value
Gender			
Female	2209 (68.67%)	19,130 (48.97%)	<0.001
Male	1008 (31.33%)	19,933 (51.03%)	
Age group			
16–24 years old	52 (1.61%)	3726 (9.54%)	<0.001
25–44 years old	846 (26.30%)	17,535 (44.89%)	
45–64 years old	2319 (72.09%)	17,802 (45.57%)	
Marital status			
Single	779 (24.21%)	13,041 (33.38%)	
Married	1627 (50.58%)	22,207 (56.85%)	<0.001
Widowed	265 (8.24%)	799 (2.05%)	
Separated/Divorced	546 (16.97%)	3016 (7.72%)	
Level of education			
Without studies	272 (8.46%)	1361 (3.48%)	
Primary	636 (19.77%)	4023 (10.30%)	<0.001
Secondary or PT	1948 (60.55%)	24,672 (63.16%)	
University	361 (11.22%)	9007 (23.06%)	
Nationality			
Spanish	3068 (95.37%)	35,789 (91.62%)	<0.001
Foreign	149 (4.63%)	3274 (8.38%)	
Size of town of residence			
<10,000 inhabitants	693 (21.54%)	8527 (21.83%)	0.71
≥10,000 inhabitants	2524 (78.46%)	30,536 (78.17%)	
Social class			
Classes I and II	384 (11.94%)	8531 (21.84%)	
Classes III and IV	967 (30.06%)	13,561 (34.72%)	<0.001
Classes V and VI	1866 (58.00%)	16,971 (43.44%)	
Body Mass Index			
Underweight	64 (1.99%)	917 (2.35%)	
Normal weight	1221 (37.95%)	18,922 (48.44%)	<0.001
Overweight	1189 (36.96%)	13,448 (34.43%)	
Obese	743 (23.10%)	5776 (14.78%)	
Current smoking habit			
Yes	1198 (37.24%)	12,146 (31.09%)	<0.001
No	2019 (62.76%)	26,917 (68.91%)	
Consumption of alcoholic beverages in the past 12 months prior to the survey			<0.001
Yes	1638 (50.92%)	26,911 (68.89%)	
No	1579 (49.08%)	12,152 (31.11%)	
Physical activity in main activity			<0.001
Physically active	443 (13.77%)	7647 (19.58%)	
Not physically active	2774 (86.23%)	31,416 (80.42%)	
Number of days in the last 7 days when the respondent had walked for at least 10 min at a time (maximum 7 days)	M 4.29 / SD 2.92	M 4.64 / SD 2.81	<0.001

PT = Professional Training; M = mean; SD = Standard Deviation.

3.2. Diet Quality

As can be seen in Table 2, the prevalence of daily consumption of leafy greens, salads and vegetables, and fresh fruit was higher among participants with a self-reported diagnosis of depression (44.33% vs. 43.67% $p < 0.001$; 61.95% vs. 60.72% $p < 0.001$, respectively). Nonetheless, the daily consumption of bread was lower in that population (82.47% vs. 83.28% $p < 0.001$). Regarding diet quality, the prevalence of poor and good diet quality was higher in individuals with depression (3.05% vs. 2.71% $p < 0.001$; 31.24% vs. 27.02% $p < 0.001$, respectively). In addition, a diet in need of improvement was more prevalent in participants without a diagnosis of depression (70.27% vs. 65.71% $p < 0.001$).

Table 2. Frequency of food consumption and diet quality according to depressive status in participants aged from 16 to 64 years (N = 42,280) (2011–2017).

Variables	Participants with a Self-Reported Diagnosis of Depression n = 3217 (%)	Participants without a Self-Reported Diagnosis of Depression n = 39,063 (%)	p-Value
Frequency of consumption of bread or grains			
Never or hardly ever	108 (3.36)	718 (1.84)	
Less than once a week	73 (2.27)	671 (1.72)	
Once or twice a week	129 (4.00)	1564 (4.00)	<0.001
Three or more times a week, but not daily	254 (7.90)	3579 (9.16)	
Daily	2653 (82.47)	32,531 (83.28)	
Frequency of consumption of leafy greens, salads and vegetables			
Never or hardly ever	61 (1.90)	469 (1.20)	
Less than once a week	99 (3.07)	925 (2.37)	
Once or twice a week	403 (12.53)	4548 (11.64)	<0.001
Three or more times a week, but not daily	1228 (38.17)	16,061 (41.12)	
Daily	1426 (44.33)	438 (43.67)	
Frequency of fresh fruit (excluding juices) consumption			
Never or hardly ever	156 (4.85)	1315 (3.37)	
Less than once a week	166 (5.16)	1491 (3.82)	
Once or twice a week	305 (9.48)	4017 (10.28)	<0.001
Three or more times a week, but not daily	597 (18.56)	8519 (21.81)	
Daily	1993 (61.95)	23,721 (60.72)	
Frequency of consumption of dairy products (milk, cheese, yoghurt)			
Never or hardly ever	124 (3.85)	990 (2.54)	
Less than once a week	76 (2.36)	803 (2.06)	
Once or twice a week	125 (3.89)	1525 (3.90)	<0.001
Three or more times a week, but not daily	240 (7.46)	3497 (8.95)	
Daily	2652 (82.44)	32,248 (82.55)	
Frequency of meat (chicken, beef, pork, lamb, etc.) consumption			
Never or hardly ever	56 (1.74)	443 (1.13)	
Less than once a week	130 (4.04)	693 (1.77)	
Once or twice a week	972 (30.22)	9585 (24.54)	<0.001
Three or more times a week, but not daily	1807 (56.17)	24,380 (62.41)	
Daily	252 (7.83)	3962 (10.15)	

Table 2. *Cont.*

Variables	Participants with a Self-Reported Diagnosis of Depression n = 3217 (%)	Participants without a Self-Reported Diagnosis of Depression n = 39,063 (%)	p-Value
Frequency of legumes consumption			
Never or hardly ever	91 (2.83)	956 (2.45)	
Less than once a week	370 (11.50)	4236 (10.85)	
Once or twice a week	1890 (58.75)	23,970 (61.36)	0.01
Three or more times a week, but not daily	820 (25.49)	9507 (24.34)	
Daily	46 (1.43)	394 (1.00)	
Frequency of consumption of cold meats and cuts			
Never or hardly ever	449 (13.96)	3868 (9.90)	
Less than once a week	647 (20.11)	6305 (16.14)	
Once or twice a week	951 (29.56)	11,627 (29.76)	<0.001
Three or more times a week, but not daily	784 (24.37)	11,694 (29.94)	
Daily	386 (12.00)	5569 (14.26)	
Frequency of consumption of sweets (biscuits, pastries, jams, cereals with sugar, sweets, etc.)			
Never or hardly ever	574 (17.84)	5528 (14.15)	
Less than once a week	596 (18.53)	6550 (16.77)	<0.001
Once or twice a week	626 (19.46)	8453 (21.64)	
Three or more times a week, but not daily	515 (16.01)	7596 (19.44)	
Daily	906 (28.16)	10,936 (28.00)	
Frequency of consumption of soft drinks with sugar			
Never or hardly ever	1606 (49.92)	15,503 (39.69)	
Less than once a week	643 (19.99)	7911 (20.25)	
Once or twice a week	383 (11.91)	6920 (17.72)	<0.001
Three or more times a week, but not daily	261 (8.11)	4247 (10.87)	
Daily	324 (10.07)	4482 (11.47)	
Diet quality			
Poor diet quality	98 (3.05)	1060 (2.71)	
Diet in need of improvement	2114 (65.71)	27,448 (70.27)	<0.001
Good diet quality	1005 (31.24)	10,555 (27.02)	

According to the year of the survey (Table 3), there was a decrease in the number of people with a self-reported diagnosis of depression who never or hardly ever consumed legumes ($\beta = -0.42$, $R^2 = 1.00$, $p = 0.03$). In the same way, the percentage of people with depression who consumed soft drinks with sugar on a daily basis decreased ($\beta = -0.44$, $R^2 = 1.00$, $p = 0.02$).

Table 3. Frequency of food consumption by people with a self-reported diagnosis of depression in Spain aged from 16 to 64 years by year of survey (N = 3217) (2011–2017).

Variables	2011/2012 n = 930 (%)	2014 n = 1168 (%)	2017 n = 1119 (%)	B	R^2	p-Value
Frequency of consumption of bread or grains						
Never or hardly ever	35 (3.76)	40 (3.43)	33 (2.95)	−0.14	0.99	0.07
Less than once a week	24 (2.58)	30 (2.57)	19 (1.70)	−0.15	0.76	0.33
Once or twice a week	47 (5.06)	38 (3.25)	44 (3.93)	−0.19	0.38	0.58
Three or more times a week, but not daily	57 (6.13)	109 (9.33)	88 (7.86)	0.29	0.29	0.64
Daily	767 (82.47)	951 (81.42)	935 (83.56)	0.18	0.26	0.66

Table 3. *Cont.*

Variables	2011/2012 n = 930 (%)	2014 n = 1168 (%)	2017 n = 1119 (%)	*B*	R²	*p*-Value
Frequency of consumption of leafy greens, salads and vegetables						
Never or hardly ever	22 (2.36)	24 (2.05)	15 (1.34)	−0.17	0.95	0.14
Less than once a week	36 (3.87)	31 (2.65)	32 (2.86)	−0.17	0.60	0.44
Once or twice a week	125 (13.44)	149 (12.76)	129 (11.53)	−0.32	0.97	0.10
Three or more times a week, but not daily	309 (33.23)	452 (38.70)	467 (41.73)	1.42	0.97	0.10
Daily	438 (47.10)	512 (43.84)	476 (42.54)	−0.76	0.94	0.15
Frequency of fresh fruit (excluding juices) consumption						
Never or hardly ever	67 (7.21)	41 (3.51)	48 (4.29)	−0.49	0.56	0.46
Less than once a week	45 (4.84)	49 (4.19)	72 (6.43)	0.27	0.48	0.52
Once or twice a week	88 (9.46)	103 (8.82)	114 (10.19)	0.12	0.28	0.64
Three or more times a week, but not daily	136 (14.62)	242 (20.72)	219 (19.57)	0.83	0.58	0.45
Daily	594 (63.87)	733 (62.76)	666 (59.52)	−0.72	0.93	0.18
Frequency of consumption of dairy products (milk, cheese, yoghurt)						
Never or hardly ever	43 (4.62)	43 (3.68)	38 (3.40)	−0.20	0.91	0.19
Less than once a week	17 (1.83)	32 (2.74)	27 (2.41)	0.10	0.40	0.57
Once or twice a week	30 (3.23)	50 (4.28)	45 (4.02)	0.13	0.52	0.49
Three or more times a week, but not daily	47 (5.05)	105 (8.99)	88 (7.86)	0.47	0.48	0.51
Daily	793 (85.27)	938 (80.31)	921 (82.31)	−0.49	0.35	0.60
Frequency of meat (chicken, beef, pork, lamb, etc.) consumption						
Never or hardly ever	22 (2.37)	13 (1.11)	21 (1.88)	−0.08	0.15	0.75
Less than once a week	40 (4.30)	50 (4.28)	40 (3.57)	−0.12	0.77	0.32
Once or twice a week	304 (32.69)	346 (29.62)	322 (28.78)	−0.65	0.90	0.20
Three or more times a week, but not daily	493 (53.01)	671 (57.45)	643 (57.46)	0.74	0.75	0.33
Daily	71 (7.63)	88 (7.54)	93 (8.31)	0.11	0.65	0.40
Frequency of consumption of legumes						
Never or hardly ever	39 (4.19)	33 (2.83)	19 (1.70)	−0.42	1.00	0.03
Less than once a week	113 (12.15)	131 (11.21)	126 (11.26)	−0.15	0.71	0.36
Once or twice a week	538 (57.85)	662 (56.68)	690 (61.66)	0.63	0.54	0.48
Three or more times a week, but not daily	222 (23.87)	330 (28.25)	268 (23.95)	0.01	0.00	0.99
Daily	18 (1.94)	12 (1.03)	16 (1.43)	−0.09	0.31	0.62
Frequency of consumption of cold meats and cuts						
Never or hardly ever	195 (20.96)	132 (11.30)	122 (10.90)	−1.68	0.78	0.31
Less than once a week	198 (21.29)	250 (21.41)	199 (17.79)	−0.58	0.72	0.35
Once or twice a week	255 (27.42)	367 (31.42)	329 (29.40)	0.33	0.25	0.67
Three or more times a week, but not daily	151 (16.24)	289 (24.74)	344 (30.74)	2.42	0.99	0.06
Daily	131 (14.09)	130 (11.13)	125 (11.17)	−0.49	0.74	0.34
Frequency of consumption of sweets (biscuits, pastries, jams, cereals with sugar, sweets, etc.)						
Never or hardly ever	245 (26.34)	180 (15.41)	149 (13.31)	−2.17	0.87	0.24
Less than once a week	158 (16.99)	212 (18.15)	226 (20.20)	0.54	0.98	0.10
Once or twice a week	131 (14.09)	238 (20.38)	257 (22.97)	1.48	0.95	0.15
Three or more times a week, but not daily	99 (10.64)	217 (18.58)	199 (17.78)	1.19	0.67	0.39
Daily	297 (31.94)	321 (27.48)	288 (25.74)	−1.03	0.94	0.16
Frequency of consumption of soft drinks with sugar						
Never or hardly ever	527 (56.67)	539 (46.15)	540 (48.26)	−1.40	0.57	0.45
Less than once a week	139 (14.95)	256 (21.92)	248 (22.16)	1.20	0.77	0.31
Once or twice a week	94 (10.11)	140 (11.99)	149 (13.31)	0.53	0.99	0.06
Three or more times a week, but not daily	63 (6.77)	115 (9.84)	83 (7.42)	0.11	0.04	0.87
Daily	107 (11.50)	118 (10.10)	99 (8.85)	−0.44	1.00	0.02

Table 3. *Cont.*

Variables	2011/2012 n = 930 (%)	2014 n = 1168 (%)	2017 n = 1119 (%)	B	R^2	*p*-Value
Diet quality						
Poor diet quality	25 (2.69)	45 (3.85)	28 (2.50)	−0.03	0.02	0.92
Diet in need of improvement	529 (56.88)	798 (68.32)	787 (70.33)	2.24	0.86	0.24
Good diet quality	376 (40.43)	325 (27.83)	304 (27.17)	−2.21	0.79	0.31

p-value is for trend.

3.3. Association between Sociodemographic, Lifestyle, and Health-Related Characteristics and Diet Quality

As regards the adjusted logistic regression model, Table 4 showed that the probability of having a poor or improvable diet quality was higher in males (OR = 1.47, 95% CI 1.23–1.76), people aged 16–24 years old (OR = 3.05, 95% CI 1.24–6.95) and 25–44 years old (OR = 2.32, 95% CI 1.89–2.86), separated or divorced (OR = 1.41, 95% CI 1.13–1.75), and people who currently smoked (OR = 1.70, 95% CI 1.43–2.02). In addition, the probability of having poor or improvable diet quality was lower in people who had not consumed alcoholic beverages in the past 12 months (OR = 0.80, 95% CI 0.69–0.94). Moreover, walking in the last 7 days for at least 10 min at a time was associated with diet quality (OR = 0.95, 95% CI 0.92–0.97).

Table 4. Association between diet quality and sociodemographic, lifestyle, and health-related variables in people with a self-reported diagnosis of depression in Spain aged from 16 to 64 years (N = 3217) (2011–2017).

Variables	Individuals with a Self-Reported Diagnosis of Depression (N = 3217)				
	Poor/Need Improvement Diet (n = 2212)				
	n (%)	OR (CI 95%)	*p*-Value	ORa (CI 95%) [1]	*p*-Value
Gender					
Female	1444 (65.37%)	Reference		Reference	
Male	768 (76.19%)	1.70 (1.43–2.01)	<0.001	1.47 (1.23–1.76)	<0.01
Age group (years)					
16–24	45 (86.54%)	3.71 (1.67–8.27)	<0.01	3.05 (1.24–6.95)	<0.01
25–44	697 (82.39%)	2.70 (2.22–3.29)	<0.001	2.32 (1.89–2.86)	<0.001
45–64	1470 (63.39%)	Reference		Reference	
Marital status					
Single	621 (79.72%)	0.72 (0.56–0.93)	0.01	0.88 (0.67–1.15)	0.34
Married	1061 (65.21%)	Reference		Reference	0.27
Widowed	152 (57.36%)	1.20 (0.97–1.48)	0.09	1.13 (0.91–1.41)	<0.01
Separated/divorced	378 (69.23%)	2.10 (1.71–2.57)	<0.001	1.41 (1.13–1.75)	
Social class					
Social classes I and II	265 (69.01%)	0.99 (0.78–1.26)	0.94		
Social classes III and IV	656 (67.84%)	0.93 (0.80–1.11)	0.46		
Social classes V and VI	1291 (69.19%)	Reference			
Level of education					
Without studies	188 (69.12%)	0.94 (0.71–1.23)	0.63		
Primary	407 (63.99%)	0.74 (0.62–0.90)	<0.01		
Secondary or PT	1374 (70.53%)	Reference			
University	243 (67.31%)	0.86 (0.68–1.10)	0.22		
Nationality					
Spanish	2094 (68.25%)	Reference	<0.01		
Foreigner	118 (79.19%)	1.78 (1.18–2.65)			
Size of town of residence					
≤10,000 inhabitants	462 (66.67%)	0.89 (0.74–1.06)	0.18		
>10,000 inhabitants	1750 (69.33%)	Reference			

Table 4. *Cont.*

Variables	Individuals with a Self-Reported Diagnosis of Depression (N = 3217)				
	Poor/Need Improvement Diet (n = 2212)				
	n (%)	OR (CI 95%)	*p*-Value	ORa (CI 95%) [1]	*p*-Value
Body mass index					
Underweight	52 (81.25%)	1.75 (0.92–3.32)	0.09		
Normal weight	870 (71.25%)	Reference			
Overweight	797 (67.03%)	0.80 (0.65–0.97)	0.02		
Obesity	493 (66.35%)	0.82 (0.69–0.98)	0.03		
Self-perceived health status					
Very good	90 (74.38%)	1.28 (0.83–1.95)	0.26		
Good	599 (67.68%)	0.92 (0.77–1.11)	0.37		
Fair	920 (69.49%)	Reference			
Poor	541 (69.38%)	0.99 (0.81–1.22)	0.96		
Very poor	152 (64.14%)	0.79 (0.59–1.06)	0.10		
Current smoking habit					
Yes	931 (77.71%)	2.01 (1.71–2.37)	<0.001	1.70 (1.43–2.02)	<0.001
No	1281 (63.45%)	Reference		Reference	
Consumption of alcoholic beverages in the past 12 months prior to the survey					<0.01
Yes	1184 (72.28%)	Reference		Reference	
No	1028 (65.10%)	0.72 (0.32–0.83)	<0.001	0.80 (0.69–0.94)	
Physical activity in main activity					
Physically active in main activity	299 (67.49%)	0.94 (0.75–1.16)			
Not physically active in main activity	1913 (68.96%)	Reference	0.54		
Physical activity during leisure time					
Yes	1130 (66.90%)	Reference			
No	1082 (70.81%)	1.20 (1.03–1.40)	0.02		
Number of days in the last 7 days when the respondent walked for at least 10 min at a time	M: 4.17 SD: 2.95	0.96 (0.93–0.98)	<0.01	0.95 (0.92–0.97)	<0.001

PT = Professional Training; M = mean; SD = Standard Deviation; OR = Odds Ratio; ORa = Odds Ratio Adjusted for all sociodemographic, lifestyle and health-related variables; CI95% = Confidence Interval; n = number of people with a poor or improvable diet quality; [1] the variables included in the final multivariate-adjusted model were: gender, age group, marital status, current smoking habit, consumption of alcoholic beverages in the past 12 months prior to the survey and number of days in the last 7 days when the respondent had walked for at least 10 min at a time; Hosmer–Lemeshow test χ^2 = 3.31, *p* = 091; Nagelkerke's R^2: 0.10; *p*-value < 0.001.

4. Discussion

4.1. Main Findings

The present study, based on a large, representative population with a self-reported diagnosis of depression in Spain, between 16–64 years old, is the first to show the relationship between sociodemographic, lifestyle and health-related characteristics and diet quality from 2011 to 2017.

The results showed that diet quality among people with a self-reported diagnosis of depression living in Spain was largely improvable. This supports the view that people with depression have lower scores on healthy dietary pattern surveys [10,45,46]. For example, Spanish people belonging to the fast food consumption quintiles Q2 to Q5 showed an increased risk of depression compared to those participants belonging to the lowest level of fast food consumption [47]. These findings help improve our understanding of whether diet quality should be a novel intervention target for the primary prevention of depression [48]. Numerous meta-analyses and systematic reviews showed the connection between adherence to good diet quality and as much as a 33% lower risk of incident depressive outcomes [31,49–52]. As part of the SMILES trial, Jacka et al. [53] showed substantial improvements in symptoms of depression following seven consultations on healthy dieting. Nevertheless, it seems that selectively-induced expectancy and a loss of blinding may have contributed to the observed effect [54].

In the present study, it was found that the male gender was associated with an increased probability of having poor or improvable diet quality than women, an outcome which is consistent with other research [55–57]. One reason for this might be that women are more likely than men to make food choices for their health benefits or to maintain a lower body weight [58]. In addition, some studies reporting lower values associated with diet quality in men could be explained by a social perception that healthy eating is an inherently feminine habit [59–62]. Tailored dietary interventions targeted specifically towards men are needed to alter these social and gender norms that link masculinity with less healthy eating [63]. In particular, it is necessary for young men to learn healthy eating habits [64].

Young people are less likely to consume healthy food compared to other age groups [65,66]. This study confirmed that the younger the subject, the greater the risk of having a poor or improvable diet quality. For instance, Nour et al. [67] reported that young people aged from 18 to 24 years old reported less variety in the consumption of vegetables than people aged between 25 and 34. Moreover, older people are more likely to achieve the recommended daily consumption of fruit and vegetables than young people [68]. Interestingly, the literature shows that young people with lower diet quality scores were more likely to report depressive symptoms [69,70].

Confirming the findings from previous studies [71,72], our results showed that being divorced or separated was associated with a lower dietary diversity score. As shown in this study, the probability of having a poor or improvable diet quality was higher in this group. This may be due to limited financial resources and lack of family support, which may restrict their access to a variety of food choices [71]. Another possible explanation might be food insecurity, which is more prevalent in divorced or separated people [73].

Among the people who met the physical activity guidelines, people who had depression had a significantly lower probability of having a higher diet quality than people without [74]. This study found that having walked more days in the last 7 for at least 10 min at a time was associated with diet quality. The reasons for this could include personal and environmental factors, such as social support, accessibility, and the availability of healthy food choices, as well as the availability of physical exercise facilities and the opportunities for walking in the neighborhood [75,76]. It should be noted that exercise could be effective psychotherapy or alternative treatment for depression [77–79]. In fact, aerobic exercise at least 3 times per week, at a moderate to high-intensity, can significantly reduce depressive symptoms [80,81]. Therefore, healthy eating habits and increased physical activity are particularly promising targets [82], which have progressively featured in the clinical practice guidelines for managing depression [83].

According to population studies, smokers and non-smokers differ in the type of food they consume [84–86]. In fact, a meta-analysis that analyzed the links between smoking and diet has revealed that the dietary habits of smokers are characterized by higher intakes of energy, saturated fat, cholesterol, and alcohol and by lower intakes of vitamins, antioxidants, and fiber, in comparison with non-smokers [87]. Moreover, a number of studies have found that less fruit and vegetables were consumed by smokers than non-smokers [88,89]. The findings from this study also showed that the probability of having a poor or improvable diet quality was higher in people who currently smoked, as is also reflected in the extensive body of literature [88,90–92]. As regards alcohol consumption, the probability of having a poor or improvable diet quality was lower in people who had not consumed alcoholic beverages in the past 12 months. This difference in diet quality among consumers and non-consumers of alcoholic beverages was also found in other studies [93,94]. Alcohol is commonly consumed around mealtimes [95], and different habits of alcoholic beverage consumption were regularly associated with less varied diet quality [96] and its increased consumption associated with depression [97–99]. Therefore, this consumption behavior may act as a confounder, which may account for the links observed between diet quality and depression [100].

The scientific literature has found an association between soft drinks and depressive symptoms from adolescence to adulthood [23,101,102]. In addition, soft drink consumption has been linked to an increased risk of type 2 diabetes [103], cardiovascular disease [104], dental caries [105,106], and weight gain [107]. Reducing this type of consumption is, therefore, a high public health priority [108]. This study revealed that the percentage of people with a self-reported diagnosis of depression who consumed soft drinks with sugar daily had decreased. This decrease could be explained by the World Health Organization's recommendation [109] to governments to reduce the consumption of products that are harmful to health through taxation and other policies in developed countries, including Spain [110]. This study also revealed that people with a self-reported diagnosis of depression who never or hardly ever consumed legumes had also decreased. For example, when legume consumption decreased among US adults, improved communication about their benefits was introduced [111].

We also identified some differences in dietary habits between depressed and non-depressed individuals. In that sense, the consumption of legumes once or twice a week was more frequent in individuals with no depression. Another study found a similar result [20]. This food group is rich in tryptophan, inositol, magnesium, and other important nutrients, such as fiber, folate, and omega-3 fatty acids. A previous study established a beneficial effect of the consumption of tryptophan, inositol, and magnesium on the mental well-being of individuals [112]. Additionally, this study showed that participants with depression had significantly higher daily consumption of sweets than their non-depressed counterparts. This finding is in line with the results of another study [113], which may be attributable to the sugar contents of this group of food. Sweets contain large amounts of sugars, which are associated with a high glycemic load [114]. Actually, research shows that high glycemic load diets are associated with a high level of pro-inflammatory cytokines and a worse lipid profile, which have already been proven to be related to high depressive symptoms [115]. In the present study, the prevalence of daily consumption of leafy greens, salads and vegetables, and fresh fruit was higher among participants with a self-reported diagnosis of depression. However, a case-control study carried out by Payne et al. [19] showed that depressed individuals consumed less fruit and vegetables than non-depressed. Regarding diet quality, observational studies have shown poorer diet quality in depressed versus non-depressed individuals, although null findings are common as well [116]. This result is similar to that found in the current study. The association of depression with poorer diets could be due to the appetite modification that frequently occurred after the disease development. Modification of appetite is a common symptom among those diagnosed with major depression, and it is one of the diagnostic criteria of depression in the DSM-V [45].

4.2. Strengths and Limitations

This study has certain limitations. Firstly, due to the cross-sectional design, it was not possible to assign causality between the sociodemographic, lifestyle, and health-related factors and diet quality. Secondly, a self-reported diagnosis of depression was used as a proxy for a confirmed diagnosis. Thirdly, it should be noted that no distinctions have been made between patients with different subtypes of depression. Moreover, people aged over 65 years were not included in this research, and therefore, the sample was not representative of all people living in Spain. Due to the fact that data from SNHS and EHSS are stored anonymously, it is impossible to know if a participant has taken part in more than one survey. Finally, it was not possible to separate remitted and current depressed subjects because neither SNHS nor EHSS took this aspect into account. On the other hand, one strength of our study is that since the data were derived from a national survey, they were obtained using a carefully planned methodology, including sampling, well-designed forms, preparation of the survey participants, supervision of the survey, and filtering of the data, all of which guarantee a representative sample of the population between 16–64 years old and lead to a greater understanding of this problem in today's society. Moreover, the data information was collected by a trained interviewer from a personal interview, which avoids the other potential biases commonly found in telephone surveys.

4.3. Implications for Research and Practice

This large, representative sample of people with a self-reported diagnosis of depression in Spain between 16 and 64 years old enabled us to evaluate a vast number of associations with factors from different domains simultaneously. Thus, this study provides valuable insights that will be useful for conducting future research. Our results of the overall prevalence of diet quality revealed that 31.24% had a good diet quality and 65.71% were in need of improvement. It is vital for health authorities to take these findings into consideration when designing strategies to improve diet quality among individuals with depression. Although this research showed that the number of people who never or hardly ever consumed legumes and people who consumed soft drinks with sugar on a daily basis declined from 2011 to 2017, government agencies should persevere with their efforts to reduce the consumption of soft drinks with sugar due to its potential dangers for general health [117] and encourage people to consume more legumes for their health benefits [111]. Additionally, our findings of depressive people suggest that males, people aged 16–24 years old and 25–44 years, separated or divorced, and also smokers were more likely to have a poor or improvable diet quality. Therefore, Spanish mental health policies should be specially adapted to take these characteristics of the population into account in order to implement, for example, programs promoting a healthy diet [5]. Finally, further studies are needed to focus on how diet quality is mechanistically connected to depression, and on how to set up controls for the commonest confounders, such as exposure to stress; new experimental methods are also needed to study the effects of diet quality and their consequences for a population with depression [31].

5. Conclusions

The overall prevalence of diet quality among individuals with a self-reported diagnosis of depression in Spain showed that 65.71% were in need of improvement and 31.24% had a good diet quality. Among the individuals suffering from depression, there was a decrease from 2011 to 2017 in the number of people who never or hardly ever consumed legumes and people who consumed soft drinks with sugar on a daily basis. Having a poor or improvable diet quality is associated with male gender, people aged 16–24 years old and 25–44 years old, separated or divorced, and also in smokers. However, the likelihood of having a poor or improvable diet quality decreases in people who had not consumed alcoholic beverages in the past 12 months. Finally, walking in the last 7 days for at least 10 min at a time is associated with diet quality.

Supplementary Materials: The following are available online at https://www.mdpi.com/2072-6643/13/1/106/s1, Table S1: Criteria to define the score for each item of the Spanish Health Eating Index (SHEI), File S1: Research Data.

Author Contributions: Conceptualization, S.P.d.l.C. and J.C.; methodology, S.P.d.l.C. and J.C.; software, S.P.d.l.C. and J.C.; validation, S.P.d.l.C. and J.C.; formal analysis, J.C.; investigation, S.P.d.l.C. and J.C.; resources, S.P.d.l.C. and J.C.; data curation, S.P.d.l.C. and J.C.; writing—original draft preparation, S.P.d.l.C. and J.C.; writing—review and editing, S.P.d.l.C. and J.C.; visualization, S.P.d.l.C. and J.C.; supervision, S.P.d.l.C.; project administration, S.P.d.l.C. and J.C. All authors have read and agreed to the published version of the manuscript.

Funding: This research received no specific grant from any funding agency.

Institutional Review Board Statement: Ethical review and approval were waived for this study, due to according with Spanish legislation, when secondary data are used, there is no need for approval from an Ethics Committee.

Informed Consent Statement: Informed consent was obtained from all subjects involved in the study.

Data Availability Statement: The data presented in this study are available as Supplementary Material (File S1: Research data).

Acknowledgments: The authors would like to express special thanks to P. Díaz-Baltanar for her assistance.

Conflicts of Interest: The authors declare no conflict of interest.

References

1. World Health Organization (WHO). Investing in Mental Health: Evidence for Action (2013). Available online: https://www.mhinnovation.net/sites/default/files/downloads/resource/WHO_Investing%20in%20Mental%20Health_eng.pdf (accessed on 25 March 2020).
2. GBD 2017 DALYs and HALE Collaborators. Global, regional, and national disability-adjusted life-years (DALYs) for 359 diseases and injuries and healthy life expectancy (HALE) for 195 countries and territories, 1990–2017: A systematic analysis for the Global Burden of Disease Study 2017. *Lancet* **2018**, *392*, 1859–1922. [CrossRef]
3. Kessler, R.C.; Bromet, E.J. The epidemiology of depression across cultures. *Annu. Rev. Public Health* **2013**, *34*, 119–138. [CrossRef] [PubMed]
4. Penninx, B.W.; Milaneschi, Y.; Lamers, F.; Vogelzangs, N. Understanding the somatic consequences of depression: Biological mechanisms and the role of depression symptom profile. *BMC Med.* **2013**, *11*, 129. [CrossRef] [PubMed]
5. World Health Organization (WHO). Mental Health Action Plan 2013–2020. Available online: https://apps.who.int/iris/bitstream/handle/10665/89966/9789241506021_eng.pdf?sequence=1 (accessed on 25 March 2020).
6. Adjibade, M.; Assmann, K.E.; Andreeva, V.A.; Lemogne, C.; Hercberg, S.; Galán, P.; Kesse-Guyot, E. Prospective association between adherence to the Mediterranean diet and risk of depressive symptoms in the French SU.VI.MAX cohort. *Eur. J. Nutr.* **2018**, *57*, 1225–1235. [CrossRef] [PubMed]
7. Dipnall, J.F.; Pasco, J.A.; Meyer, D.; Berk, M.; Williams, L.J.; Dodd, S.; Jacka, F.N. The association between dietary patterns, diabetes and depression. *J. Affect. Disord.* **2015**, *174*, 215–224. [CrossRef] [PubMed]
8. Gougeon, L.; Payette, H.; Morais, J.; Gaudreau, P.; Shatenstein, B.; Gray-Donald, K. Dietary patterns and incidence of depression in a cohort of community-dwelling older Canadians. *J. Nutr. Health Aging* **2015**, *19*, 431–436. [CrossRef]
9. Tsai, H.-J. Dietary patterns and depressive symptoms in a Taiwanese population aged 53 years and over: Results from the Taiwan Longitudinal Study of Aging. *Geriatr. Gerontol. Int.* **2016**, *16*, 1289–1295. [CrossRef]
10. Elstgeest, L.E.M.; Winkens, L.H.H.; Penninx, B.W.J.H.; Brouwer, I.A.; Visser, M. Associations of depressive symptoms and history with three a priori diet quality indices in middle-aged and older adults. *J. Affect Disord.* **2019**, *249*, 394–403. [CrossRef]
11. Ruusunen, A.; Lehto, S.M.; Mursu, J.; Tolmunen, T.; Tuomainen, T.-P.; Kauhanen, J.; Voutilainen, S. Dietary patterns are associated with the prevalence of elevated depressive symptoms and the risk of getting a hospital discharge diagnosis of depression in middle-aged or older Finnish men. *J. Affect. Disord.* **2014**, *159*, 1–6. [CrossRef]
12. Flórez, K.R.; Dubowitz, T.; Ghosh-Dastidar, M.B.; Beckman, R.; Collins, R.L. Associations between depressive symptomatology, diet, and body mass index among participants in the supplemental nutrition assistance program. *J. Acad. Nutr. Diet.* **2015**, *115*, 1102–1108. [CrossRef]
13. Gibson-Smith, D.; Bot, M.; Brouwer, I.A.; Visser, M.; Penninx, B.W. Diet quality in persons with and without depressive and anxiety disorders. *J. Psychiatr. Res.* **2018**, *106*, 1–7. [CrossRef] [PubMed]
14. Thomas-Odenthal, F.; Molero, P.; van der Does, W.; Molendijk, M. Impact of review method on the conclusions of clinical reviews: A systematic review on dietary interventions in depression as a case in point. *PLoS ONE* **2020**, *15*, e0238131. [CrossRef] [PubMed]
15. Appelhans, B.M.; Whited, M.C.; Schneider, K.L.; Ma, Y.; Oleski, J.L.; Merriam, P.A.; Waring, M.E.; Olendzki, B.C.; Mann, D.M.; Ockene, I.S.; et al. Depression severity, diet quality, and physical activity in women with obesity and depression. *J. Acad. Nutr. Diet.* **2012**, *112*, 693–698. [CrossRef]
16. Whitaker, K.M.; Sharpe, P.A.; Wilcox, S.; Hutto, B.E. Depressive symptoms are associated with dietary intake but not physical activity among overweight and obese women from disadvantaged neighborhoods. *Nutr. Res.* **2014**, *34*, 294–301. [CrossRef] [PubMed]
17. Nucci, D.; Fatigoni, C.; Amerio, A.; Odone, A.; Gianfredi, V. Red and processed meat consumption and risk of depression: A systematic review and meta-analysis. *Int. J. Environ. Res. Public Health* **2020**, *17*, 6686. [CrossRef]
18. Jeffery, R.W.; Linde, J.A.; Simon, G.E.; Ludman, E.J.; Rohde, P.; Ichikawa, L.E.; Finch, E.A. Reported food choices in older women in relation to body mass index and depressive symptoms. *Appetite* **2009**, *52*, 238–240. [CrossRef]
19. Payne, M.E.; Steck, S.E.; George, R.R.; Steffens, D.C. Fruit, vegetable, and antioxidant intakes are lower in older adults with depression. *J. Acad. Nutr. Diet.* **2012**, *112*, 2022–2027. [CrossRef]
20. Grases, G.; Colom, M.A.; Sanchis, P.; Grases, F. Possible relation between consumption of different food groups and depression. *BMC Psychol.* **2019**, *7*, 14. [CrossRef]

21. Akbaraly, T.N.; Sabia, S.; Shipley, M.J.; Batty, G.D.; Kivimaki, M. Adherence to healthy dietary guidelines and future depressive symptoms: Evidence for sex differentials in the Whitehall II Study. *Am. J. Clin. Nutr.* **2013**, *97*, 419–427. [CrossRef]
22. Yu, B.; He, H.; Zhang, Q.; Wu, H.; Du, H.; Liu, L.; Wang, C.; Shi, H.; Xia, Y.; Guo, X.; et al. Soft drink consumption is associated with depressive symptoms among adults in China. *J. Affect. Disord.* **2015**, *172*, 422–427. [CrossRef]
23. Kang, D.; Kim, Y.; Je, Y. Non-alcoholic beverage consumption and risk of depression: Epidemiological evidence from observational studies. *Eur. J. Clin. Nutr.* **2018**, *72*, 1506–1516. [CrossRef] [PubMed]
24. Hu, D.; Cheng, L.; Jiang, W. Sugar-sweetened beverages consumption and the risk of depression: A meta-analysis of observational studies. *J. Affect. Disord.* **2019**, *245*, 348–355. [CrossRef] [PubMed]
25. Lorant, V.; Deliège, D.; Eaton, W.; Robert, A.; Philippot, P.; Ansseau, M. Socioeconomic inequalities in depression: A meta-analysis. *Am. J. Epidemiol.* **2003**, *157*, 98–112. [CrossRef] [PubMed]
26. Boone-Heinonen, J.; Diez Roux, A.V.; Kiefe, C.I.; Lewis, C.E.; Guilkey, D.K.; Gordon-Larsen, P. Neighborhood socioeconomic status predictors of physical activity through young to middle adulthood: The CARDIA study. *Soc. Sci. Med.* **2011**, *72*, 641–649. [CrossRef]
27. Larson, N.I.; Story, M.T.; Nelson, M.C. Neighborhood environments: Disparities in access to healthy foods in the US. *Am. J. Prev. Med.* **2009**, *36*, 74–81. [CrossRef]
28. Bernstein, A.M.; Bloom, D.E.; Rosner, B.A.; Franz, M.; Willett, W.C. Relation of food cost to healthfulness of diet among US women. *Am. J. Clin. Nutr.* **2010**, *92*, 1197–1203. [CrossRef]
29. Wise, L.A.; Adams-Campbell, L.L.; Palmer, J.R.; Rosenberg, L. Leisure time physical activity in relation to depressive symptoms in the Black Women's Health Study. *Ann. Behav. Med.* **2006**, *32*, 68–76. [CrossRef]
30. Beydoun, M.A.; Wang, Y. Pathways linking socioeconomic status to obesity through depression and lifestyle factors among young US adults. *J. Affect. Disord.* **2010**, *123*, 52–63. [CrossRef]
31. Molendijk, M.; Molero, P.; Ortuño Sánchez-Pedreño, F.; Van der Does, W.; Martínez González, M.A. Diet quality and depression risk: A systematic review and dose-response meta-analysis of prospective studies. *J. Affect. Disord.* **2018**, *226*, 346–354. [CrossRef]
32. van Zoonen, K.; Buntrock, C.; Ebert, D.D.; Smit, F.; Reynolds, C.F.; Beekman, A.T.F.; Cuijpers, P. Preventing the onset of major depressive disorder: A meta-analytic review of psychological interventions. *Int. J. Epidemiol.* **2014**, *43*, 318–329. [CrossRef]
33. Fournier, J.C.; DeRubeis, R.J.; Hollon, S.D.; Dimidjian, S.; Amsterdam, J.D.; Shelton, R.C.; Fawcett, J. Antidepressant drug effects and depression severity: A patient-level meta-analysis. *JAMA* **2010**, *303*, 47–53. [CrossRef] [PubMed]
34. Lim, G.Y.; Tam, W.W.; Lu, Y.; Ho, C.S.; Zhang, M.W.; Ho, R.C. Prevalence of depression in the community from 30 countries between 1994 and 2014. *Sci. Rep.* **2018**, *8*, 2861. [CrossRef] [PubMed]
35. Commonwealth Department of Health and Aged Care & Australian Institute of Health and Welfare (AIHW). NHPA Report on Mental Health: A Report Focusing on Depression 1998, Summary. Available online: https://www.aihw.gov.au/reports/mental-health-services/nhpa-report-mental-health-focus-depression-1998/contents/table-of-contents (accessed on 2 April 2020).
36. Lai, J.S.; Oldmeadow, C.; Hure, A.J.; McEvoy, M.; Byles, J.; Attia, J. Longitudinal diet quality is not associated with depressive symptoms in a cohort of middle-aged Australian women. *Br. J. Nutr.* **2016**, *115*, 842–850. [CrossRef] [PubMed]
37. McNaughton, S.A. Dietary patterns and diet quality: Approaches to assessing complex exposures in nutrition. *Australas. Epidemiol.* **2010**, *17*, 35–37.
38. Spanish Society of Community Nutrition (SSCN). Healthy Dietary Guidelines (2014). Available online: http://www.nutricioncomunitaria.org/es/otras-publicaciones (accessed on 2 April 2020).
39. Ministerio de Sanidad Servicios Sociales e Igualdad, Instituto Nacional de Estadística. *Encuesta Nacional de Salud España ENSE 2011/12*; Ministerio de Sanidad, Servicios Sociales e Igualdad: Madrid, Spain, 2013. Available online: https://www.mscbs.gob.es/estadEstudios/estadisticas/encuestaNacional/encuesta2011.htm (accessed on 25 May 2020).
40. Ministerio de Sanidad Servicios Sociales e Igualdad, Instituto Nacional de Estadística. *Encuesta Europea de Salud en España EESE 2014*; Ministerio de Sanidad, Servicios Sociales e Igualdad: Madrid, Spain, 2015. Available online: https://www.mscbs.gob.es/estadEstudios/estadisticas/EncuestaEuropea/Enc_Eur_Salud_en_Esp_2014.htm (accessed on 25 May 2020).
41. Ministerio de Sanidad Servicios Sociales e Igualdad, Instituto Nacional de Estadística. *Encuesta Nacional de Salud España ENSE 2017*; Ministerio de Sanidad, Servicios Sociales e Igualdad: Madrid, Spain, 2018. Available online: https://www.mscbs.gob.es/estadEstudios/estadisticas/encuestaNacional/encuesta2017.htm (accessed on 25 May 2020).
42. Norte Navarro, A.; Ortiz Moncada, R. Spanish diet quality according to the healthy eating index. *Nutr. Hosp.* **2011**, *26*, 330–336. [CrossRef] [PubMed]
43. Domingo-Salvany, A.; Bacigalupe, A.; Carrasco, J.M.; Espelt, A.; Ferrando, J.; Borrell, C. Proposals for social class classification based on the Spanish National Classification of Occupations 2011 using neo-Weberian and neo-Marxist approaches. *Gac. Sanit.* **2011**, *27*, 263–272. [CrossRef]
44. World Health Organization (WHO). Body Mass Index (BMI). Available online: http://www.euro.who.int/en/health-topics/disease-prevention/nutrition/a-healthy-lifestyle/body-mass-index-bmi (accessed on 10 June 2020).
45. Jacka, F.N.; Cherbuin, N.; Anstey, K.J.; Butterworth, P. Does reverse causality explain the relationship between diet and depression? *J. Affect. Disord.* **2015**, *175*, 248–250. [CrossRef]
46. Bayes, J.; Schloss, J.; Sibbritt, D. Investigation into the diets and nutritional knowledge of young men with depression: The MENDDS survey. *Nutrition* **2020**, *78*, 110946. [CrossRef]

47. Sánchez Villegas, A.; Toledo, E.; de Irala, J.; Ruiz Canela, M.; Pla Vidal, J.; Martínez González, M.A. Fast-food and commercial baked good consumption and the risk of depression. *Public Health Nutr.* **2012**, *15*, 424–432. [CrossRef]
48. Marozoff, S.; Veugelers, P.J.; Dabravolskaj, J.; Eurich, D.T.; Ye, M.; Maximova, K. Diet quality and health service utilization for depression: A prospective investigation of adults in Alberta's Tomorrow Project. *Nutrients* **2020**, *12*, 2437. [CrossRef]
49. Lai, J.S.; Hiles, S.; Bisquera, A.; Hure, A.J.; McEvoy, M.; Attia, J. A systematic review and meta-analysis of dietary patterns and depression in community-dwelling adults. *Am. J. Clin. Nutr.* **2014**, *99*, 181–197. [CrossRef] [PubMed]
50. Li, Y.; Lv, M.-R.; Wei, Y.J.; Sun, L.; Zhang, J.-X.; Zhang, H.-G.; Li, B. Dietary patterns and depression risk: A meta-analysis. *Psychiatry Res.* **2017**, *253*, 373–382. [CrossRef] [PubMed]
51. Lassale, C.; Batty, G.D.; Baghdadli, A.; Jacka, F.; Sánchez Villegas, A.; Kivimäki, M.; Akbaraly, T. Healthy dietary indices and risk of depressive outcomes: A systematic review and meta-analysis of observational studies. *Mol. Psychiatry* **2019**, *24*, 965–986. [CrossRef] [PubMed]
52. Nicolaou, M.; Colpo, M.; Vermeulen, E.; Elstgeest, L.E.M.; Cabout, M.; Gibson-Smith, D.; Knuppel, A.; Sini, G.; Schoenaker, D.A.; Mishra, G.D. Association of *a priori* dietary patterns with depressive symptoms: A harmonized meta-analysis of observational studies. *Psychol. Med.* **2019**, *50*, 1872–1883. [CrossRef] [PubMed]
53. Jacka, F.N.; O'Neil, A.; Opie, R.; Itsiopoulos, C.; Cotton, S.; Mohebbi, M.; Castle, D.; Dash, S.; Mihalopoulos, C.; Chatterton, M.L.; et al. A randomised controlled trial of dietary improvement for adults with major depression (the 'SMILES' trial). *BMC Med.* **2017**, *15*, 23. [CrossRef] [PubMed]
54. Molendijk, M.L.; Fried, E.I.; van der Does, W. The SMILES trial: Do undisclosed recruitment practices explain the remarkably large effect? *BMC Med.* **2018**, *16*, 243. [CrossRef] [PubMed]
55. Hiza, H.A.B.; Casavale, K.O.; Guenther, P.M.; Davis, C.A. Diet quality of Americans differs by age, sex, race/ethnicity, income, and education level. *J. Acad. Nutr. Diet.* **2013**, *113*, 297–306. [CrossRef]
56. Wang, D.D.; Leung, C.W.; Li, Y.; Ding, E.L.; Chiuve, S.E.; Hu, F.B.; Willett, W.C. Trends in dietary quality among adults in the United States, 1999 through 2010. *JAMA Intern. Med.* **2014**, *174*, 1587–1595. [CrossRef]
57. van Lee, L.; Geelen, A.; Kiefte-de Jong, J.C.; Witteman, J.C.M.; Hofman, A.; Vonk, N.; Jankovic, N.; van Huysduynen, E.H.; de Vries, J.H.M.; van't Veer, P.; et al. Adherence to the Dutch dietary guidelines is inversely associated with 20-year mortality in a large prospective cohort study. *Eur. J. Clin. Nutr.* **2016**, *70*, 262–268. [CrossRef]
58. Munt, A.; Partridge, S.; Allman-Farinelli, M. The barriers and enablers of healthy eating among young adults: A missing piece of the obesity puzzle: A scoping review. *Obes. Rev.* **2017**, *18*, 1–17. [CrossRef]
59. Rothgerber, H. Real men don't eat (vegetable) quiche: Masculinity and the justification of meat consumption. *Psychol. Men Masc.* **2013**, *14*, 363–375. [CrossRef]
60. Valdez, L.A.; Amezquita, A.; Hooker, S.P.; Garcia, D.O. Mexican-origin male perspectives of diet-related behaviors associated with weight management. *Int. J. Obes.* **2017**, *41*, 1824–1830. [CrossRef] [PubMed]
61. Robertson, C.; Avenell, A.; Boachie, C.; Stewart, F.; Archibald, D.; Douglas, F.; Hoddinott, P.; van Teijlingen, E.; Boyers, D. Should weight loss and maintenance programmes be designed differently for men? A systematic review of long-term randomised controlled trials presenting data for men and women: The ROMEO project. *Obes. Res. Clin. Pract.* **2016**, *10*, 70–84. [CrossRef] [PubMed]
62. Campos, L.; Bernardes, S.; Godinho, C. Food as a way to convey masculinities: How conformity to hegemonic masculinity norms influences men's and women's food consumption. *J. Health Psychol.* **2020**, *25*, 1842–1856. [CrossRef]
63. VanKim, N.A.; Corliss, H.L.; Jun, H.-J.; Calzo, J.P.; AlAwadhi, M.; Austin, S.B. Gender expression and sexual orientation differences in diet quality and eating habits from adolescence to young adulthood. *J. Acad. Nutr. Diet.* **2019**, *119*, 2028–2040. [CrossRef]
64. Lee, J.; Allen, J. Gender differences in healthy and unhealthy food consumption and its relationship with depression in young adulthood. *Community Ment. Health J.* **2020**. [CrossRef]
65. Kumar, G.S.; Pan, L.; Park, S.; Lee-Kwan, S.H.; Onufrak, S.; Blanck, H.M. Sugar-sweetened beverage consumption among adults 18 states. *MMWR. Morb. Mortal. Wkly. Rep.* **2014**, *63*, 686–690.
66. Park, S.; Pan, L.; Sherry, B.; Blanck, H.M. Consumption of sugar-sweetened beverages among US adults in 6 states: Behavioral Risk Factor Surveillance System, 2011. *Prev. Chronic Dis.* **2014**, *11*, E65. [CrossRef]
67. Nour, M.; Sui, Z.; Grech, A.; Rangan, A.; McGeechan, K.; Allman-Farinelli, M. The fruit and vegetable intake of young Australian adults: A population perspective. *Public Health Nutr.* **2017**, *20*, 2499–2512. [CrossRef]
68. Stark Casagrande, S.; Wang, Y.; Anderson, C.; Gary, T.L. Have Americans increased their fruit and vegetable intake? The trends between 1988 and 2002. *Am. J. Prev. Med.* **2007**, *32*, 257–263. [CrossRef]
69. Sakai, H.; Murakami, K.; Kobayashi, S.; Suga, H.; Sasaki, S. Food-based diet quality score in relation to depressive symptoms in young and middle-aged Japanese women. *Br. J. Nutr.* **2017**, *117*, 1674–1681. [CrossRef] [PubMed]
70. Yang, S.-Y.; Fu, S.-H.; Chen, K.-L.; Hsieh, P.-L.; Lin, P.-H. Relationships between depression, health-related behaviors, and internet addiction in female junior college students. *PLoS ONE* **2019**, *14*, e0220784. [CrossRef] [PubMed]
71. Alkerwi, A.A.; Vernier, C.; Sauvageot, N.; Crichton, G.E.; Elias, M.F. Demographic and socioeconomic disparity in nutrition: Application of a novel Correlated Component Regression approach. *BMJ Open* **2015**, *5*, e006814. [CrossRef]
72. Díaz Méndez, C.; García Espejo, I. Social inequalities in following official guidelines on healthy diet during the period of economic crisis in Spain. *Int. J. Health Serv.* **2019**, *49*, 582–605. [CrossRef] [PubMed]

73. Grimaccia, E.; Naccarato, A. Food insecurity in Europe: A gender perspective. *Soc. Indic. Res.* **2020**, 1–19. [CrossRef] [PubMed]

74. Errisuriz, V.L.; Delfausse, L.; Villatoro, A.P.; McDaniel, M.D.; Esparza, L.; Parra Medina, D. Depression and physical activity affect diet quality of foreign-born latina women living on the U.S.-Mexico Border. *Nutrients* **2019**, *11*, 1254. [CrossRef]

75. Lee, C.; Ory, M.G.; Yoon, J.; Forjuoh, S.N. Neighborhood walking among overweight and obese adults: Age variations in barriers and motivators. *J. Community Health* **2013**, *38*, 12–22. [CrossRef]

76. Vaughan, C.A.; Ghosh-Dastidar, M.; Dubowitz, T. Attitudes and barriers to healthy diet and physical activity: A latent profile analysis. *Health Educ. Behav.* **2018**, *45*, 381–393. [CrossRef]

77. Cleare, A.; Pariante, C.M.; Young, A.H.; Anderson, I.M.; Christmas, D.; Cowen, P.J.; Dickens, C.; Ferrier, I.N.; Geddes, J.; Gilbody, S.; et al. Evidence-based guidelines for treating depressive disorders with antidepressants: A revision of the 2008 British Association for Psychopharmacology guidelines. *J. Psychopharmacol.* **2015**, *29*, 459–525. [CrossRef]

78. Knapen, J.; Vancampfort, D.; Moriën, Y.; Marchal, Y. Exercise therapy improves both mental and physical health in patients with major depression. *Disabil. Rehabil.* **2015**, *37*, 1490–1495. [CrossRef]

79. Rebar, A.L.; Stanton, R.; Geard, D.; Short, C.; Duncan, M.J.; Vandelanotte, C. A meta-meta-analysis of the effect of physical activity on depression and anxiety in non-clinical adult populations. *Health Psychol. Rev.* **2015**, *9*, 366–378. [CrossRef] [PubMed]

80. Stanton, R.; Reaburn, P. Exercise and the treatment of depression: A review of the exercise program variables. *J. Sci. Med. Sport* **2014**, *17*, 177–182. [CrossRef] [PubMed]

81. Schuch, F.B.; Vancampfort, D.; Richards, J.; Rosenbaum, S.; Ward, P.B.; Stubbs, B. Exercise as a treatment for depression: A meta-analysis adjusting for publication bias. *J. Psychiatr. Res.* **2016**, *77*, 42–51. [CrossRef]

82. Jacka, F.N.; Rothon, C.; Taylor, S.; Berk, M.; Stansfeld, S.A. Diet quality and mental health problems in adolescents from East London: A prospective study. *Soc. Psychiatry Psychiatr. Epidemiol.* **2013**, *48*, 1297–1306. [CrossRef] [PubMed]

83. Malhi, G.S.; Bassett, D.; Boyce, P.; Bryant, R.; Fitzgerald, P.B.; Fritz, K.; Hopwood, M.; Lyndon, B.; Mulder, R.; Murray, G.; et al. Royal Australian and New Zealand College of Psychiatrists clinical practice guidelines for mood disorders. *Aust. N. Z. J. Psychiatry* **2015**, *49*, 1–185. [CrossRef] [PubMed]

84. Preston, A.M. Cigarette smoking-nutritional implications. *Prog. Food Nutr. Sci.* **1991**, *15*, 183–217.

85. Midgette, A.S.; Baron, J.A.; Rohan, T.E. Do cigarette smokers have diets that increase their risks of coronary heart disease and cancer? *Am. J. Epidemiol.* **1993**, *137*, 521–529. [CrossRef]

86. Subar, A.F.; Harlan, L.C. Nutrient and food group intake by tobacco use status: The 1987 National Health Interview Survey. *Ann. N. Y. Acad. Sci.* **1993**, *686*, 310–321. [CrossRef]

87. Dallongeville, J.; Marécaux, N.; Fruchart, J.C.; Amouyel, P. Cigarette smoking is associated with unhealthy patterns of nutrient intake: A meta-analysis. *J. Nutr.* **1998**, *128*, 1450–1457. [CrossRef]

88. Dyer, A.R.; Elliott, P.; Stamler, J.; Chan, Q.; Ueshima, H.; Zhou, B.F. Dietary intake in male and female smokers, ex-smokers, and never smokers: The INTERMAP study. *J. Hum. Hypertens.* **2003**, *17*, 641–654. [CrossRef]

89. Alkerwi, A.; Sauvageot, N.; Nau, A.; Lair, M.-L.; Donneau, A.-F.; Albert, A.; Guillaume, M. Population compliance with national dietary recommendations and its determinants: Findings from the ORISCAV-LUX study. *Br. J. Nutr.* **2012**, *108*, 2083–2092. [CrossRef] [PubMed]

90. Northrop-Clewes, C.A.; Thurnham, D.I. Monitoring micronutrients in cigarette smokers. *Clin. Chim. Acta.* **2007**, *377*, 14–38. [CrossRef] [PubMed]

91. Pot, G.K.; Richards, M.; Prynne, C.J.; Stephen, A.M. Development of the Eating Choices Index (ECI): A four-item index to measure healthiness of diet. *Public Health Nutr.* **2014**, *17*, 2660–2666. [CrossRef]

92. Alkerwi, A.; Baydarlioglu, B.; Sauvageot, N.; Stranges, S.; Lemmens, P.; Shivappa, N.; Hébert, J.R. Smoking status is inversely associated with overall diet quality: Findings from the ORISCAV-LUX study. *Clin. Nutr.* **2017**, *36*, 1275–1282. [CrossRef] [PubMed]

93. Breslow, R.A.; Chen, C.M.; Graubard, B.I.; Jacobovits, T.; Kant, A.K. Diets of drinkers on drinking and nondrinking days: NHANES 2003–2008. *Am. J. Clin. Nutr.* **2013**, *97*, 1068–1075. [CrossRef] [PubMed]

94. De Andrade, S.C.; Nogueira Previdelli, Á.; Galvão Cesar, C.L.; Lobo Marchioni, D.M.; Fisberg, R.M. Trends in diet quality among adolescents, adults and older adults: A population-based study. *Prev. Med. Rep.* **2016**, *4*, 391–396. [CrossRef]

95. Yeomans, M.R.; Caton, S.; Hetherington, M.M. Alcohol and food intake. *Curr. Opin. Clin. Nutr. Metab. Care.* **2003**, *6*, 639–644. [CrossRef]

96. Kesse, E.; Clavel–Chapelon, F.; Slimani, N.; van Liere, M. Do eating habits differ according to alcohol consumption? Results of a study of the French cohort of the European Prospective Investigation into Cancer and Nutrition (E3N-EPIC). *Am. J. Clin. Nutr.* **2001**, *74*, 322–327. [CrossRef]

97. Boden, J.M.; Fergusson, D.M. Alcohol and depression. *Addiction* **2011**, *106*, 906–914. [CrossRef]

98. Awaworyi Churchill, S.; Farrell, L. Alcohol and depression: Evidence from the 2014 health survey for England. *Drug Alcohol Depend.* **2017**, *180*, 86–92. [CrossRef]

99. Gémes, K.; Forsell, Y.; Janszky, I.; László, K.D.; Lundin, A.; Ponce de León, A.; Mukamal, K.J.; Moller, J. Moderate alcohol consumption and depression—A longitudinal population-based study in Sweden. *Acta Psychiatr. Scand.* **2019**, *139*, 526–535. [CrossRef] [PubMed]

100. Winpenny, E.M.; van Harmelen, A.-L.; White, M.; van Sluijs, E.M.; Goodyer, I.M. Diet quality and depressive symptoms in adolescence: No cross-sectional or prospective associations following adjustment for covariates. *Public Health Nutr.* **2018**, *21*, 2376–2384. [CrossRef] [PubMed]

101. Pabayo, R.; Dias, J.; Hemenway, D.; Molnar, B.E. Sweetened beverage consumption is a risk factor for depressive symptoms among adolescents living in Boston, Massachusetts, USA. *Public Health Nutr.* **2016**, *19*, 3062–3069. [CrossRef] [PubMed]
102. Zhang, X.; Huang, X.; Xiao, Y.; Jing, D.; Huang, Y.; Chen, L.; Luo, D.; Chen, X.; Shen, M. Daily intake of soft drinks is associated with symptoms of anxiety and depression in Chinese adolescents. *Public Health Nutr.* **2019**, *22*, 2553–2560. [CrossRef] [PubMed]
103. Imamura, F.; O'Connor, L.; Ye, Z.; Mursu, J.; Hayashino, Y.; Bhupathiraju, S.N.; Forouhi, N.G. Consumption of sugar sweetened beverages, artificially sweetened beverages, and fruit juice and incidence of type 2 diabetes: Systematic review, meta-analysis, and estimation of population attributable fraction. *BMJ* **2015**, *351*, h3576. [CrossRef] [PubMed]
104. Kim, Y.; Je, Y. Prospective association of sugar-sweetened and artificially sweetened beverage intake with risk of hypertension. *Arch. Cardiovasc. Dis.* **2016**, *109*, 242–253. [CrossRef]
105. Bernabé, E.; Vehkalahti, M.M.; Sheiham, A.; Aromaa, A.; Suominen, A.L. Sugar-sweetened beverages and dental caries in adults: A 4-year prospective study. *J. Dent.* **2014**, *42*, 952–958. [CrossRef]
106. Moynihan, P.J.; Kelly, S.A.M. Effect on caries of restricting sugars intake: Systematic review to inform WHO guidelines. *J. Dent. Res.* **2014**, *93*, 8–18. [CrossRef]
107. Luger, M.; Lafontan, M.; Bes-Rastrollo, M.; Winzer, E.; Yumuk, V.; Farpour-Lambert, N. Sugar-sweetened beverages and weight gain in children and adults: A systematic review from 2013 to 2015 and a comparison with previous studies. *Obes. Facts* **2017**, *10*, 674–693. [CrossRef]
108. Sisti, J.S.; Mezzacca, T.A.; Anekwe, A.; Farley, S.M. Examining trends in beverage sales in New York City during comprehensive efforts to reduce sugary drink consumption, 2010–2015. *J. Community Health* **2020**. [CrossRef]
109. World Health Organization (WHO). Together Let's Beat NCDs. Taxes on Sugary Drinks: Why Do It? 2017. Available online: https://apps.who.int/iris/bitstream/handle/10665/260253/WHO-NMH-PND-16.5Rev.1-eng.pdf?sequence=1&isAllowed=y (accessed on 10 October 2020).
110. Vall Castelló, J.; López Casasnovas, G. *Impact of SSB Taxes on Consumption*; Universitat Pompeu Fabra: Barcelona, Spain, 2018.
111. Perera, T.; Russo, C.; Takata, Y.; Bobe, G. Legume consumption patterns in US Adults: National Health and Nutrition Examination Survey (NHANES) 2011-2014 and Bean, Lentils, Peas (BLP) 2017 Survey. *Nutrients* **2020**, *12*, 1237. [CrossRef] [PubMed]
112. Suga, H.; Asakura, K.; Kobayashi, S.; Nojima, M.; Sasaki, S.; the Three-generation Study of Women on Diets and Health Study Group. Association between habitual tryptophan intake and depressive symptoms in young and middle-aged women. *J. Affect. Disord.* **2018**, *231*, 44–50. [CrossRef] [PubMed]
113. Seo, Y.; Je, Y. A comparative study of dietary habits and nutritional intakes among Korean adults according to current depression status. *Asia Pac. Psychiatry* **2017**, *10*, e12321. [CrossRef] [PubMed]
114. Yusta Boyo, M.J.; Bermejo, L.M.; García Solano, M.; López Sobaler, A.M.; Ortega, R.M.; García Pérez, M.; Dal-Re Saavedra, M.Á. Sugar content in processed foods in Spain and a comparison of mandatory nutrition labelling and laboratory values. *Nutrients* **2020**, *12*, 1078. [CrossRef] [PubMed]
115. Xia, Y.; Wang, N.; Yu, B.; Zhang, Q.; Liu, L.; Meng, G.; Wu, H.; Du, H.; Shi, H.; Guo, X.; et al. Dietary patterns are associated with depressive symptoms among Chinese adults: A case–control study with propensity score matching. *Eur. J. Nutr.* **2017**, *56*, 2577–2587. [CrossRef] [PubMed]
116. Quirk, S.E.; Williams, L.J.; O'Neil, A.; Pasco, J.A.; Jacka, F.N.; Housden, S.; Berk, M.; Brennan, S.L. The association between diet quality, dietary patterns and depression in adults: A systematic review. *BMC Psychiatry* **2013**, *13*, 175. [CrossRef]
117. Tahmassebi, J.F.; BaniHani, A. Impact of soft drinks to health and economy: A critical review. *Eur. Arch. Paediatr. Dent.* **2020**, *21*, 109–117. [CrossRef]

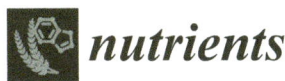 *nutrients*

Review

Passiflora incarnata in Neuropsychiatric Disorders—A Systematic Review

Katarzyna Janda 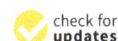, Karolina Wojtkowska, Karolina Jakubczyk *, Justyna Antoniewicz and Karolina Skonieczna-Żydecka

Department of Human Nutrition and Metabolomics, Pomeranian Medical University in Szczecin, 71-460 Szczecin, Poland; Katarzyna.Janda@pum.edu.pl (K.J.); lottecharlotte23@gmail.com (K.W.); kaldunskajustyna@gmail.com (J.A.); karzyd@pum.edu.pl (K.S.-Ż.)
* Correspondence: jakubczyk.kar@gmail.com; Tel.: +48-790-233-164

Received: 25 November 2020; Accepted: 16 December 2020; Published: 19 December 2020

Abstract: Background: Stress is a natural response of the body, induced by factors of a physical (hunger, thirst, and infection) and/or psychological (perceived threat, anxiety, or concern) nature. Chronic, long-term stress may cause problems with sleep, concentration, and memory, as well as affective disorders. The passionflower (*Passiflora incarnata*) is a perennial plant with documented therapeutic properties. The literature data suggest that the passionflower itself, as well as its preparations, helps reduce stress and can therefore be helpful in the treatment of insomnia, anxiety, and depression. The objective of this systematic review was to evaluate *Passiflora incarnata* in terms of its neuropsychiatric effects. Methods: The scientific databases PubMed, ClinTrials.gov, and Embase were searched up to 22 October 2019. The search identified randomized clinical trials describing the effects of *Passiflora incarnata* in neuropsychiatric disorders. Results: The systematic review included nine clinical trials. The duration of the studies included in the analysis varied widely, from one day up to 30 days. Study participants were no less than 18 years old. In each of the papers, the effects of passionflower were measured by using a number of different tests and scales. The majority of studies reported reduced anxiety levels following the administration of *Passiflora incarnata* preparations, with the effect less evident in people with mild anxiety symptoms. No adverse effects, including memory loss or collapse of psychometric functions, were observed. Conclusion: *Passiflora incarnata* may be helpful in treating some symptoms in neuropsychiatric patients.

Keywords: *Passiflora incarnata*; neuropsychiatric disorders; stress; anxiety; depression

1. Introduction

The passionflower (*Passiflora incarnata* L.) is a perennial plant which that can grow up to 10 m, with egg-shaped edible fruit. The low-calorie fruit (41–53 kcal/100 g) is a rich source of vitamins A, C, B1, and B2, as well as calcium, phosphorus, and iron. The species is native to South America, Australia, and South East Asia, and today is cultivated to source raw material for pharmaceutical use [1]. *Passiflora incarnata* is one of the best-documented species of the *Passiflora* genus with therapeutic properties. The aerial parts of the plant, flowers, and fruits are used for medicinal purposes. They are credited with anthelmintic, antispasmodic, and anxiolytic effects. The passionflower is also used as a remedy for burns, diarrhea, painful menstruation, hemorrhoids, in neurotic disorders, insomnia, to treat morphine dependence, and can be helpful in convulsions or neuralgia, too. *Passiflora incarnata* is a source of alkaloids, phenolic compounds, flavonoid, and cyanogenic glycosides. The primary phytochemicals found in the passionflower are flavonoids (apigenin, luteolin, quercetin, and kaempferol) and flavonoid glycosides (vitexin, isovitexin, orientin, and isoorientin) [1,2]. The species has the highest overall isovitexin content [3]. On 25 March 2014, the European Medicines Agency published a herbal monograph on *Passiflora incarnata*, thus recognizing its status as a medicinal product [4]. Clinical trials found no threats to human health in relation to the use of *Passiflora incarnata* [5,6].

Stress is a natural response of the body. It can be induced by factors of a physical (hunger, thirst, infection) and/or psychological (perceived threat, anxiety or concern) nature—namely stressors. Stress has been linked to cellular inflammation. Physiologically, the body's response to stress causes an immediate activation of the adrenergic system and the sympathetic–adrenomedullary axis (SAM axis), followed by the hypothalamic–pituitary–adrenal axis (HPA axis). Chronic, long-term stress is a pathological condition, which may impair concentration and memory, as well as lead to affective disorders, such as depression, schizophrenia, and the post-traumatic stress disorder [7]. *Passiflora incarnata* is one of the herbal remedies used to alleviate the effects of stress [2]. A rat study demonstrated that long-term use of passionflower was correlated with reduced stress levels and, consequently, increased motivation to act and improved motor activity [8]. The beneficial effects of passionflower on memory function have also been confirmed [9]. The use of *P. incarnata* in people with chronic insomnia may produce a therapeutic effect in the management of sleep disorders, memory loss, and degenerative brain diseases. *Passiflora* may be helpful in the treatment of insomnia, through its sedative action, as a result of which the person experiencing difficulty sleeping will be more likely to get to sleep [10]. *Passiflora* demonstrates positive effects in episodes of anxiety, restlessness, sleeplessness, and in depressive states [11].

The objective of this systematic review was to evaluate the efficacy of *Passiflora incarnata* preparations in the treatment of neuropsychiatric disorders. The systematic review included randomized controlled trials (RCT) which investigated the relationship between the use of *Passiflora incarnata* and a range of disorders of the nervous system.

2. Materials and Methods

2.1. Search Strategy, Inclusion Criteria

At least two independent authors (K.W., J.A. and K.S.Z.) searched PubMed/MEDLINE/Embase, from database inception until 22 October 2019, without language restrictions. Randomized clinical trials have been found to describe the effect of the use of passion flower in neuropsychiatric disorders. The following search string in Pub Med was used: ("passiflora" OR "passion fruit" OR "passion" OR "passion flower") AND (anxiety OR depression OR insomnia OR somatoform); Embase ("passiflora"/exp OR "passiflora") AND ("depression"/exp OR "central depression" OR "clinical depression" OR "depression" OR "depressive disease" OR "depressive disorder" OR "depressive episode" OR "depressive illness" OR "depressive personality disorder" OR "depressive state" OR "depressive symptom" OR "depressive syndrome" OR "mental depression" OR "parental depression" OR "anxiety disorder"/exp OR "anxiety disorder" OR "anxiety disorders" OR "insomnia"/exp OR "agrypnia" OR "hyposomnia" OR "insomnia" OR "sleep initiation and maintenance disorders" OR "sleeplessness" OR" somatoform disorder"/exp OR "somatoform disorder" OR "somatoform disorders"), oraz ClinTrials.gov (*Passiflora*).

We utilized the following inclusion criteria: (i) original studies, (ii) studies with access to full text, (iii) studies in which the treatment included any products (supplements, tinctures, extracts, infusions, raw materials, etc.) containing *Passiflora incarnata*, (iv) presence of meta-analytical data (change score/endpoint) on psychiatric symptoms in the process of each neuropsychiatric disease, and (v) studies carried out in humans. Exclusion criteria were as follows: (i) intervention with products containing other psychoactive substances; (ii) meta-analyses, systematic reviews, and review works.

2.2. Data Abstraction

Data for country in which the study was conducted, information about the sponsors, type of blindness, duration of the study, and main purpose of the study, as well as the name of the preparation used during therapy, were extracted. During data abstraction, detailed data on the studied population were looked for, i.e., the average age and standard deviation of studied persons, the number and percentage of men participating in the study, and the number of people randomized to the study. Data extraction was performed based on the guidelines contained in the Preferred Reporting Items for Systematic Reviews and Meta-Analyses (PRISMA) protocol, but with no study protocol registration. If data were missing, authors were contacted via email, to ask for additional information. Inconsistencies were resolved by consensus, with the corresponding author being involved. The results that were compared in the systematic review involved various scales and tests, such as the Hamilton Rating Scale for Depression (HRSD), Visual Analogue Scale (VAS), Numerical Rating Scale (NRS), Observers Assessment of Alertness and Sedation Scale (OAA/S), Corah's Dental Anxiety Scale, Revised (DAS-R), Ramsey Scale, Digit symbol substitution test (DSST), Concentration Endurance Test, (The d2 test), Memory test, Continuous Performance Task/Test (CPT), Trieger Dot Test (TDT), Perceptive Accuracy Test (PAT), Finger Tapping Test (FTT), and State-Trait Anxiety Inventory (STAI-S, STAI-T). Data from charts and figures were extracted by means of WebPlotDigitizer software (https://automeris.io/WebPlotDigitizer/) in order to detect the risk of bias, the Cochrane Collaboration's tool for assessing risk of bias was used.

2.3. Outcomes

The primary outcome was to evaluate the effects of a *Passiflora incarnata* on neuropsychiatric symptoms, namely depressive/anxious phenotype and reactivity to stress. Co-secondary outcomes were insomnia, somatoform and psychomotor functions, sedation, and nervous restlessness.

3. Results

3.1. Search Results

The first search in PubMed and Embase databases resulted in 417 hits. Among them, 305 studies were excluded as duplicates and/or after evaluation at the title/abstract level. After excluding 305 studies, 112 full-text articles were eventually reviewed, 103 of which were excluded due to the failure to meet previously established inclusion criteria. The main reasons for exclusion were as follows: review ($n = 31$), intervention with multi-herbal preparations ($n = 21$), an article published in a language other than Polish or English ($n = 11$), lack of access to full text ($n = 8$), intervention with other psychoactive substances ($n = 3$), supplementation during pregnancy ($n = 1$), review of the substance isolated from *Passiflora incarnata* ($n = 1$), lack of availability of final results ($n = 1$), a study in which a comparison group was missing ($n = 1$), and a study that did not focus on neuropsychiatric disorders ($n = 1$). Finally, nine studies were included in the systematic review. The scheme of searching databases is included in Figure 1.

3.2. Study Characteristics

Nine studies carried out between 2017 and 2019 were included in this systematic review.

The objective of this systematic review was to evaluate *Passiflora incarnata* in terms of its neuropsychiatric effects. More than half of the studies (five) were carried out in Iran, and the others in Brazil, Turkey, Germany, and Australia. The vast majority of study participants was healthy [6,12–18]. There was only one study [19] in which the participants had a diagnosis of Generalized Anxiety Disorder (GAD). The duration of the studies included in the analysis varied widely—from one day up to 30 days. Predominantly, the aim of the reviewed papers ($n = 4$) was to assess the effects of passionflower use on the anxiety experienced by patients during spinal anesthesia, dental procedures, or surgery. Studies investigating the effects of *P. incarnata* administration on sleep quality and cognitive functions were also included in the analysis. The majority of the analyzed studies ($n = 7$) were double-blind (DB), with one cross-over study. The other trials ($n = 2$) were single-blind (SB), and one ($n = 1$) was a cross-over study. In all the papers included in the review, the participants were no less than 18 years old. Details of the studies included in the systematic review are presented in Table 1.

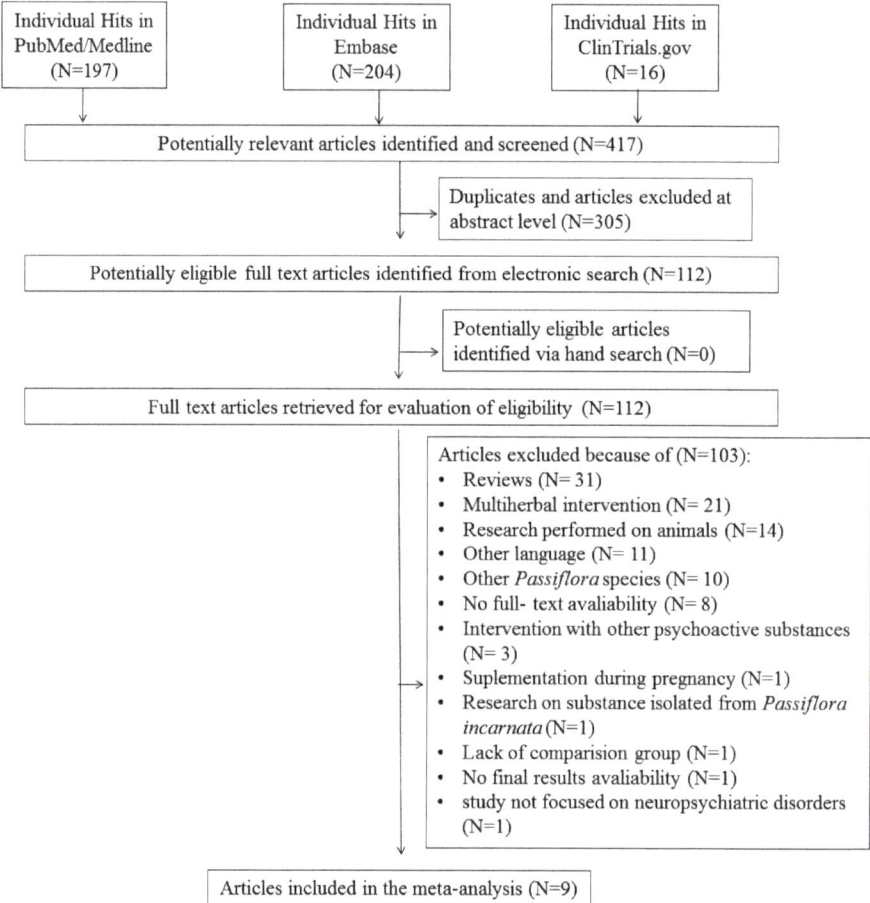

Figure 1. Study flowchart.

3.3. Effect of Passiflora Treatments on Neuropsychiatric Parameters

The systematic review included nine studies. In each of the works, different criteria were taken into account: the Hamilton Rating Scale for Depression (HRSD), Observers Assessment of Alertness and Sedation Scale (OAA/S), Corah's Dental Anxiety Scale, Revised (DAS-R), Ramsey Scale, Digit symbol substitution test (DSST), Continuous Performance Task/Test (CPT), Trieger Dot Test (TDT), Perceptive Accuracy Test (PAT), Finger Tapping Test (FTT), State-Trait Anxiety Inventory (STAI), Visual Analogue Scale (VAS), memory test, and Concentration Endurance Test (d2 test). The results of the use of the *Passiflora* preparations are presented in Tables 2 and 3.

Table 1. Characteristics of studies included in the systematic review.

	Description of Treatment				Characteristics of The Intervention and of the Study Group					
Reference/Year/Country	Study Objective	Blinding	Duration of Administration (Days)	ROB *	Commercial Name of Product Containing *P. Incarnata*	*Passiflora* Dose	Comparator	*n* Total Randomized/Analyzed	Age Years (Mean)	Males (%)
Akhondzadeh et al., 2001 (Iran) [12]	Comparative efficacy of *Passiflora incarnata* extract with oxazepam in the treatment of systemic anxiety disorder	DB	28	5	Passipay (Iran, Darouk)	45 drops/day	Placebo + oxazepam (30 mg/day)	36/32	19–47 #	44.4
Aslanargun et al., 2012 (Turkey) [13]	Effects of preoperative oral administration of *Passiflora incarnata* on anxiety, psychomotor functions, sedation and hemodynamics in patients undergoing spinal anesthesia	DB	1	4	*Passiflora* Syrup (Sandoz, Kocaeli, Turkey)	700 mg/5 mL	Placebo	60/60	25–55 #	86.6
Azimaraghi et al., 2017 (Iran) [14]	The efficacy of *Passiflora incarnata* to reduce preoperative anxiety in comparison to oxazepam	DB	NA	7	Passipy™ (Iran Darouk)	500 mg	Oxazepam (10 mg)	128/128	36.77	57.8

Table 1. *Cont.*

	Description of Treatment				Characteristics of The Intervention and of the Study Group				
Reference/ Year/Country	Study Objective	Blinding	Duration of Administration (Days)	ROB *	Commercial Name of Product Containing P. Incarnata	Passiflora Dose	Comparator	n Total Randomized/ Analyzed	Age Years (Mean)	Males (%)
Dantas et al., 2017 (Brazil) [15]	The influence of Passiflora incarnata and midazolam on the control of anxiety in patients exposed to the extraction of the third mandibular molar tooth	DB, CO	15-30	7	Passiflora incarnata	260 mg	Midazolam (15 mg)	40/40	23.94	32.5
Dimpfel et al., 2011 (Germany) [16]	Explanation of the effectiveness of the preparation by analysis of current density (CfD) of brain activity in the presence of various mental challenges	SB, CO	1	4	NEURAPAS®	192 mg of P. incarnata extract	Placebo	16/16	47.85	50
Kaviani et al., 2013 (Iran) [17]	Determining the effectiveness of passion flower application in reducing anxiety during dental procedures	SB	2	4	Passipay (Iran, Darouk)	40 drops/day	Placebo	63/63	34.07	38.1

Table 1. Cont.

Reference/ Year/Country	Description of Treatment				Characteristics of The Intervention and of the Study Group				
	Study Objective	Blinding	Duration of Administration (Days)	ROB *	Commercial Name of Product Containing P. Incarnata	Passiflora Dose	Comparator	n Total Randomized/ Analyzed	Age Years (Mean)	Males (%)
Kaviani et al., 2013 (Iran) [17]	Determining the effectiveness of passion flower application in reducing anxiety during dental procedures	SB	2	4	Passipay (Iran, Darouk)	40 drops/day	Negative group	63/63	34.07	38.1
Movafegh et al., 2008 (Iran) [6]	Effectiveness of Passiflora in reducing preoperative anxiety	DB	1	7	Passipy™ (Iran Darouk)	500 mg	Placebo	60/60	31.85	50
Ngan and Conduit, 2011 (Australia) [18]	To test the effectiveness of the Passiflora infusion on human sleep, measured by means of sleep logs approved by polysomnography	DB	22	6	Tea bags (Hilde Hemmes' HerbalSupplies Pty Ltd.; SA, Australia)	infusion (2 g in 250 mL water; concentration 0.8%)	Placebo	41/41	22.73	34.1

57

Table 1. *Cont.*

Reference/ Year/Country	Description of Treatment				Characteristics of The Intervention and of the Study Group				
	Study Objective	Blinding	Duration of Administration (Days)	ROB *	Commercial Name of Product Containing *P. Incarnata*	*Passiflora* Dose	Comparator	*n* Total Randomized/ Analyzed	Age Years (Mean)	Males (%)
Rokhtabnak et al., 2017 (Iran) [19]	Effects of *Passiflora incarnata* and melatonin on cognitive functions and sedative effect without causing cognitive disturbance	DB	1	7	*Passiflora incarnata*	1000 mg (prepared and packed by Department of Pharmacy, Shahid Beheshti University of Medical Sciences, Iran)	Melatonin (6 mg)	64/52	20–60 #	44.2

Notes: #—range; *—the risk of bias (ROB), shown in numbers; DB—double blind; SB—single blind; CO—cross-over; NA—not available.

Table 2. Results of the systematic review.

Reference/Year/Country	Comparator	Control Group		Tested Group		Conclusions
		Baseline Data	Endpoint Data	Baseline Data	Endpoint Data	
Akhondzadeh et al., 2001 (Iran) [12]	Placebo + oxazepam (30 mg/day)	Hamilton scale: 19.74 ± 0.83	Hamilton scale: 5.1 ± 1.28	Hamilton scale: 19.74 ± 0.83	Hamilton scale: 5.5 ± 0.75	*Passiflora* extract is effective in the treatment of systemic anxiety; additionally, there is a low incidence of impairment of work efficiency with *Passiflora* extract, as compared to oxazepam. There is a need for further research on the use of *Passiflora* in the treatment of systemic anxiety.
Aslanargun et al., 2012 (Turkey) [13]	Placebo	STAI-S: 34.8 ± 8.4; STAI-T: 35.3 ± 8.3; PAT: 95.2 ± 16.4; FTT: 72.3 ± 14.1; OAA/S: 5 ± 0; NRS: 6.6 ± 1; TDTmm: 0.8 ± 0.2; TDTnr: 0.9 ± 0.7; DSST: 30.8 ± 5;	STAI-S: 36.6 ± 7.6; STAI-T: 38.1 ± 9.2; PAT: 99.1 ± 1.4; FTT: 72.3 ± 13.1; OAA/S: 5 ± 0.15; NRS: 6.1 ± 1.3; TDTmm:1.1 ± 0.3; TDTnr: 1.2 ± 1; DSST: 29.1± 4.8;	STAI-S: 36.4 ± 10.9; STAI-T: 32.5 ± 9.5; PAT: 98.0 ± 2.6; FTT:67.4 ± 18.9; OAA/S: 5 ± 0; NRS:7.6 ± 0.9; TDTmm: 0.9 ± 0.2; TDTnr: 0.8 ± 0.8; DSST: 31.1 ± 5.1;	STAI-S: 35.7 ± 10.8; STAI-T: 33.4 ± 8.7; PAT: 99.1 ± 1.7; FTT: 67.6 ± 19.8; OAA/S: 5 ± 0.15; NRS: 4.4 ± 1.2; TDTmm: 1.2 ± 0.4; TDTnr: 1 ± 0.9; DSST: 28.6 ± 5;	Preoperative oral administration of 700 mg/5 mL of *Passiflora* water extract reduces the level of anxiety in patients before spinal anesthesia without changing their sedation level, psychomotor function test results, or hemodynamics.
Azimaraghi et al., 2017 (Iran) [14]	Oxazepam (10 mg)	NRS: 6 6 ± 1; TDTmm: 3.8 ± 0.2; TDTnr: 0.9 ± 0.7; DSST: 30.8 ± 5;	NRS: 6.1 ± 1.3; TDTmm: 1.1 ± 0.3; TDTnr: 1.2 ± 1; DSST: 29.1 ± 4.8;	NRS: 7.6 ± 0.9; TDTmm: 0.9 ± 0.2; TDTnr: 0.8 ± 0.8; DSST: 31.1 ± 5.1;	NRS: 4.4 ± 1.2; TDTmm: 1.2 ± 0.4; TDTnr: 1 ± 0.9; DSST: 28.6 ± 5;	In outpatient surgery, oral administration of *Passiflora* as a premedication reduces preoperative anxiety with comparable dysfunction of psychomotor functions, as compared to preoperative oral intake of oxazepam.

Table 2. *Cont.*

Reference/Year/Country	Comparator	Control Group		Tested Group		Conclusions
		Baseline Data	Endpoint Data	Baseline Data	Endpoint Data	
Dimpfel et al., 2011 (Germany) [16]	Midazolam (15 mg)	d2 test: 12.32 ± 4.02; memory test: 10.77 ± 3.98; ccCPT: 6.57 ± 6.17;	d2 test: 13.59 ± 3.77; memory test: 11.51 ± 3.74; CPT: 6.87 ± 7.3;	d2 test: 12.14 ± 3.06; memory test: 11.37 ± 3.64; CPT: 5.59 ± 5.85;	d2 test: 13.53 ± 3.13; memory test: 11.95 ± 3.65; CPT: 7.86 ± 5.76;	Analysis of neurophysiological changes after NEURAPAS® intake showed similarity of changes compared to sedatives and antidepressants, in EEG, without cognitive function impairment.
Kaviani et al., 2013 (Iran) [17]	Placebo	Corah DAS-R: 12 ± 2.66;	Corah DAS-R: 10.52 ± 2.11;	Corah DAS-R: 13.09 ± 2.42;	Corah DAS-R: 8.47 ± 2.08;	The serving of the passion flower as a premeditation is effective in reducing anxiety. Further trials with more people are needed to confirm the results.
	Placebo	Corah DAS-R: 11.66 ± 2.39	Corah DAS-R: 11.23 ± 2.34	Corah DAS-R: 13.09 ± 2.42;	Corah DAS-R: 8.47 ± 2.08;	
Movafegh et al., 2008 (Iran) [6]	Negative group	NRS: 5.1 ± 2; TDImm: 0.6 ± 1; TDInr: 0.8 ± 0.9; DSST: 24.3 ± 6.2;	NRS: 3.88 ± 0.81; TDImm: 0.6 ± 0.3; TDInr: 0.9 ± 0.8; DSST: 21.5 ± 7.1;	NRS: 4.6 ± 1.7; TDImm: 0.7 ± 1.1; TDInr: 0.7 ± 0.62; DSST: 23.6 ± 7.2;	NRS: 0.97 ± 0.72; TDImm: 0.7 ± 0.2; TDInr: 8 ± 0.5; DSST: 22.4 ± 6.5;	In outpatient surgery, oral administration of *Passiflora* as premeditation reduces anxiety without sedation.
Ngan and Conduit, 2011 (Australia) [18]	Placebo	NA	NA	NA	NA	Consumption of a small dose of *Passiflora* infusion brings short-term subjective benefits to healthy adults with mild fluctuations in sleep quality.
Rokhtabnak et al., 2017 (Iran) [19]	Placebo	DSST: 30.67 ± nd; Ramsy scale: 1.81 ± nd; VAS: 26.5 ± nd;	DSST: 27.5 ± nd; Ramsey scale: 1.95 ± nd; VAS: 26.5 ± nd;	DSST: 22.33 ± nd; Ramsey scale: 1.85 ± nd; VAS: 26.5 ± nd;	DSST: 25.5 ± nd; Ramsey scale: 1.95 ± nd; VAS: 26.5 ± nd;	*Passiflora* premedication reduces anxiety, as does melatonin, but melatonin causes less cognitive disorders compared to *Passiflora*.

VAS (Visual Analogue Scale), NRS (Numerical Rating Scale), OAA/S (Observers Assessment of Alertness and Sedation Scale), DAS-R (Corah's Dental Anxiety Scale, Revised), DSST (Digit Symbol Substitution Test), CPT (Continuous Performance Task/Test), TDT (Trieger Dot Test), PAT (Perceptive Accuracy Test), FTT (Finger Tapping Test), STAI (State-Trait Anxiety Inventory), NA—not available, nd—no data

Table 3. Results of the systematic review. The following table refers to the results of the cross-review [15].

What Did You Feel during the Surgery?	Protocol 1 (Midazolam)		Protocol 2 (Passiflora)		Results
	Midazolam (1)	Passiflora (2)	Passiflora (2)	Midazolam (1)	
Calm	5 (33.3%)	17 (68%)	13 (52%)	3 (20%)	*Passiflora* showed an anti-anxiety effect similar to midazolam; it was safe and effective in the case of conscious sedation in adult patients having their third mandibular molar tooth extracted
Slight anxiety	6 (40%)	7 (28%)	10 (40%)	8 (55.3%)	
Serious anxiety or fear	3 (20%)	1 (4%)	2 (8%)	3 (20%)	
Bad feeling caused by anxiety	1 (6.7%)	0	0	1 (6.7%)	
Total	15	25	25	15	

The Hamilton Depression (HAM-D) Scale is a numerical scale consisting of 21 points (or 17 points in some cases). It is a tool used in general psychiatry, to assess the diagnosis of depression and to clinically evaluate the use of antidepressants. The HAM-D score level of depression is as follows: 10–13, mild; 14–17, mild to moderate; and >17, moderate to severe [20]. The numerical and analog-visual scales belong to pain scales with scores ranging from 0 to 10, with score 0 reflecting no pain and 10 the strongest imaginable pain. The four-stage OAA/S scale is a useful tool in assessing the awareness of patients who have received midazolam. The scale has been used for sedation-related drugs, to assess a person's level of sedation, since the 1990s [21]. The Corah Dental Anxiety Scale has been used since the 1970s [22]. It consists of four items (questions) on dental anxiety. Each answer is scored from 1 to 5. A total of 20 points can be obtained, with a score above 15 suggesting the presence of a dental phobia [23]. The Corah scale is another Dental Anxiety Scale which can be used in children [24]. The Ramsey scale is one of the most widely used scales to assess the level of sedation. Scores are recorded from 0 to 6, with 0 being conscious and 6 being deeply coma [25]. The DSST test is primarily used in clinical neuropsychology. Initially, it helped scientists to understand how a person learns. Currently, it is used in the assessment of cognitive disorders, such as schizophrenia and major depression [26]. The concentration strength test concerns the diagnosis in the context of concentration, as well as the perception and possible correction of errors [27]. The memory test mainly focuses on visual memory. It informs about possible alterations within the central nervous system, and it can also be used to assess the attention/concentration disorders. The continuous exercise test is a neuropsychological test that is used in the diagnosis of ADHD and epilepsy, as well as in patients with brain damage. It focuses mainly on the patient's constant attention, while allowing us to measure the degree of impulsiveness during the test. It helps to collect quantitative data about the patient [28,29]. Measurement of perceptual-motor skills is performed by using the Trieger point tests (e.g., TDT) or the exact perception tests (e.g., PAT) [30,31]. TDT is also a useful tool for assessing the level of anesthesia and recovery [32]. The finger tapping test is one of the standard neuropsychological assessments that examines motor functioning, specifically, motor speed and lateralized coordination. The inventory of the state and trait of anxiety allows the assessment of the severity of anxiety and its characteristics [33].

3.4. Risk of Bias Assessment

The bias analysis showed that the three studies were of low quality and received less than 5 points in the risk of bias (ROB) evaluation [13,16,17]. In the last six [6,12,14,15,18,19], the number of points was higher than 5. The average number of points in all studies is 5.66 The results of the bias risk analysis are presented in Table 4.

Table 4. Risk of bias (ROB).

Reference/Country	Publication Year	Random Generation of The Error Sequence (Selection Error)	Hiding the Allocation (Selection Variation)	Blinding of Participants and Staff (Biased Evaluation)	Performance Evaluation Blindness (Detection Error)	Incomplete Result Data	Selective Reporting (Reporting Error)	Other Biases	Number of Indications with Low Risk of Bias
Akhondzadeh et al. (Iran) [12]	2001	L	?	L	?	L	L	L	5
Aslanargun et al. (Turkey) [13]	2012	?	?	L	?	L	L	L	4
Azimaraghi et al. (Iran) [14]	2017	L	L	L	L	L	L	L	7
Dantas et al. (Brazil) [15]	2017	L	L	L	L	L	L	L	7
Dimpfel et al. (Germany) [16]	2011	L	?	?	?	L	L	L	4
Kaviani et al. (Iran) [17]	2013	L	?	H	?	L	L	L	4
Movafegh et al. (Iran) [6]	2008	L	L	L	L	L	L	L	7
Ngan and Conduit (Australia) [18]	2011	?	L	L	L	L	L	L	6
Rokhtabnaket al. (Iran) [19]	2017	L	L	L	L	L	L	L	7

L—low risk of bias; H—high risk of bias; ?—unclear risk of bias.

4. Discussion

Neuropsychiatric disorders, such as schizophrenia, bipolar affective disorder, major depressive disorder, and attention-deficit hyperactivity disorder, are a common and, regrettably, increasingly prevalent problem. Around the world, depression affects some 322 million people, while 264 million live with anxiety [34]. Mild dysfunctions of the nervous system can be treated with psychotherapy, but more severe disorders require pharmacological treatment alongside therapy [35]. In the past year, the academic interest in these disorders has been growing due to the COVID-19 pandemic and the related upsurge in anxiety and depression [36]. Pharmacotherapy is effective, but, at the same time, it carries the risk of side effects and dependence [37]. Hence, the search for herbal remedies for neuropsychiatric disorders continues to go on [38]. *Passiflora incarnata* is a perennial plant containing precious phytochemicals with health-promoting properties. The most important among them would appear to be chrysin, due to its neuroprotective effects [39]. The systematic review method used in this study made it possible to assess the efficacy of passionflower with respect to neurological disorders, by synthesizing the results of nine clinical trials included herein. This is the first systematic review evaluating the effects of *Passiflora incarnata* in neuropsychiatric disorders.

Nine clinical trials were included in this paper. The reviewed studies analyzed the effects of passionflower preparations on anxiety levels experienced by patients during medical interventions, including spinal anesthesia, dental procedures, or surgery, as well as on sleep quality and cognitive functions. In eight papers, the study subjects were healthy, and, in one, *P. incarnata* was given to patients with a diagnosis of Generalized Anxiety Disorder (GAD). Various commercial products containing passionflower preparations were administered in the analyzed trials, including drops, tablets, and syrup. Detailed information, including the type of preparation and dosage, is presented in Table 1.

Akhondzadeh et al. [12], in their study of people with Generalized Anxiety Disorder (GAD), compared the effects of passionflower extract with oxazepam over a period of 28 days. To this end, they used the Hamilton Rating Scale for Depression. Study participants receiving either passionflower extract (45 drops/day) or oxazepam were evaluated each day, prior to, during, and after taking the relevant substance (Table 2). The authors demonstrated that there were no significant differences between taking passionflower vs. oxazepam, and the former did not cause an impairment of job performance in the subjects. A follow-up large-scale trial was recommended.

Aslanargun et al. [13] investigated the effects of administering passionflower syrup (700 mg/5 mL, 30 min before anesthesia) on anxiety, psychomotor function, sedation, and hemodynamics in patients before spinal anesthesia. The effects of passionflower were examined in awake patients after surgery (Table 2). The authors demonstrated that *P. incarnata* significantly contributed to reducing preoperative anxiety. Even though it was reported that psychomotor functions were impaired 30 min after extubation, the preoperative values were restored by 90 min. Side effects, including cutaneous vasculitis, urticaria, asthma, or rhinitis, were not observed. Hemodynamic parameters did not change after the administration of *Passiflora*, as compared to the placebo. Additional advantages included the lack of intraoperative sedation and respiratory depression. According to the authors, *P. incarnata* is a safe and effective anxiolytic which can be used before spinal anesthesia.

The objective of the study by Azimaraghi et al. [14] was to compare the efficacy of passionflower and oxazepam in reducing patients' preoperative anxiety. The authors demonstrated that patients who were given *Passiflora* tablets (500 mg for premedication) had lower preoperative anxiety levels, as compared to the group receiving oxazepam, and the effects of both medications on postoperative psychomotor function were similar. Recovery time was, likewise, comparable in both groups (Table 2). The authors suggest that *Passiflora incarnata* is safe and definitely more effective for reducing preoperative anxiety in comparison to oxazepam. They also point out that it can be included in the treatment of preoperative anxiety in children and adolescents.

To compare the anxiolytic action of *Passiflora incarnata* with that of midazolam, Dantas et al. [15] employed an experimental model involving bilateral extraction of the mandibular third molars.

The participants received 15 mg of midazolam (one pill) or 260 mg of *Passiflora incarnata* (one pill) administered orally 30 min before the start of the surgical procedure. In a cross-over design, participants were randomly assigned an extraction side (right or left) and a protocol (midazolam or *Passiflora*) at the first procedure. The researcher delivered the drugs to the participants, in encoded form, as "Protocol 1" (midazolam) or "Protocol 2" (*Passiflora*). The patients were asked to specify whether they felt calm, a little anxious, very anxious, or so anxious that they felt bad. Detailed results are presented in Table 3. Higher levels of anxiety were observed in women than in men. The anxiolytic action of both substances used in the study was similar. Among the participants in the midazolam group, 20% reported they did not remember anything, while none of the patients receiving passionflower reported such an experience. In terms of adverse effects, somnolence was reported by 82.5% of the participants who received midazolam, and 50% in the Passiflora group. When given the choice, 52% of the participants would opt for surgery with midazolam, and 27.5% for the *P. incarnata* treatment, while the remainder found no difference between these interventions. The authors suggest that the higher preference for midazolam among the participants was related to the effect of amnesia, which prevented the formation of negative memories.

Dimpfel et al. [16] evaluated the effects of NEURAPAS® (192 mg of *P. incarnata* extract) on brain electric activity. Electroencephalogram (EEG) recordings were made at 30 min and 1.5, 3, and 4 h after administering the preparation. EEG tests were performed during the Concentration Endurance Test, memory test, and Continuous Performance Task/Test. Results are presented in Table 2. No differences were observed in the analyzed psychometric parameters between NEURAPAS® vs. placebo. Sixteen participants receiving NEURAPAS® obtained higher values in the Continuous Performance Task/Test. The analysis of neurophysiological alterations after taking NEURAPAS® revealed frequency changes in EEG that were similar to those of sedative and antidepressant medications, without impairing cognitive function.

The objective of the study by Kaviani et al. [17] was to evaluate the effects of the passionflower extract on anxiety levels in psychiatrically healthy patients undergoing dental treatment. No differences were observed in mean anxiety scores before taking the medication (Table 2). The authors emphasize their important finding of very effective anxiety-reducing action of the passionflower. They also acknowledge the need for further research on *P. incarnata*.

Movafegh et al. [6] investigated the effects of passionflower (500 mg) on anxiety in surgery patients. The results of their tests are presented in Table 2. The authors conclude that *P. incarnata* at 500 mg/day provides a safe and effective anxiolytic effect, without impairing psychomotor function. At the same time, they strongly stress that their sample was too small ($n = 60$) and urge that research should be continued with a larger group.

Ngan and Conduit [18] analyzed the effects of *Passiflora incarnata* herbal tea on sleep quality over a period of seven days, as measured by using sleep diaries and polysomnography. The participants drank 250 mL of the herbal tea once a day, in the evening (to avoid the sedative effect during the day), and the measurements were performed in the morning, upon rising. The State-Trait Anxiety Inventory (STAI-S) was used to evaluate the efficacy of passionflower infusions, but the results were not included in the report from the study. An attempt was made to contact the authors to obtain their results, but there was no answer. In terms of subjective sleep-quality parameters, a significant improvement of the reported sleep quality (SQ) was observed in the *Passiflora* treatment, with a mean increase of 5.2%, compared to the placebo. The authors highlight that passionflower may have a limited impact on sleep quality in people with low anxiety levels. Their findings may also have been affected by the long interval between drinking the herbal tea and the measurement of anxiety.

The objective of the study by Rokhtabnak et al. [19] was to compare the effects of premedication with melatonin vs. *Passiflora incarnata* on the cognitive function in adult patients undergoing elective surgery. No significant differences in pain scores were observed between the groups, either before or after surgery. The Digital Symbol Substitution Test revealed better postoperative results for melatonin than *Passiflora*. Both groups showed reduced anxiety and increased sedation scores in the Ramsey test.

Detailed results are presented in Table 2. The authors report positive effects of both interventions on reducing patient anxiety.

Passiflora incarnata is important in herbal medicine for treating anxiety or nervousness, Generalized Anxiety Disorder (GAD), symptoms of opiate withdrawal, insomnia, neuralgia, convulsion, spasmodic asthma, ADHD, palpitations, cardiac rhythm abnormalities, hypertension, sexual dysfunction, and menopause. However, the mechanism of action is still under discussion. Despite gaps in our understanding of neurophysiological processes, it is increasingly being recognized that dysfunction of the GABA system is implicated in many neuropsychiatric conditions, including anxiety and depressive disorders. Therefore, the in vitro effects of a dry extract of *P. incarnata* on the GABA system were investigated. The extract inhibited [3H]-GABA uptake into rat cortical synaptosomes but had no effect on GABA release and GABA transaminase activity. *P. incarnata* inhibited concentration dependently on the binding of [3H]-SR95531 to GABAA-receptors and of [3H]-CGP 54626 to GABAB-receptors. Using the [35S]-GTPγS binding assay, *Passiflora* could be classified as an antagonist of the GABAB receptor. In contrast, the ethanol- and the benzodiazepine-site of the GABAA-receptor were not affected by this extract. In conclusion, the first evidence was shown that numerous pharmacological effects of *P. incarnata* are mediated via modulation of the GABA system, including affinity to GABAA and GABAB receptors, and effects on GABA uptake [40]. Aman et al. carried out research on mice which indicated that *P. incarnata* may be useful in treating neuropathic pain. The authors suggested that these properties may result from underlying opioid and GABA-ergic mechanisms, but also pointed to the potential involvement of oleamid-based cannabimimetics [41]. The mechanism of action cannot, at present, be regarded as clarified; however, more recent studies imply that the anxiolytic effects may be mediated via modulation of the GABA system [42–44]

This systematic review has some limitations. First, there are few studies on the effects of *Passiflora incarnata* in neuropsychiatric disorders. Taking into account the inclusion and exclusion criteria, only nine works were qualified for the present synthesis. Secondly, almost all authors postulate to continue research in large-scale populations. In the analyzed publications, the study groups ranged from only 16 to 128 persons. Moreover, it has been proposed to include populations of different ethnicities in continuing the research. Due to the high heterogeneity, it was impossible to perform a meta-analysis, which further suggests that research in this area should be continued.

Another limitation may be the lack of information on which part of the plant was used in the research. Traditional medicine uses the leaves, stamps, seeds, and flowers (aerial parts) of *P. incarnate* [4]. Unfortunately, the authors usually do not specify in their publications what part of the plant was used by them. Ngan and Conduit [18] indicated that they used leaves, stamps, seeds, and flowers. Perhaps all the others also used all the aboveground parts as a mixture. It seems advisable, therefore, for the authors to indicate what part of the plant they used in their research, as this may be relevant for the interpretation of the results and discussion.

In conclusion, the authors of the works included in this systematic review all agree that *Passiflora incarnata* may be an effective, cheap, and safe drug used in counteracting at least some of the symptoms of neuropsychiatric origin. At the same time, they indicate the advisability of continuing research on a large population of people from various geographical regions.

5. Conclusions

Passionflower has the potential to alleviate some symptoms of neuropsychiatric origin. No adverse effects, including memory loss or collapse of psychometric functions, have been linked to passionflower administration. The anti-anxiety effect of *Passiflora incarnata* is comparable to drugs such as oxazepam or midazolam. Consequently, it seems to be an effective and safe pharmaceutical to reduce stress reactivity, insomnia, anxiety, and depression-like behaviors.

Author Contributions: Conceptualization, K.S.-Ż. and K.W.; data curation, K.W., K.J. (Karolina Jakubczyk), and J.A.; formal analysis, K.S.-Ż.; investigation, K.W., K.J. (Karolina Jakubczyk), and K.S.-Ż.; methodology, K.S.-Ż.; project administration, K.J. (Katarzyna Janda); resources, K.W. and K.J. (Katarzyna Janda); software, K.S.-Ż.;

supervision, K.S.-Ż.; visualization, K.S.-Ż., writing—original draft, K.W.; writing—review and editing, K.S.-Ż. and K.J. (Karolina Jakubczyk) All authors have read and agreed to the published version of the manuscript.

Funding: The project was financed from the program of the Minister of Science and Higher Education, under the name "Regional Initiative of Excellence", in 2019–2022, project number 002/RID/2018/19, amount of financing 12 000 000 PLN.

Conflicts of Interest: The authors declare no conflict of interest.

References

1. Patel, S. Passiflora Incarnata Linn: A phytopharmacological review. *Int. J. Green Pharm.* **2009**, *3*, 277–280. [CrossRef]

2. Da Fonseca, L.R.; de Rodrigues, R.A.; de Ramos, A.S.; da Cruz, J.D.; Ferreira, J.L.P.; de Silva, J.R.A.; Amaral, A.C.F. Herbal Medicinal Products from Passiflora for Anxiety: An Unexploited Potential. Available online: https://www.hindawi.com/journals/tswj/2020/6598434/ (accessed on 17 November 2020).

3. Dhawan, K.; Dhawan, S.; Sharma, A. Passiflora: A review update. *J. Ethnopharmacol.* **2004**, *94*, 1–23. [CrossRef] [PubMed]

4. European Medicines Agency. *Assessment Report on Passiflora Incarnata L. herba*; European Medicines Agency: Amsterdam, The Netherlands, 2014; Volume 22.

5. Miyasaka, L.S.; Atallah, A.N.; Soares, B.G.O. Passiflora for anxiety disorder. *Cochrane Database Syst. Rev.* **2007**, CD004518. [CrossRef] [PubMed]

6. Movafegh, A.; Alizadeh, R.; Hajimohamadi, F.; Esfehani, F.; Nejatfar, M. Preoperative oral *Passiflora Incarnata* reduces anxiety in ambulatory surgery patients: A double-blind, placebo-controlled study. *Anesth. Analg.* **2008**, *106*, 1728–1732. [CrossRef]

7. Lupien, S.J.; McEwen, B.S.; Gunnar, M.R.; Heim, C. Effects of stress throughout the lifespan on the brain, behaviour and cognition. *Nat. Rev. Neurosci.* **2009**, *10*, 434–445. [CrossRef] [PubMed]

8. Jawna-Zboińska, K.; Blecharz-Klin, K.; Joniec-Maciejak, I.; Wawer, A.; Pyrzanowska, J.; Piechal, A.; Mirowska-Guzel, D.; Widy-Tyszkiewicz, E. *Passiflora Incarnata* L. Improves Spatial Memory, Reduces Stress, and Affects Neurotransmission in Rats. *Phytother. Res.* **2016**, *30*, 781–789. [CrossRef]

9. Kim, G.-H.; Lim, K.; Yang, H.S.; Lee, J.-K.; Kim, Y.; Park, S.-K.; Kim, S.-H.; Park, S.; Kim, T.-H.; Moon, J.-S.; et al. Improvement in neurogenesis and memory function by administration of *Passiflora Incarnata* L. extract applied to sleep disorder in rodent models. *J. Chem. Neuroanat.* **2019**, *98*, 27–40. [CrossRef]

10. Miroddi, M.; Calapai, G.; Navarra, M.; Minciullo, P.L.; Gangemi, S. *Passiflora Incarnata* L.: Ethnopharmacology, clinical application, safety and evaluation of clinical trials. *J. Ethnopharmacol.* **2013**, *150*, 791–804. [CrossRef]

11. Kim, M.; Lim, H.-S.; Lee, H.-H.; Kim, T.-H. Role Identification of *Passiflora Incarnata* Linnaeus: A Mini Review. *J. Menopausal. Med.* **2017**, *23*, 156–159. [CrossRef]

12. Makara-Studzińska, M.; Pyłypczuk, A.; Madej, A. Nasilenie objawów depresji i lęku wśród osób uzależnionych od alkoholu i hazardu. *EJMT* **2015**, *2*, 7.

13. Sohn, H.-M.; Ryu, J.-H. Monitored anesthesia care in and outside the operating room. *Korean J. Anesthesiol.* **2016**, *69*, 319–326. [CrossRef] [PubMed]

14. Freeman, R.; Clarke, H.M.M.; Humphris, G.M. Conversion tables for the Corah and Modified Dental Anxiety Scales. *Community Dent. Health* **2007**, *24*, 49–54. [PubMed]

15. Corah, N.L.; Gale, E.N.; Illig, S.J. Assessment of a dental anxiety scale. *J. Am. Dent. Assoc.* **1978**, *97*, 816–819. [CrossRef]

16. Murray, P.; Liddell, A.; Donohue, J. A longitudinal study of the contribution of dental experience to dental anxiety in children between 9 and 12 years of age. *J. Behav. Med.* **1989**, *12*, 309–320. [CrossRef]

17. Cravero, J.P.; Kaplan, R.F.; Landrigan-Ossar, M.; Coté, C.J. 48—Sedation for Diagnostic and Therapeutic Procedures outside the Operating Room. In *A Practice of Anesthesia for Infants and Children*, 6th ed.; Coté, C.J., Lerman, J., Anderson, B.J., Eds.; Elsevier: Philadelphia, PA, USA, 2019; pp. 1109–1128.e7, ISBN 978-0-323-42974-0.

18. Jaeger, J. Digit Symbol Substitution Test: The Case for Sensitivity over Specificity in Neuropsychological Testing. *J. Clin. Psychopharmacol.* **2018**, *38*, 513–519. [CrossRef] [PubMed]

19. Bates, M.E.; Lemay, E.P. The d2 Test of attention: Construct validity and extensions in scoring techniques. *J. Int. Neuropsychol. Soc.* **2004**, *10*, 392–400. [CrossRef]

20. Gualtieri, C.T.; Johnson, L.G. ADHD: Is Objective Diagnosis Possible? *Psychiatry (Edgmont)* **2005**, *2*, 44–53.
21. Rodríguez, C.; Areces, D.; García, T.; Cueli, M.; González-Castro, P. Comparison between two continuous performance tests for identifying ADHD: Traditional vs. virtual reality. *Int. J. Clin. Health Psychol.* **2018**, *18*, 254–263. [CrossRef]
22. Tsai, S.K.; Lee, C.; Kwan, W.F.; Chen, B.J. Recovery of cognitive functions after anaesthesia with desflurane or isoflurane and nitrous oxide. *Br. J. Anaesth.* **1992**, *69*, 255–258. [CrossRef]
23. Gupta, A.; Lind, S.; Eklund, A.; Lennmarken, C. The effects of midazolam and flumazenil on psychomotor function. *J. Clin. Anesth.* **1997**, *9*, 21–25. [CrossRef]
24. Hentzen, S.; Haret, D.; Ward, C.; Peterson, A.R. King Device Test as a Monitor of Anesthetic Recovery. A validation study. *Pediatr. Anesth. Crit. Care J. PACCJ* **2019**, 31–36. [CrossRef]
25. Axelrod, B.N.; Meyers, J.E.; Davis, J.J. Finger Tapping Test performance as a measure of performance validity. *Clin. Neuropsychol.* **2014**, *28*, 876–888. [CrossRef] [PubMed]
26. Dantas, L.-P.; de Oliveira-Ribeiro, A.; de Almeida-Souza, L.-M.; Groppo, F.-C. Effects of *Passiflora Incarnata* and midazolam for control of anxiety in patients undergoing dental extraction. *Med. Oral Patol. Oral Cir. Bucal* **2017**, *22*, e95–e101. [CrossRef]
27. Aslanargun, P.; Cuvas, O.; Dikmen, B.; Aslan, E.; Yuksel, M.U. *Passiflora Incarnata* Linneaus as an anxiolytic before spinal anesthesia. *J. Anesth.* **2012**, *26*, 39–44. [CrossRef] [PubMed]
28. Dimpfel, W.; Koch, K.; Weiss, G. Early effect of NEURAPAS®balance on current source density (CSD) of human EEG. *BMC Psychiatry* **2011**, *11*, 123. [CrossRef]
29. Kaviani, N.; Tavakoli, M.; Tabanmehr, M.; Havaei, R. The efficacy of *Passiflora Incarnata* linnaeus in reducing dental anxiety in patients undergoing periodontal treatment. *J. Dent. (Shiraz)* **2013**, *14*, 68–72.
30. Akhondzadeh, S.; Naghavi, H.R.; Vazirian, M.; Shayeganpour, A.; Rashidi, H.; Khani, M. Passionflower in the treatment of generalized anxiety: A pilot double-blind randomized controlled trial with oxazepam. *J. Clin. Pharm. Ther.* **2001**, *26*, 363–367. [CrossRef]
31. Azimaraghi, O.; Yousefshahi, F.; Khatavi, F.; Zamani, M.M.; Movafegh, A. Both Oral *Passiflora Incarnata* and Oxazepam Can Reduce Pre-Operative Anxiety in Ambulatory Surgery Patients: A Double-Blind, Placebo-Controlled Study. *Asian J. Pharm. Clin. Res.* **2017**, *10*, 331–334. [CrossRef]
32. Ngan, A.; Conduit, R. A double-blind, placebo-controlled investigation of the effects of *Passiflora Incarnata* (passionflower) herbal tea on subjective sleep quality. *Phytother. Res.* **2011**, *25*, 1153–1159. [CrossRef]
33. Rokhtabnak, F.; Ghodraty, M.R.; Kholdebarin, A.; Khatibi, A.; Seyed Alizadeh, S.S.; Koleini, Z.S.; Zamani, M.M.; Pournajafian, A. Comparing the Effect of Preoperative Administration of Melatonin and *Passiflora Incarnata* on Postoperative Cognitive Disorders in Adult Patients Undergoing Elective Surgery. *Anesth. Pain Med.* **2017**, *7*, e41238. [CrossRef]
34. WHO. Depression and other Common Mental Disorders. Available online: http://www.who.int/mental_health/management/depression/prevalence_global_health_estimates/en/ (accessed on 17 November 2020).
35. Cuijpers, P.; Stringaris, A.; Wolpert, M. Treatment outcomes for depression: Challenges and opportunities. *Lancet Psychiatry* **2020**, *7*, 925–927. [CrossRef]
36. Rogers, J.P.; Chesney, E.; Oliver, D.; Pollak, T.A.; McGuire, P.; Fusar-Poli, P.; Zandi, M.S.; Lewis, G.; David, A.S. Psychiatric and neuropsychiatric presentations associated with severe coronavirus infections: A systematic review and meta-analysis with comparison to the COVID-19 pandemic. *Lancet Psychiatry* **2020**, *7*, 611–627. [CrossRef]
37. Vasileva, L.V.; Ivanovska, M.V.; Murdjeva, M.A.; Saracheva, K.E.; Georgiev, M.I. Immunoregulatory natural compounds in stress-induced depression: An alternative or an adjunct to conventional antidepressant therapy? *Food Chem. Toxicol.* **2019**, *127*, 81–88. [CrossRef] [PubMed]
38. Liu, L.; Liu, C.; Wang, Y.; Wang, P.; Li, Y.; Li, B. Herbal Medicine for Anxiety, Depression and Insomnia. *Curr. Neuropharmacol.* **2015**, *13*. [CrossRef]
39. Al-kuraishy, H.; Alwindy, S.; Al-Gareeb, A. Beneficial Neuro-Pharmacological Effect of Passionflower (*Passiflora Incarnate* L). *Online J. Neurol. Brain Disord.* **2020**, *3*, 285–289. [CrossRef]
40. Appel, K.; Rose, T.; Fiebich, B.; Kammler, T.; Hoffmann, C.; Weiss, G. Modulation of the γ-aminobutyric acid (GABA) system by *Passiflora Incarnata* L. *Phytother. Res. PTR* **2011**, *25*, 838–843. [CrossRef]
41. Aman, U.; Subhan, F.; Shahid, M.; Akbar, S.; Ahmad, N.; Ali, G.; Fawad, K.; Sewell, R.D.E. *Passiflora Incarnata* attenuation of neuropathic allodynia and vulvodynia apropos GABA-ergic and opioidergic antinociceptive and behavioural mechanisms. *BMC Complement. Altern. Med.* **2016**, *16*, 77. [CrossRef]

42. Grundmann, O.; Wang, J.; McGregor, G.P.; Butterweck, V. Anxiolytic activity of a phytochemically characterized *Passiflora Incarnata* extract is mediated via the GABAergic system. *Planta Med.* **2008**, *74*, 1769–1773. [CrossRef]

43. Nassiri-Asl, M.; Zamansoltani, F.; Shariatirad, S. Possible role of GABAA—Benzodiazepine receptor in anticonvulsant effects of Pasipay in rats. *J. Chin. Integr. Med.* **2008**, *6*, 1170–1173. [CrossRef]

44. Elsas, S.-M.; Rossi, D.J.; Raber, J.; White, G.; Seeley, C.-A.; Gregory, W.L.; Mohr, C.; Pfankuch, T.; Soumyanath, A. *Passiflora incarnata* L. (Passionflower) extracts elicit GABA currents in hippocampal neurons in vitro, and show anxiogenic and anticonvulsant effects in vivo, varying with extraction method. *Phytomedicine* **2010**, *17*, 940–949. [CrossRef]

Publisher's Note: MDPI stays neutral with regard to jurisdictional claims in published maps and institutional affiliations.

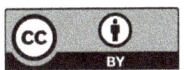

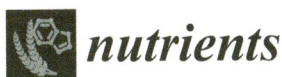

Article

Evaluating the Effects of Grain of Isogenic Wheat Lines Differing in the Content of Anthocyanins in Mouse Models of Neurodegenerative Disorders

Maria A. Tikhonova [1,2,*], Olesya Yu. Shoeva [1], Michael V. Tenditnik [2], Marina V. Ovsyukova [2], Anna A. Akopyan [2], Nina I. Dubrovina [2], Tamara G. Amstislavskaya [1,2] and Elena K. Khlestkina [1,3]

1   Federal Research Center "Institute of Cytology and Genetics", Siberian Branch of the Russian Academy of Sciences, 630090 Novosibirsk, Russia; olesya_ter@bionet.nsc.ru (O.Y.S.); AmstislavskayaTG@physiol.ru (T.G.A.); khlest@bionet.nsc.ru (E.K.K.)
2   Federal State Budgetary Scientific Institution "Scientific Research Institute of Neurosciences and Medicine" (SRINM), 630117 Novosibirsk, Russia; m.v.tenditnik@physiol.ru (M.V.T.); maryov@ngs.ru (M.V.O.); annaaleksanovna@mail.ru (A.A.A.); dubrov@physiol.ru (N.I.D.)
3   N.I. Vavilov All-Russian Research Institute of Plant Genetic Resources, 190000 St. Petersburg, Russia
*   Correspondence: tikhonovama@physiol.ru

Received: 25 October 2020; Accepted: 16 December 2020; Published: 18 December 2020

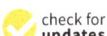

Abstract: Functional foods enriched with plant polyphenols and anthocyanins in particular attract special attention due to multiple beneficial bioactive properties of the latter. We evaluated the effects of a grain diet rich in anthocyanins in a mouse model of Alzheimer's disease induced by amyloid-beta (Aβ) and a transgenic mouse model of Parkinson's disease (PD) with overexpression of human alpha-synuclein. The mice were kept at a diet that consisted of the wheat grain of near isogenic lines differing in anthocyanin content for five–six months. The anthocyanin-rich diet was safe and possessed positive effects on cognitive function. Anthocyanins prevented deficits in working memory induced by Aβ or a long-term grain mono-diet; they partially reversed episodic memory alterations. Both types of grain diets prolonged memory extinction and rescued its facilitation in the PD model. The dynamics of the extinction in the group fed with the anthocyanin-rich wheat was closer to that in a group of wild-type mice given standard chow. The anthocyanin rich diet reduced alpha-synuclein accumulation and modulated microglial response in the brain of the transgenic mice including the elevated expression of arginase1 that marks M2 microglia. Thus, anthocyanin-rich wheat is suggested as a promising source of functional nutrition at the early stages of neurodegenerative disorders.

Keywords: bioflavonoids; functional food; neurodegeneration; cognitive; T-maze; Barnes test; passive avoidance; animal models; alpha-synuclein; neuroinflammation

---

1. Introduction

Due to global population aging, dementia caused by neurodegeneration has received increasing attention. Dementia is among the priority health problems of the World Health Organization (WHO) Mental Health Gap Program (mhGAP). The WHO estimates that there are currently 35.6 million people with dementia all over the world. Cognitive impairment (dementia) in the elderly leads to their disability and requires large financial and moral costs in caring for this category of patients from relatives and medical personnel, thus bringing considerable damage and suffering to individuals and the whole society. The most common cause of dementia at old age is Alzheimer's disease (AD) (60–70% of all cases). Parkinson's disease (PD) is the second most common neurodegenerative disorder. Similar to AD, the main risk factor for the development of PD is aging. It should be noted that the classical notion of PD as a motor disorder has changed significantly over the past few years. According to the latest publications, practically all patients suffering from PD have cognitive impairments with the progression of the disease, while in many patients mild deficits are detected even a few years before the manifestation of motor symptoms [1,2].

To date, there are no approved methods or drugs for the effective treatment of neurodegenerative disorders. The current methods for AD and PD treatment are symptomatic (e.g., AChEI for AD or dopaminergic substitution (L-DOPA) for PD), they do not halt the progression of the disease, nor ameliorate cognitive deficits [3,4]. Hence, major efforts are aimed at the discovery of a novel, effective pathogenesis-relevant therapy. Neurodegenerative disorders have a multifactorial etiology and involve various pathological processes in addition to neurotoxicity of protein aggregates (e.g., oxidative stress, neuroinflammatory response, disturbed neurotrophic function and neurogenesis, synaptic and neurotransmission dysfunction, ion disbalance, etc.) that often closely interact and overlap. Multipurpose or multi-target therapy aimed at various important pathogenetic hubs in the course of AD and PD is regarded currently as a relevant and promising approach [5]. Another important point is choosing the appropriate treatment approaches according to the stage of a disease. Since pathological perturbations of the cellular proteostasis network responsible for the maintenance of protein homeostasis with the accumulation of neurotoxic protein aggregates precedes the initial signs of cognitive impairment and clinical manifestation in patients with AD or PD by at least 10–20 years, a preventive long-term intervention at the asymptomatic preclinical and early stages of the disease progression is considered the most prospective [6].

Currently, functional nutrition has developed intensively. Functional foods enriched with biologically active substances are an essential part of dietary therapy. Plant polyphenols attract particular attention as components of functional nutrition due to their multiple beneficial properties. One of the promising classes of compounds that can be included in the diet for long courses and contribute to the prevention and reduction of risk of chronic diseases is anthocyanins [7]. They are water-soluble plant pigments belonging to a group of polyphenolic compounds flavonoids, naturally occurring in fruits, vegetables, and cereal grains [8]. Both human and animal studies have shown that anthocyanins and, concomitant to them, phenolic phytochemicals have wide biological activities ranging from cytoprotective, antimicrobial, and antitumor effects to anti-obesity and cardio- and neuroprotective potential [9–11]. The health-promoting effects of the flavonoids are based on their ability to interact with cells proteins like receptors, kinases, or transcription factors and modulate signaling pathways, and their antioxidant properties [11,12]. It should be noted that no cases of overdose or toxicity have been identified with the consumption of foods rich in anthocyanins [13]. Currently, due to the potential benefits of anthocyanins for human health, there is a strong tendency to increase anthocyanin content in agricultural plants including cereal grains. The latter has gained especial attention because of widespread consumption of grains and their availability throughout the year [14,15]. However, the information on the health-promoting effects of cereal anthocyanins including their role in protection against neurodegenerative diseases, especially in vivo, is very scant [15].

This study aimed to evaluate the effects of a grain diet rich in anthocyanins in a mouse model of AD induced by central amyloid-beta administration and a transgenic model of PD in mice with overexpression of human alpha-synuclein. We used two wheat lines that have similar genomes with the exception of a small part of chromosome 2A, which contains a gene regulating anthocyanin biosynthesis [16]. Wheat near isogenic lines differing in grain anthocyanin content applied in the current study allowed establishing the role of the *Pp3* gene that marks the line with anthocyanin-rich grains in protection against neurodegenerative disorders and evaluated the potential of the gene in breeding of wheat cultivars with high anthocyanin content intended for dietary nutrition.

2. Materials and Methods

2.1. Experimental Animals and Procedures Involving Animals

Experiments were performed using male mice of: (1) C57Bl/6J strain born and reared at SPF (Specified Pathogen Free) conditions that were purchased from the SPF-vivarium of the Institute of Cytology and Genetics SB RAS (Novosibirsk, Russia); and (2) B6.Cg-Tg(Prnp-SNCA*A53T)23Mkle/J) strain and control wild-type strain that were purchased from the SPF-vivarium of the Institute of Cytology and Genetics SB RAS (Novosibirsk, Russia). Transgenic hemizygous mice were produced by the insertion of human A53T missense mutant form of alpha-synuclein cDNA in the mouse genome downstream of a mouse prion Prnp promoter (https://www.jax.org/strain/006823). Wild-type controls are the littermates of the transgenic mice, transgene noncarriers.

Animals were housed in groups of five–six per cage ($40 \times 25 \times 15$ cm) under standard conditions (light–dark cycle: 14 h light and 10 h dark (lights off at 3 p.m.); temperature: 18–22 °C; relative humidity: 50–60%). All the experimental procedures were carried out in accordance with the guidelines of the NIH Guide for the Care and Use of Laboratory Animals and were approved by the Institutional Animal Care and Use Committee of the Federal State Budgetary Scientific Institution "Scientific Research Institute of Neurosciences and Medicine" (SRINM; formerly "Scientific Research Institute of Physiology and Basic Medicine") (Novosibirsk, Russia). Every effort was made to minimize the number of animals used and their suffering.

2.1.1. Experimental Design and Treatment (Diets)

Mus musculus is by nature an omnivore but has evolved and adapted to be a primary consumer of a wide range of seeds. Its wild/feral populations can adapt to agricultural landscapes, especially those involving annual cereal production. They are common pests in granaries. Hence, a grain diet is a natural food for mice. Moreover, under conditions of free choice, mice preferred the soft white wheat over laboratory pellets by about 4 to 1 [17]. However, wheat contains less protein and fewer calories [18] than the balanced laboratory chow. Prolonged treatment with only grain per se might result in nutritional deficit and behavioral changes. Hence, the effects of the wheat grain with high content of anthocyanins were compared both with those of standard chow and control wheat grain of near isogenic line.

In each experiment, mice were subdivided into three groups and prescribed one of the following diets. The mice of "St. diet" groups received a standard granulated chow for laboratory mice (Ssniff R/M-H V1534-300, Soest, Germany) and pure water (Rosinka, Novosibirsk, Russia) ad libitum. The mice of "CGr" and "Gr_HCA" groups were subjected to a mono-diet which consisted of wheat grain of isogenic lines (i:S29*Pp-A1Pp-D1pp3*^{P} (Control Grain, CG) or i:S29*Pp-A1Pp-D1Pp3*^{P} (grain with high content of anthocyanins, Gr_HCA), respectively) and pure water ad libitum. i:S29*Pp-A1Pp-D1Pp3*^{P} line (Gr_HCA) marked by a dominant allele of the *Pp3* gene accumulates anthocyanins in a grain pericarp, whereas isogenic i:S29*Pp-A1Pp-D1pp3*^{P} line (CGr) characterized by a recessive allele of the *Pp3* gene does not; the lines were developed at the Institute of Cytology and Genetics SB RAS (Novosibirsk, Russia) [16]. The content of anthocyanins in the Gr_HCA was 140 mM/g. The remaining elemental composition and amino acid content in whole wheat flour obtained from the wheat lines were similar [19]. It should be noted that food intake was significantly affected by grain diet ($F(2, 3) = 25.1$, $p < 0.05$). In C57Bl/6J mice, food intake per mouse during the six-month-long feeding period was substantially reduced in mice given control grain (503.7 ± 6.5 g) or grain with high content of anthocyanins (507.8 ± 33.4 g) in comparison with mice fed with standard chow and given water (705.6 ± 20.8 g, $p < 0.01$). Mice given different types of grain did not vary significantly in the parameter ($p > 0.05$).

To evaluate the general effects and tolerance of a grain diet, we fed the mice of the C57Bl/6J strain with grain or standard chow since the age of one month (early after weaning) up to the age of eight months ($n = 16–20$ animals in each group). Body weight gain and food intake were registered. After six months of treatment, blood samples for further biochemical assay were collected from five randomly selected animals of each group. Mice of the C57Bl/6J strain born and reared in SPF conditions bore both types of grain diet well up to six months of feeding. However, prolonged grain diet (up to eight months of feeding) caused death of 40% of mice while all mice fed with standard chow were alive. Average life expectancy at grain mono-diet of those dead mice was 8.5 months (252.3 ± 18.8 days in a group given control grain and 266.3 ± 13.3 days in a group given grain with high content of anthocyanins). Thus, we limited the duration of the experiments by six months of feeding with grain mono-diets. Mice of B6.Cg-Tg(Prnp-SNCA*A53T)23Mkle/J strain (further–mut(PD)), a genetic model of PD, and control wild-type (WT) mice were also born and reared in SPF conditions but bore the grain diet much worse if started feeding with grain at the age of one month. Almost all mut(PD) mice and WT controls died after two weeks of grain diet. Hence, we fed mice of those strains with standard chow from weaning up to the age of 2.5 months and started feeding the adult 2.5-month-old mice with grain diets. A later start of feeding with grain allowed us to hold the five-month-long experiment with mut(PD) mice at grain diets without significant loss of animals.

In the series on a model of AD, experiments were conducted using a pharmacological model of neurodegeneration caused by central injection of an amyloid beta ($A\beta$) fragment 25–35. Mice of C57Bl/6J strain were subdivided into six groups ($n = 5$–6 animals in each group): (1) standard diet and bilateral injections of sterile water into the lateral ventricles of the brain (i.c.v.) (Control+St.diet); (2) control grain diet and bilateral i.c.v. injections of sterile water (Control+CGr); (3) grain with high content of anthocyanins and bilateral i.c.v. injections of sterile water (Control+Gr_HCA); (4) standard diet and bilateral i.c.v. injection of $A\beta$25–35 ($A\beta$+St.diet); (5) control grain diet and bilateral i.c.v. injection of $A\beta$25–35 ($A\beta$+CGr); or (6) grain with high content of anthocyanins and bilateral i.c.v. injection of $A\beta$25–35 ($A\beta$+Gr_HCA). The experiment started early after weaning when mice were one month old. Mice were fed with grain or standard chow for five months. Then all animals underwent stereotaxic surgery. During the 2nd to 5th weeks after the introduction of $A\beta$ or vehicle into cerebral ventricles, behavioral testing was performed since the behavioral deficits induced by $A\beta$25-35 are pronounced during this period [20–22]. Mut(PD) mice, a genetic model of PD, and control WT mice were subjected to different diets from the age of 2.5 months ($n = 8$–11 animals in each group). After four months of treatment, mut(PD) and WT mice were tested for behavior and then sacrificed for further immunohistochemical (IHC) analysis of their brains.

2.1.2. The Model of AD

$A\beta$25–35 was dissolved in sterile water at a concentration of 1 mg/mL and stored at $-20°C$ until use. Before administration to the animals, the prepared $A\beta$ solution was thawed and incubated for 4 days at 37 °C to form aggregates. Injections into cerebral ventricles were performed according to previously published protocols [20,22] with minor modifications. The mice were anesthetized by administration of a 2.5% solution of avertin (2,2,2-tribromoethanol and 2-methyl-2-butanol; 100 µL/10 g, i.p.; Sigma–Aldrich Co.). The $A\beta$ solution or sterile water was injected bilaterally with a Hamilton syringe (25 µL, model 1702 RN SYR, with a 22s ga needle, 2 inches), using a micropump (injection rate 0.8 µL/min). The needle was left at the injection site for 2 min after the injection. A total of 10 µL (9.43 nmole) of the solution was injected. The following coordinates adapted from the mouse brain atlas were used [23]: AP: -0.5 mm, ML: ± 1 mm, DV: -3 mm from the bregma, midline, and skull surface, respectively.

2.2. Behavioral Tests

Each animal was handled for 5 min/day on three consecutive days before being taken into experiment. Open field and passive avoidance tests were performed. Observations were performed during the dark phase between 15:00 and 22:00 h. For behavioral testing, the animals were placed individually in a clean cage (25 × 40 × 20 cm), and transported to a dim observation room (28 lux of the red light) with sound isolation reinforced by a masking white noise of 70 dB. Performance in the behavioral tests was monitored using a video camera Panasonic WV-CL930 (Panasonic System Networks Suzhou Co. Ltd., Suzhou, China) positioned above an apparatus and processed with original

EthoVision XT software (Noldus, The Netherlands). The test equipment was cleaned using 20% ethanol and thoroughly dried before each test trial.

2.2.1. The Open Field Test

This test was carried out in an apparatus with a square arena (40 × 40 cm) and plastic walls 37.5 cm high brightly lit from above (1000 lux). A mouse was placed in the center of the arena, and its movements were recorded for 10 min. The following parameters were determined: general locomotion (the distance traveled in cm); vertical locomotor and exploratory activity (rearing number); anxiety (time spent in the central part of the arena); and emotionality (defecation number).

2.2.2. The Passive Avoidance Test

Training on the passive avoidance reaction was performed by a standard single-session method in an experimental chamber with dark and light compartments and an automated Gemini Avoidance System apparatus (San Diego Instruments, CA, USA) as described in detail earlier [24]. The Gemini software automatically recorded the latency of the transfer to the dark compartment and the data of testing served as a measure of acquisition of the conditioned passive avoidance reaction. Memory extinction was measured during the next ten days.

2.2.3. The T-Maze Test

The test was conducted according to the spontaneous alteration protocol at red lighting of 28 lux [25]. The T-shaped apparatus consisted of a start arm (30 × 7 cm) and two side arms (37 × 7 cm) with plastic walls of 20 cm high. The start zone in the start arm was 18 × 7 cm while central zone between the side arms was 7 × 7 cm. All compartments were separated by automatic slide doors controlled remotely by the EthoVision XT software (Noldus, The Netherlands). The test consisted of three trials per day during three consecutive days for each mouse. Each trial included two choice runs. At the beginning of each run, a mouse was placed in the start zone. During each run, the mouse made a choice of a side arm by entering into it. In the first run, right after the choice was made, a slide door separating the side arm with the mouse shut down and the mouse stayed in the selected arm for 30 s until the second run. In the second run, a mouse should have chosen a side arm opposite to that chosen in the first run (correct choice). Correct responses in the nine trials were recorded. The percentage of correct choices was regarded as an index of working memory [25,26]. The duration of each run was restricted to 90 s.

2.2.4. Barnes Maze Test

The test assesses spatial learning and memory. A mouse was placed on an elevated open circular arena (d = 120 cm, height from the floor = 90 cm) with 40 holes (d = 5 cm, distance between holes = 8 cm). An escape box was placed beneath one of the holes and its location was randomly assigned of four positions for each mouse. Aversive bright lighting (1000 lux) and the stress of being in the open space motivated an animal to search for the escape box to hide. Visual cues placed in the testing room provided spatial orientation. Testing was conducted according to the standard protocol [26,27] and consisted of three phases: habituation (one day, two sessions of 3 min), acquisition (four days, four sessions of 3 min per day), and testing trial (one day, one session of 60 s). Habituation: a mouse was placed near the hole with the escape box attached ("goal hole"); if the animal did not find the goal hole within 3 min, it was gently guided to the escape box and left there for 60 s. Acquisition: the animal was placed in the center of a platform and was free to explore the platform and search for the goal hole and escape box; if the animal did not find the goal hole within 3 min, it was gently guided to the escape box and left there for 60 s. The latency of finding the goal hole was recorded. Episodic memory was assessed as the dynamics of the latency in the four consecutive sessions on the first training day. Long-term spatial memory and learning were assessed as the dynamics of the latency in the first sessions of each training day. During the testing trial, the escape box was removed and mice moved freely for 60 s. Exploratory activity (by the total number of nose pokes and percentage of visited holes) and long-term memory and learning (by the percentage of mice that found a target hole during 60 s of the test, latency to find the target hole, target hole nose pokes, the percentage of non-target holes nose pokes (error rate), and a weighted mean distance to the target hole) were evaluated. The weighted mean distance was calculated according to the formula: $\Sigma[de] \times ne/\Sigma ntotal$, where de = distance moved to the escape hole; ne = number of nose pokes into the escape hole; and ntotal = total number of nose pokes into all holes [28].

2.3. IHC Analysis

On the day of euthanasia, mice were culled with CO_2. The animals were perfused transcardially with phosphate-buffered saline (PBS) followed by 4% paraformaldehyde in PBS, then the brains were rapidly excised and postfixed in PBS containing 30% sucrose at 4 °C until further neuromorphological analysis. The IHC analysis was performed on 30-μm-thick cryosections according to a protocol described in detail previously [24]. Coronal slices along the frontal cortex (AP: 2.93 to 2.45 mm), striatum (AP: 1.21 to 0.73 mm), hippocampus (AP: −2.03 to −2.15 mm), or substantia nigra (s. nigra) (AP: −2.91 to −3.15 mm) of each mouse brain were made. We applied a rabbit polyclonal antibody (NB110-61645, 1:1000 dilution, Novus Biologicals, Littleton, CO, USA) as a primary antibody to detect human α-synuclein, a rabbit polyclonal antibody (NBP1-32731, 1:1000 dilution, Novus Biologicals, Littleton, CO, USA) as the primary antibody to detect M2 microglial marker arginase 1, or a goat polyclonal antibody (NB100-1028, 1:200 dilution, Novus Biologicals, USA) as the primary antibody to detect microglial marker AIF-1/IBA1. A fluorescently labeled (Alexa Fluor 488–conjugated) goat anti-rabbit IgG antibody (ab150077, 1:600 dilution, Abcam, UK) or Alexa Fluor 488–conjugated donkey anti-goat IgG antibody (ab150129, 1:200 dilution, Abcam, UK) served as the secondary antibodies, respectively. Fluorescent images were finally obtained by means of an Axioplan 2 (Carl Zeiss) imaging microscope and a confocal laser scanning microscope LSM 510 META (Carl Zeiss) and then analyzed in Image Pro Plus Software 6.0 (Media Cybernetics, MD, USA). Fluorescence intensity was measured as background-corrected optical density (OD) with subtraction of staining signals of the non-immunoreactive regions in the images converted to grayscale. The area of interest was: 7423 μm² (IBA1 or arginase 1) or 30,014 μm² (alpha-synuclein) in the frontal cortex; 19,353 μm², 26,100 μm², or 50,868 μm² in the hippocampal CA1 area, CA3 area, or dentate gyrus (DG), respectively; 18,208 μm² in the striatum; and 103,985 μm² in s. nigra.

2.4. Biochemical Assays

Trunk blood of a mouse was collected into sterile Eppendorf tubes right after sacrifice, then in 30 min the bio-samples were centrifuged for 20 min at 3000 rpm and +4 °C, serum was stored at −24 °C until assay. Serum was three times diluted with PBS. Serum levels of the uric acid, creatinine, total cholesterol, low-density lipoprotein cholesterol (LDL-C), triglycerides, and high-density lipoproteins (HDL), as well as the activity of aminotransferases (aspartate aminotransferase (AST), alanine aminotransferase (ALT)) and the levels of total bilirubin were measured using clinical chemistry analyzer Konelab 30i and Konelab kits (Thermo Fisher Scientific Inc., USA) according to the manufacturer's instructions [29].

2.5. Data Analysis

All results are presented as mean ± SEM and compared using one or two-way ANOVA followed by post-hoc Fisher's Least Significant Difference (LSD) test. The independent variables for the two-way ANOVA were treatment duration (six- or eight-month-long), Aβ administration (control or Aβ-treated mice), or genotype (WT or mut(PD)) and diet (St. diet, CGR, or Gr_HCA). Repeated measures ANOVA followed by Fisher LSD post-hoc comparison was applied to analyze the data of the passive avoidance test/Barnes test with genotype/Aβ administration and diet as between-subject variables and time (training, test, or extinction days/number of a session on the 1st day of training; number of a day of training) as a repeated measure. The level of significance was defined as $p < 0.05$. STATISTICA 10.0 software (StatSoft, Tulsa, OK, USA) was used to perform all the statistical analyses.

3. Results

3.1. Effects of Grain Diet on Body Weight Gain

Body weight gain was significantly influenced by grain diet (Figure 1). Two-way ANOVA showed a significant effect of the type of diet ($F_{(2, 58)}$ = 234.1, $p < 0.001$), duration of feeding ($F_{(1, 58)}$ = 20.6, $p < 0.001$) as well as of the interaction between the factors ($F_{(2, 58)}$ = 18.6, $p < 0.001$) on mouse body weight (Figure 1a). Mice of C57Bl/6J strain that were given grain had lighter body mass than mice of groups given standard chow ($p < 0.001$), both after six and eight months of the experiment. It is worth noting that mice fed with standard chow gained body mass by the eight months of the experiment as compared to mice that had been fed with standard chow during six months ($p < 0.001$), while no significant body weight gain was observed in mice exposed to grain diets. Mice given different types of grain did not vary significantly in body mass at both time points of the experiment (Figure 1a). No significant effect of Aβ25-35 central injection on body mass of mice was found ($F_{(1, 49)} < 1$; data not shown). In the experiment with a PD model, two-way ANOVA revealed a significant effect of the type of diet ($F_{(2, 41)}$ = 110.8, $p < 0.001$), but not of the genotype ($F_{(1, 41)} < 1$) or of the interaction between the factors ($F_{(2, 41)}$ = 1.1, $p > 0.05$) on mouse body weight gain. As in the experiment with mice of C57Bl/6J strain, mice of both mutant and WT genotypes that were given grain had lighter body mass than mice of groups given standard chow ($p < 0.001$). No significant differences were found between the groups given different types of grain ($p > 0.05$) (Figure 1b).

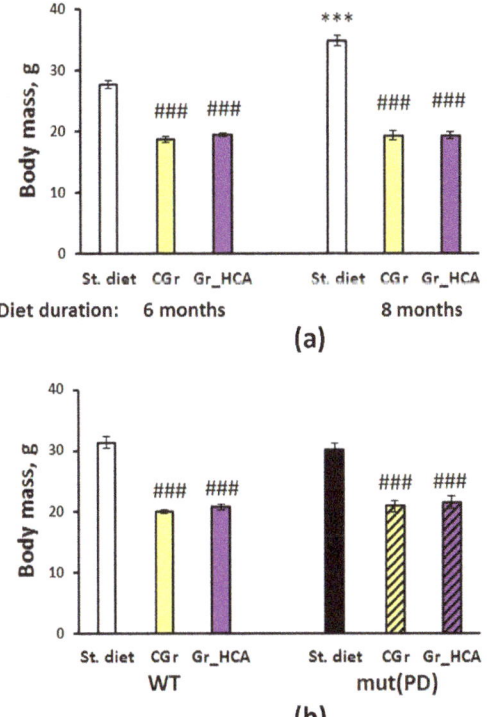

(a)

(b)

Figure 1. Effects of the type of diet and treatment duration (**a**) or of the type of diet and overexpression of α-synuclein (genetic Parkinson's disease (PD) model) (**b**) on body weight gain in mice. Data are presented as the mean ± S.E.M. of the values obtained in an independent group of animals (n = 6–15 per group). Statistically significant differences: ### $p < 0.001$ vs. a respective group given the standard diet (St. diet); *** $p < 0.001$ vs. a respective group given the same type of diet for six months.

3.2. Effects on Biochemical Parameters of Serum

The effects of grain diet on the biochemical parameters of serum were assessed in mice of C57Bl/6J strain. Biochemical features of the groups are summarized in Table 1. While the activity of ALT and AST and the levels of total bilirubin, triglycerides, and creatinine were not significantly affected by the diet, significant differences were revealed in the levels of uric acid and the parameters of lipid profile. One-way ANOVA showed a significant effect of the type of diet on the levels of uric acid. However, the parameter was significantly reduced in the "CGr" group ($p < 0.05$) but not in the "Gr_HCA" group compared to the "St. diet" control group. Significant influence of the diet factor was found on the levels of total cholesterol, LDL-C, and HDL-C (α-cholesterol). All the indices were augmented in the groups fed with both types of grain. Nevertheless, atherogenic coefficient, the ratio of non-HDL cholesterol to HDL cholesterol, was even lowered in mice given both types of grain as compared to the mice fed with standard chow and given water ("St.diet").

Table 1. Effects of the type of a diet on the biochemical parameters of serum in C57Bl/6J mice.

Parameter	Group			F, p
	St. diet	CGr	Gr_HCA	
	Indices of liver function			
ALT, U/L	52.2 ± 7.68	41.6 ± 7.0	54.8 ± 8.6	$F(2, 12) < 1$
AST, U/L	272.4 ± 15.7	286.5 ± 25.8	326.1 ± 8.1	$F(2, 12) = 1.5, p > 0.05$
Total bilirubin, mmol/L	1.86 ± 0.82	2.04 ± 0.63	1.20 ± 1.05	$F(2, 12) < 1$
	Indices of kidney function and protein metabolism			
Creatinine, μmol/L	56.0 ± 3.9	55.3 ± 3.6	65.4 ± 0.6	$F(2, 12) = 1.9, p > 0.05$
Uric acid, mmol/L	191.2 ± 15.4	132.2 ± 11.9 (#)	189.1 ± 14.2 (+)	**$F(2, 12) = 5.95, p < 0.05$**
	Indices of lipid metabolism			
Total cholesterol, mmol/L	2.12 ± 0.09	4.51 ± 0.19 (###)	4.98 ± 0.34 (###)	**$F(2, 12) = 66.0, p < 0.001$**
Triglycerides, mmol/L	0.91 ± 0.09	0.73 ± 0.05	0.82 ± 0.02	$F(2, 12) = 2.0, p > 0.05$
LDL-C, mmol/L	0.43 ± 0.01	0.89 ± 0.04 (###)	1.04 ± 0.06 (###, +)	**$F(2, 12) = 73.8, p < 0.001$**
HDL, mmol/L (α-cholesterol)	0.95 ± 0.06	2.27 ± 0.12 (###)	2.51 ± 0.23 (###)	**$F(2, 12) = 47.1, p < 0.001$**
Atherogenic coefficient	1.24 ± 0.07	0.99 ± 0.03 (##)	0.99 ± 0.06 (#)	**$F(2, 12) = 7.1, p < 0.05$**

Data are presented as the mean ± S.E.M. of the values obtained in an independent group of animals ($n = 5$ per group). Statistically significant differences (bold): # $p < 0.05$, ## $p < 0.01$, ### $p < 0.001$ vs. a control group given the standard diet (St. diet); + $p < 0.05$ vs. the group given the control grain diet (CGr). ALT, alanine aminotransferase; AST, aspartate aminotransferase; LDL-C, low-density lipoprotein cholesterol; HDL, high-density lipoproteins.

3.3. Behavioral Effects

3.3.1. The Open Field Test

The open field test was performed to monitor general locomotion, vertical locomotor and exploratory activity, anxiety, and emotionality in mice (Supplementary Materials: Table S1). Aβ treatment did not affect significantly the parameters studied in mice fed with standard chow or the grain with high content of anthocyanins. High content of anthocyanins in the diet did not produce marked effects on the behavior of Aβ-treated mice in this test either. When testing a PD model, mut(PD) mice had higher horizontal locomotion than WT mice. Grain mono-diets significantly decreased horizontal and vertical activity in mice of both genotypes. The diet factor also significantly influenced the number of fecal boli. The parameter was reduced in the grain-treated mice, probably due to the diminished food intake and body mass found in those groups. It is noteworthy that no significant differences between the groups of the PD model given grain diets in the open field test were found.

3.3.2. The T-Maze Test

Two-way ANOVA did not show a significant effect of the type of diet ($F(2, 26) < 1$) or Aβ25-35 administration ($F(1, 26) = 1.9, p > 0.05$) on the index of working memory in C57Bl/6J mice but there was a marked influence of the interaction between the factors (F(2, 26) = 3.8, $p < 0.05$) (Figure 2a). Aβ25-35 treatment reduced the parameter in mice fed with standard chow but not in mice with grain diets. Mice of "Control+CGr" group that were given the control grain without Aβ25-35 had a diminished percentage of correct choices compared to mice fed with the standard chow or the grain with high content of anthocyanins ($p < 0.05$).

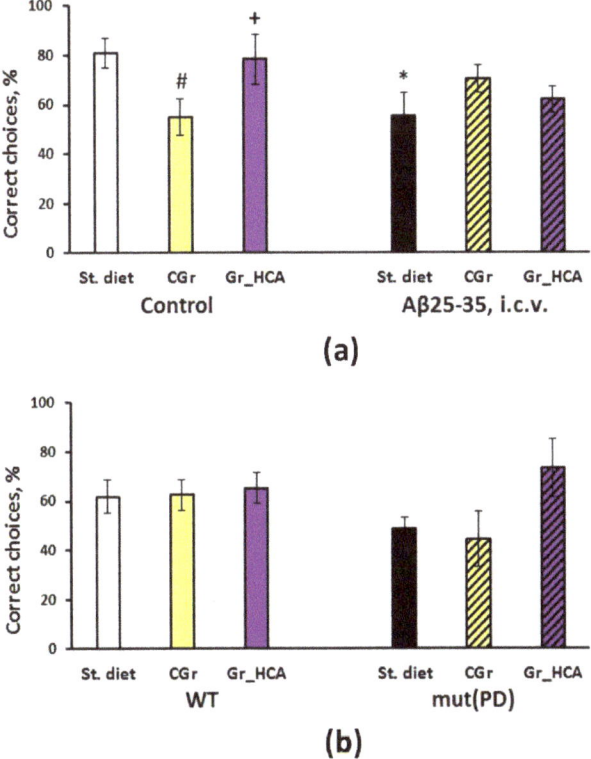

Figure 2. Effects of the type of diet and Aβ25-35 administration (Alzheimer's disease (AD) model) (**a**) or of the type of diet and overexpression of α-synuclein (genetic PD model) (**b**) on the working memory in mice evaluated in the T-maze test. Data are presented as the mean ± S.E.M. of the values obtained in an independent group of animals (n = 5–11 per group). Statistically significant differences: * $p < 0.05$ vs. a respective control group (in the experiment with AD model); # $p < 0.05$ vs. a respective group given the standard diet (St. diet); + $p < 0.05$ vs. a respective group given the control grain diet (CGr).

Although there was a tendency to decrease in the index of working spatial memory in the transgenic mice and an increase in the group fed with anthocyanin-rich grain diet in the T-maze test in the experiment with the PD model, two-way ANOVA did not reveal any significant effects of the type of diet (F(2, 39) = 1.9, $p > 0.05$), genotype (F(1, 39) = 1.2, $p > 0.05$) or the interaction between the factors (F(2, 39) = 1.3, $p > 0.05$) on the working memory in mice (Figure 2b).

3.3.3. Barnes Test

Three-way ANOVA showed a significant effect of learning (repeated measures) (F(3, 81) = 15.2, $p < 0.001$) as well as of the Aβ25-35 administration (F(1, 27) = 4.6, $p < 0.05$) on the latency to find an escape box in the Barnes test during the first training day in C57Bl/6J mice (Figure 3a) while the influence of the diet type (F(2, 27) = 2.1, $p > 0.05$) or the interaction of this factor with the other factors was insignificant. Control groups treated with the both grain diets had similar dynamics of learning, a significant decrease in the latency to find an escape box was observed since the second training session. In the control group treated with standard chow, a significant reduction of the latency was revealed after the third training session. Aβ25-35-treated groups had slightly higher latencies. Mice of the group fed with the standard chow that were administered with Aβ25-35 demonstrated a significant reduction in the latency only by the fourth session. At the same time, mice of both groups fed with the grain diets that were administered with Aβ25-35 had a significant decrease in the latency by the second ("Aβ+Gr_HCA") or third ("Aβ+CGr") session but it vanished at the fourth session. It is noteworthy that mice of the "Control+Gr_HCA" group demonstrated the shortest latencies to find the escape box during the first day of training.

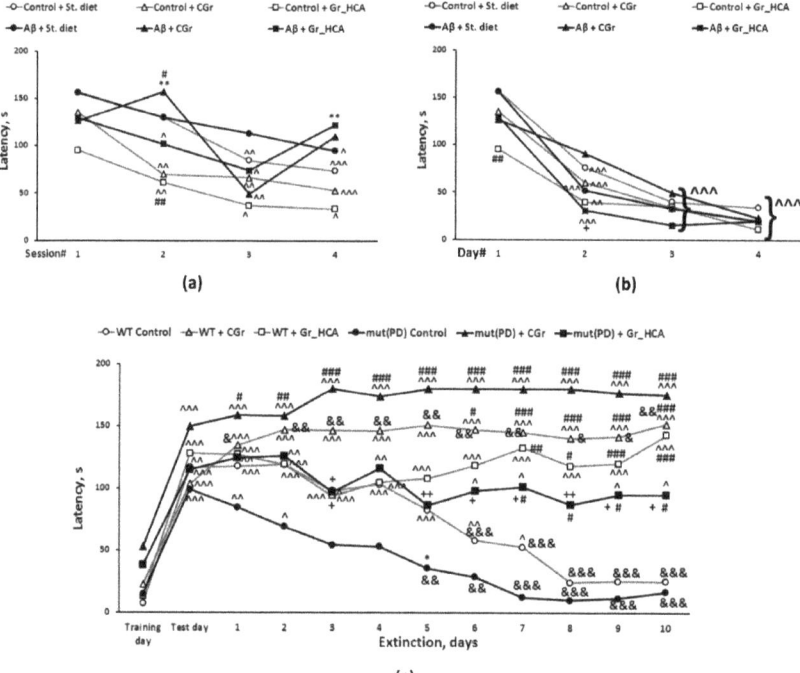

Figure 3. Effects of the type of diet and Aβ25-35 administration (AD model) on the episodic memory measured during the first day of training (**a**) or long-term spatial memory and learning estimated during four days of training (**b**) in Barnes test, or of the type of diet and overexpression of α-synuclein (genetic PD model) on the contextual memory retrieval and memory extinction evaluated in the passive avoidance test (**c**) in mice. Data are presented as the means of the values obtained in an independent group of animals (n = 5–12 per group). Statistically significant differences: ^ $p < 0.05$, ^^ $p < 0.01$, ^^^ $p < 0.001$ compared to values of the same group in the first session (**a**), on the first day of training (**b**), on the training day (**c**); & $p < 0.05$, && $p < 0.01$, &&& $p < 0.001$ compared to values of the same group on the test day; * $p < 0.05$, ** $p < 0.01$ vs. a respective control (in the experiment with AD model) or wild-type (WT) (in the experiment with PD model) group; # $p < 0.05$, ## $p < 0.01$, ### $p < 0.001$ vs. a respective group given the standard diet (St. diet); + $p < 0.05$, ++ $p < 0.01$ vs. a respective group given the control grain diet (CGr).

Three-way ANOVA showed a significant effect of learning (repeated measures) ($F(3, 81) = 66.1$, $p < 0.001$) on the latency to find an escape box in the Barnes test during four days of training in C57Bl/6J mice (Figure 3b) while the influence of the type of diet ($F(2, 27) = 3.3, p > 0.05$), Aβ25-35 administration

(F(1, 27) < 1), or the interactions between the factors was insignificant. All studied groups had similar dynamics of learning with a gradual decrease in the latency to find an escape box since the second training day. The index of learning and memory was better in mice of the "Aβ+Gr_HCA" group than in mice of the "Aβ+CGr" group on the second day of training ($p < 0.05$).

The parameters of long-term spatial memory and learning were evaluated on the next day after four days of training in the test session. The results are summarized in Supplementary Materials: Table S2. Only one parameter of exploratory activity (the total number of nose pokes) was significantly affected by the interaction between the diet type and Aβ25-35 administration in C57Bl/6J mice. Nevertheless, Aβ25-35 injections provoked a significant decrease in the total number of nose pokes only in mice of the group fed with control grain ("Aβ+CGr") as compared to the respective group without Aβ25-35 treatment ("Control+CGr", $p < 0.01$). Mice of "Control+Gr_HCA" had a decreased total number of nose pokes as compared to mice of "Control+CGr" ($p < 0.01$). Groups did not vary significantly in the indices of cognitive function.

3.3.4. The Passive Avoidance Test

We revealed a significant influence of the repeated measures (time) factor (F(11, 484) = 20.8, $p < 0.001$), diet factor (F(2, 44) = 16.7, $p < 0.001$), and interaction between the repeated measures and diet factors (F(22, 484) = 6.3, $p < 0.001$) on the step-through latency when evaluating contextual memory retrieval and memory extinction in mut(PD) and WT mice (Figure 3c). Latency to enter a dark compartment during training (before the foot shock) did not differ significantly among the experimental groups. As evidence of learning and acquisition of the conditioned passive avoidance reaction on testing day, 24 h after receiving the foot shock, mice of all groups demonstrated increased step-through latencies. With exposure to the context in the absence of additional shocks, the fear response gradually diminished, which is called memory extinction [30]. In "WT+St. diet" and "mut(PD)+St. diet" groups, the values of step-through latency stayed significantly increased for seven and two days, respectively, as compared to the training day. A significant decrease in step-through latency was determined since the 6th and 5th day of the extinction phase compared to the test day in "WT+St. diet" and "mut(PD)+St. diet" groups, respectively. Hence, extinction was more pronounced in the "mut(PD)+St. diet" group. At the same time, the values of step-through latency stayed markedly increased for ten days of the extinction phase as compared to the training day in all groups treated with grain. We did not observe a substantial reduction in step-through latency in mice of those group during ten days of the extinction phase. Control grain diet caused an exaggerated response in transgenic mice as the values of step-through latencies during the extinction phase were significantly higher than on the training day. At the same time, in the "mut(PD)+Gr_HCA" group, the dynamics of memory extinction were closer to those of the "WT+St. diet" group and the values of step-through latencies during the extinction phase were substantially lower than in the "mut(PD)+CGr" group. Thus, grain diets modulated memory extinction in mut(PD) mice.

3.4. IHC Analysis

The accumulation of human α-synuclein in the mouse brain was measured. We detected immunofluorescence against human α-synuclein only in the frontal cortex of seven-month-old transgenic mut(PD) mice (Figure 4). Both genotype (F(1, 14) = 92.3, $p < 0.001$) and diet (F(2, 14) = 5.6, $p < 0.05$) or the interaction of the factors (F(2, 14) = 4.0, $p < 0.05$) had a significant effect on the α-synuclein accumulation in the 2nd layer of the frontal cortex (Figure 4a). The treatment with grain diet with high content of anthocyanins ("mut(PD)+Gr_HCA") produced a significant decrease in the α-synuclein deposition as compared to the "mut(PD)+St. diet" ($p < 0.01$) or "mut(PD)+CGr" ($p < 0.001$) group. The neuroinflammatory marker of microglia activation IBA1 was also increased in the frontal cortex of transgenic mut(PD) mice (genotype factor: F(1, 12) = 18.3, $p < 0.01$) as well as in the striatum (genotype factor: F(1, 14) = 8.6, $p < 0.05$) and s. nigra (genotype factor: F(1, 14) = 29.3, $p < 0.001$) but not in the hippocampus. The grain with high content of anthocyanins reduced IBA1 expression in the striatum, s. nigra, and hippocampal CA1 and DG regions of mut(PD) mice (Figure 5a). Although the grain diet with high content of anthocyanins did not affect IBA1 expression in the frontal cortex of mut(PD) mice, it altered the expression of arginase 1 marking the M2 microglia that promotes tissue viability and neuronal survival in this brain structure. Mice of "mut(PD)+Gr_HCA" had elevated levels of arginase 1 in the frontal cortex as compared to the levels detected in all other groups (diet factor: $F(2, 13) = 5.8$, $p < 0.05$) (Figure 6).

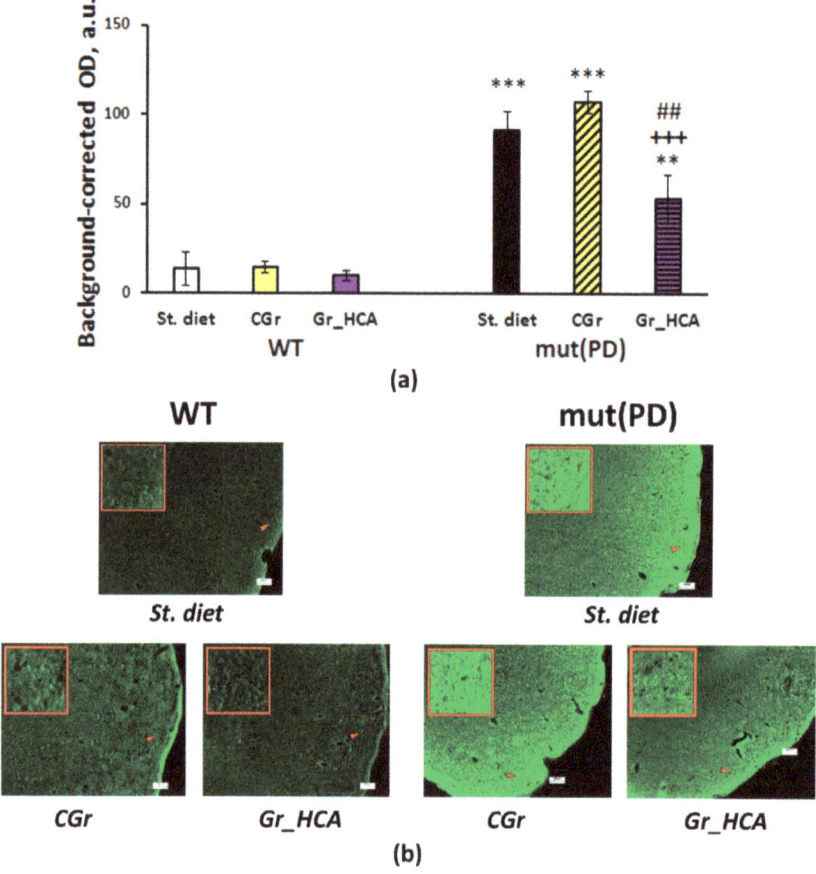

Figure 4. Effects of the type of diet and overexpression of α-synuclein (genetic PD model) on the α-synuclein accumulation in the frontal cortex in mice. (**a**) Quantitative results. The data are expressed as the means ± SEMs of the values obtained in an independent group of animals (*n* = 3–4 per group). Statistically significant differences: ** $p < 0.01$, *** $p < 0.001$ vs. a respective WT group; ## $p < 0.01$ vs. a respective group of mut(PD) mice given the standard diet ("mut(PD)+St. diet"); +++ $p < 0.001$ vs. a respective group of mut(PD) mice given the control grain diet ("mut(PD)+CGr"). (**b**) α-synuclein immunoreactivity in the frontal cortex. Magnification, 100×; bar, 100 μm.

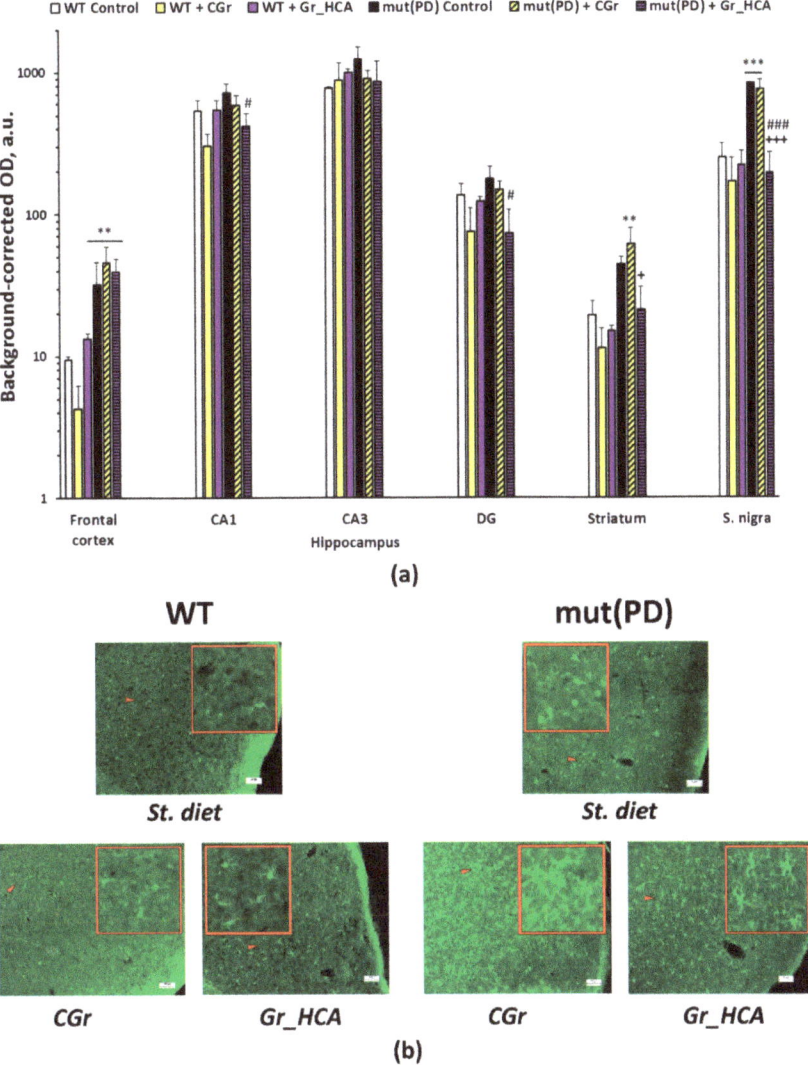

(a)

(b)

Figure 5. Effects of the type of diet and overexpression of α-synuclein (genetic PD model) on the expression of microglial marker IBA1 in the mouse brain. (**a**) Quantitative results. CA1–CA1 hippocampal area, CA3–CA3 hippocampal area, DG–dentate gyrus. The data are expressed as the means ± SEMs of the values obtained in an independent group of animals (*n* = 3–4 per group). Statistically significant differences: ** *p* < 0.01, *** *p* < 0.001 vs. respective WT groups; # *p* < 0.05, ### *p* < 0.001 vs. a respective group of mut(PD) mice given the standard diet ("mut(PD) + St. diet"); + *p* < 0.05, +++ *p* < 0.001 vs. a respective group of mut(PD) mice given the control grain diet ("mut(PD) + CGr"). (**b**) IBA1 immunoreactivity in the frontal cortex. Magnification, 200×; bar, 50 μm.

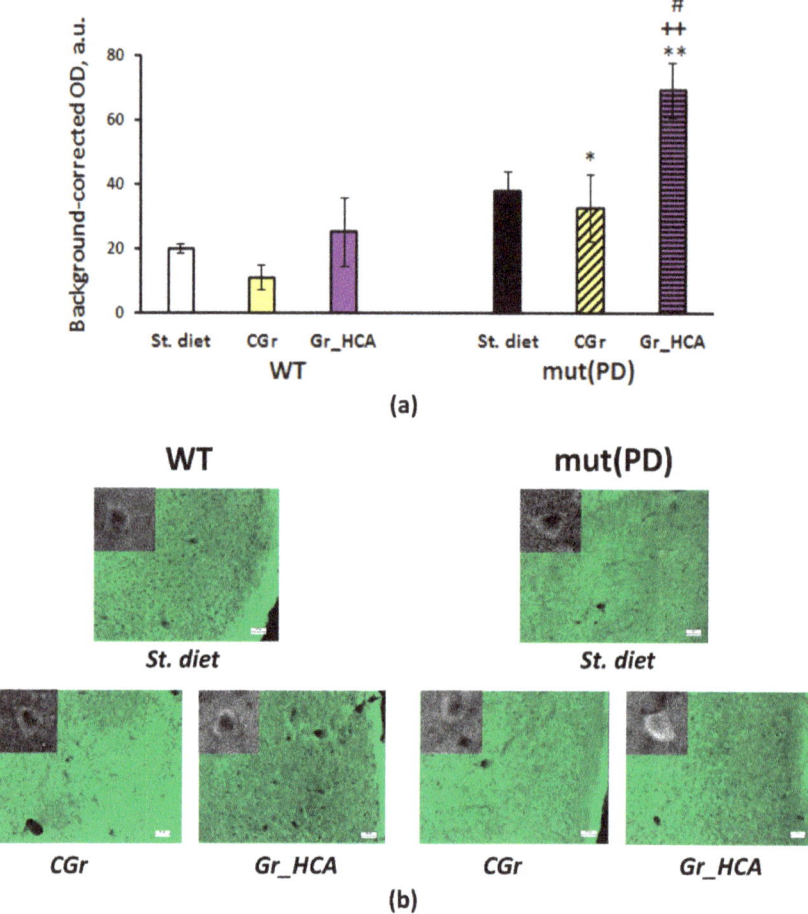

Figure 6. Effects of the type of diet and overexpression of α-synuclein (genetic PD model) on the expression of arginase 1 in the frontal cortex in mice. (**a**) Quantitative results. The data are expressed as the means ± SEMs of the values obtained in an independent group of animals (*n* = 3–4 per group). Statistically significant differences: * *p* < 0.05, ** *p* < 0.01 vs. a respective WT group; # *p* < 0.05 vs. a respective group of mut(PD) mice given the standard diet ("mut(PD)+St. diet"); ++ *p* < 0.01 vs. a respective group of mut(PD) mice given the control grain diet ("mut(PD)+CGr"). (**b**) Arginase 1 immunoreactivity in the frontal cortex. Magnification, 200×; bar, 50 μm. High magnification images (630×) of arginase 1-positive cells are shown in the insets.

4. Discussion

For a long time, the role of anthocyanins as ingredients of functional foods has been underestimated, in particular, due to the notion of their low bioavailability. However, the accumulating evidence of the positive effects of anthocyanins on the physiological functions in animals and humans has led to reconsidering this question. According to early reports, anthocyanins were characterized as the least bioavailable among all the flavonoid compounds. Only 0.4% of the initial amount of anthocyanins consumed in food was detected in the blood plasma of animals and humans [31]. Such low concentrations of anthocyanins could not explain the physiological effects observed after their consumption. Improvement of detection methods made it possible to assess the bioavailability of anthocyanins taking into account their metabolites and interaction products that was much higher than the bioavailability assessed only by the content of the parent compounds [32]. In studies on animals fed with anthocyanin-rich foods, anthocyanins have been found in almost all organs and tissues including the brain. The latter indicates an active absorption of anthocyanins and their ability to cross the blood-brain barrier [33,34]. It is important to note that the initial forms of anthocyanins prevail in animal tissues at short-term treatment while their long-term consumption causes accumulation of anthocyanin metabolites that is associated with the activity of the gut microbiota [34]. An additive and synergistic efficiency of anthocyanin compounds in providing the health benefits should be also taken into account [35]. The biological significance of native natural compound complexes may differ much from that of isolated purified substances. The effect of natural compounds is diminished when biologically active mixtures (extracts) are divided into purified components and introduced separately [36]. Thus, not only the anthocyanin pigments themselves and their health effects but natural biological plant products containing mixtures of these compounds as functional foods are of great interest.

Anthocyanin-rich fruits may have a positive effect at aging-related neuronal and behavioral deficits [37]. Both human and animal studies have demonstrated beneficial effects of the fruit-derived products on cognitive function. In a randomized controlled clinical study, daily ingestion of anthocyanin-rich cherry juice improved fluency, short-term memory, and long-term memory in aged people (70+) with dementia [38]. Anthocyanin-rich mulberry extracts corrected the cognitive impairment in mice with accelerated senescence and AD-like neurodegeneration [39]. In vitro models of PD, extracts rich in anthocyanins, and proanthocyanidins also exhibited neuroprotective activity [40]. Together with the absence of toxicity, negative side effects, or overdose [13], anthocyanin-rich products appear to be promising functional foods for neurodegeneration prevention and therapy as it requires long-term courses of treatment.

The main sources of anthocyanins are dark-colored fruits and berries [41]. However, recently crops such as cereals and potatoes have been regarded as sources of anthocyanins since their grains or tubers may also accumulate anthocyanin compounds [15,42]. Although grains and tubers contain fewer anthocyanins compared to berries, they are more attractive as functional foods due to their longer storage, availability, and daily consumption by most people compared to seasonal berries and fruits. It should be noted that anthocyanins persist in finished products made of wheat grain rich in anthocyanins [19,43–47]. Moreover, a bread made of whole-grain flour with anthocyanins had a longer shelf life compared to bread made of anthocyanin-free flour [44]. Thus, here we evaluated the effects of a diet consisted of whole wheat grain rich in anthocyanins on cognitive function using the models of neurodegenerative disorders.

First, we evaluated the diet tolerance and general effects of the grain diets. Both types of grain mono-diets caused a significant decrease in body weight gain. The body mass of mice given only grain was approximately 1.5 times less than in those fed with standard chow after six months of treatment and approximately 1.8 times less after eight months of a diet. These effects might be attributed to the lower food intake in the grain-treated groups and calorie restriction due to the lean diet containing only grain. Notably, mice treated with the grain with high content of anthocyanins did not differ in the body weight gain from mice fed with the control grain. Although anthocyanins were revealed to affect the fat and carbohydrate metabolism [9,48,49], here we did not observe further loss of body mass in mice fed with the grain with high content of anthocyanins in comparison with the effect of the control grain diet. Moreover, the effects of grain diets on the biochemical indices of blood serum were similar. Both grain mono-diets produced the marked deviations in the parameters of lipid metabolism including the elevated levels of total cholesterol, LDL-C, and HDL-C (α-cholesterol). Nevertheless, atherogenic coefficient that is related to the risk of cardio pathology was even lowered in mice given both types of grain as compared to the mice fed with standard chow.

Similar effects of the diet factor on body weight gain were found in the experiments with AD and PD models. When testing mice for general locomotion, exploratory activity, anxiety, and emotionality in the open field test, Aβ treatment did not significantly affect the behavior of mice fed with standard chow or the grain with high content of anthocyanins. High content of anthocyanins in the diet did not produce marked effects on the parameters studied in Aβ-treated mice in this test as well. In the PD model, horizontal locomotion was augmented, which is in good agreement with previous studies on this transgenic PD model [50–52]. Grain mono-diets significantly decreased horizontal and vertical activity in mice of both genotypes. Notably, no significant differences between the groups of PD model given grain diets in the open field test were found. Hence, the observed effects of anthocyanins on cognitive function were specific and did not depend on the general locomotor or exploratory behavioral changes.

Early stages of AD are associated with disturbances in amyloid metabolism and accumulation of amyloid oligomers [53]. Aβ oligomers are the most toxic forms of amyloid that lead to synaptic and neuronal dysfunctions [54,55]. It is the soluble oligomers of Aβ and not the fibrillar one in amyloid plaques that are currently attributed to the main toxic effect on neurons at the very early stages of AD and probably initiate the pathological cascade [56]. Aβ 25-35 fragment used in the work is characterized by high neurotoxicity due to the high aggregative properties [57,58]. In animal models, it causes certain impairment of cognitive function including the decline in working spatial memory, learning, short-term and long-term memory [20,22,59], along with Aβ accumulation, tau hyperphosphorylation, and neuroinflammatory responses in the brain [22]. We revealed the disturbances in working memory in the T-maze test as well as in episodic memory and retarded spatial learning during the first day of training in the Barnes test induced by Aβ 25-35 administration in mice. At the same time, the indices of long-term spatial memory in the Barnes test were not significantly affected in the "Aβ+St. diet" group. Thus, the slight alterations in cognitive function observed correspond well to the early symptoms of AD. It should be noted that the control wheat diet resulted in similar cognitive alteration in the T-maze test. Anthocyanins prevented the deficit in working spatial memory induced by Aβ 25-35 administration or prolonged grain mono-diet. In the Barnes test, Aβ treatment produced slight alterations in the episodic memory and learning during the first day of training that were partially restored by both types of grain diet. Notably, mice of the "Control+Gr_HCA" group demonstrated the shortest latencies to find the escape box during the first day of training. We may conclude that the wheat grain with high anthocyanin content improves cognitive function; its application is safe for AD-like pathology. Together with previous reports on the positive effects of anthocyanin-enriched extracts in mouse AD models [21,60,61], the results of the study confirm the potential of the anthocyanin-enriched wheat grain as a functional food for dietary supplementation against cognitive decline from the early stages of AD progression.

Pathological aggregation and accumulation of α-synuclein in neurons and Lewy bodies appear to play a core role in the pathogenesis of synucleinopathies and PD in particular [62]. Hence, overexpression of α-synuclein is a common PD model [63]. Although pronounced motor disturbances occur in the transgenic mice with overexpression of mutant human α-synuclein at the age of 9–13 months [52], certain behavioral and cognitive alterations appear at the early stages of the pathology course [51,64]. A previous study indicated spatial memory deficit in mice of this PD model at the ages of six and twelve months using Y-maze test [51]. In the present study, although there was a tendency to decrease in the index of working spatial memory in the transgenic mice and an increase in the group fed with anthocyanin-rich grain diet in the T-maze test, the influence of factors or their interaction was not significant. In the passive avoidance test, contextual memory retrieval did not differ significantly among the experimental groups while memory extinction was more pronounced in the transgenic mice fed with the standard chow. Repeated context exposure gradually reduced memory retention and stimulated extinction. A significant decrease in the step–through latency observed in mut(PD) control mice occurred much earlier than in WT control mice indicating the facilitated extinction and attenuated memory retention. These results are in a good agreement with the previous reports on the facilitation of memory extinction in MPTP-induced PD model [65,66]. Hence, the mut(PD) control mice were characterized by cognitive impairment (deficit of the fear

Nutrients **2020**, *12*, 3877

memory trace retrieval). Both types of grain diets rescued facilitation of contextual fear extinction and improved the retrieval of memory trace via enhancement of reconsolidation. Step-through latencies stayed markedly increased for ten days of the extinction phase as compared to the training day in all groups treated with grain. Prolonged memory extinction might be considered a cognitive alteration. Moreover, the control grain diet caused an exaggerated response in transgenic mice as the values of step-through latencies during the extinction phase were significantly higher than on the training day. However, the values of step-through latencies during the extinction phase were substantially lower in the transgenic mice fed with the anthocyanin-rich grain that in those fed with the control grain. Moreover, the dynamics of memory extinction in the "mut(PD)+Gr_HCA" was closer to that one of the "WT+St. diet" group.

Memory alterations were accompanied by the α-synuclein accumulation in the frontal cortex in the transgenic mice. The anthocyanin-rich grain diet but not the control grain diet significantly reduced the deposition of α-synuclein in the frontal cortex of mut(PD) mice. The results agreed with the previous findings in vitro on the capability of the major metabolite of the anthocyanins cyanidin 3-glucoside to inhibit aggregation and fibril formation of α-synuclein [67,68]. Microglia-mediated neuroinflammation is an important component in PD pathogenesis [69]. A microglial marker IBA1 was augmented in the frontal cortex as well as in the nigrostriatal brain regions of the transgenic mice. Interestingly, the effects of the anthocyanin-rich grain diet on microglia were structure-specific. The anthocyanin-rich grain diminished microglia activation in the striatum and s. nigra but not in the frontal cortex. The decreased microglial response agrees with in vitro findings on an attenuated M1 microglial phenotype after anthocyanin treatment [70]. At the same time, the transgenic mice fed with the anthocyanin-rich grain had the increased expression of arginase 1, a marker of M2 microglia, in the frontal cortex. M2 microglia promotes antiinflammation, tissue repair, and extracellular matrix reconstruction [69]. However, anthocyanins were not able to shift microglia to an M2 strict phenotype in vitro [70]. One may suggest that the modulation of microglial phenotype by anthocyanin treatment in the transgenic PD model was indirect and related to the decreased α-synuclein burden which might be further resolved by M2 microglia [71]. Thus, anthocyanin-enriched wheat grain modulated memory extinction along with the reduction in α-synuclein accumulation and modulation of the microglial response in the brain in the α-synuclein-induced transgenic PD model.

5. Conclusions

Thus, the results provide notable evidence that anthocyanin-rich wheat is a promising source for functional nutrition due to its positive effects on cognitive function and on important pathogenetic processes of neurodegenerative disorders such as accumulation of pathological protein aggregates and neuroinflammation. The diet consisted of whole wheat grain rich in anthocyanins was safe and it possessed beneficial effects on cognitive function in mouse models of early stages of AD and PD. Anthocyanins prevented the deficit in working memory induced by Aβ or prolonged grain mono-diet. Both grain diets partially reversed the retarded learning and episodic memory alterations in AD model. The transgenic PD model was also characterized by cognitive impairment, the facilitation of memory extinction (deficit of the fear memory trace retrieval), while both types of grain diets rescued facilitation of contextual fear extinction and improved the retrieval of memory trace via enhancement of reconsolidation. Both grain diets prolonged the memory extinction that might be considered a cognitive alteration as well. However, the dynamics of the extinction in the group fed with the anthocyanin-rich grain was closer to that in the group of WT mice given standard chow. The behavioral effects of the anthocyanin-rich grain diet were accompanied by the reduction of α-synuclein accumulation and modulation of the microglial response in the brain of the transgenic mice. The results confirmed the potential of the *Pp3* gene that marks the wheat line with anthocyanin-rich grains in breeding of wheat cultivars with high anthocyanin content intended for dietary nutrition.

Supplementary Materials: The following are available online at http://www.mdpi.com/2072-6643/12/12/3877/s1, Table S1: Effects of the type of diet and Aβ25-35 administration (AD model) or of the type of diet and overexpression of α-synuclein (genetic PD model) on the behavior of mice in the open field test; Table S2: Effects of the type of diet and Aβ25-35 administration (AD model) on the parameters of long-term memory and learning evaluated on the next day after four days of training in the test session of the Barnes test in C57Bl/6J mice.

Author Contributions: Conceptualization, E.K.K. and T.G.A.; methodology, M.V.T., A.A.A., M.V.O., and N.I.D.; formal analysis, M.V.T., A.A.A., M.V.O., and N.I.D.; investigation, M.V.T., A.A.A., M.V.O., and N.I.D.; data curation, M.A.T.; writing—original draft preparation, M.A.T. and O.Y.S.; writing—review and editing, M.A.T., E.K.K., and T.G.A.; visualization, M.A.T., A.A.A., and M.V.O.; supervision, M.A.T., T.G.A., and E.K.K.; project administration, E.K.K.; funding acquisition, E.K.K. All authors have read and agreed to the published version of the manuscript.

Funding: This research was funded by Russian Science Foundation (grant No. 16-14-00086).

Acknowledgments: The studies were implemented using the equipment of the Federal State Budgetary Scientific Institution "Scientific Research Institute of Neurosciences and Medicine" (theme No. AAAA-A16-116021010228-0). We thank Konstantin S. Pavlov for technical support in animal treatment and behavioral testing. Microscopy of sections was partially performed at the Microscopy Center of the Siberian Branch of the Russian Academy of Sciences at the Institute of Cytology and Genetics SB RAS (Novosibirsk, Russia); we thank Sergey I. Baiborodin for kind assistance and technical support at the Center.

Conflicts of Interest: The authors declare no conflict of interest. The funders had no role in the design of the study; in the collection, analyses, or interpretation of data; in the writing of the manuscript, or in the decision to publish the results.

References

1. Brown, E.G.; Tanner, C.M. Impaired Cognition and the Risk of Parkinson Disease: Trouble in Mind. *JAMA Neurol.* **2017**, *74*, 1398–1400. [CrossRef]

2. Jellinger, K.A. Dementia with Lewy bodies and Parkinson's disease-dementia: Current concepts and controversies. *J. Neural Transm.* **2018**, *125*, 615–650. [CrossRef]

3. Kumar, A.; Singh, A.; Ekavali. A review on Alzheimer's disease pathophysiology and its management: An update. *Pharm. Rep.* **2015**, *67*, 195–203. [CrossRef] [PubMed]

4. Poewe, W.; Antonini, A.; Zijlmans, J.C.; Burkhard, P.R.; Vingerhoets, F. Levodopa in the treatment of Parkinson's disease: An old drug still going strong. *Clin. Interv. Aging* **2010**, *5*, 229–238. [CrossRef] [PubMed]

5. Sahoo, A.K.; Dandapat, J.; Dash, U.C.; Kanhar, S. Features and outcomes of drugs for combination therapy as multi-targets strategy to combat Alzheimer's disease. *J. Ethnopharmacol.* **2018**, *215*, 42–73. [CrossRef] [PubMed]

6. Frozza, R.L.; Lourenco, M.V.; De Felice, F.G. Challenges for Alzheimer's Disease Therapy: Insights from Novel Mechanisms Beyond Memory Defects. *Front. Neurosci.* **2018**, *12*, 37. [CrossRef]

7. Khoo, H.E.; Azlan, A.; Tang, S.T.; Lim, S.M. Anthocyanidins and anthocyanins: Colored pigments as food, pharmaceutical ingredients, and the potential health benefits. *Food Nutr. Res.* **2017**, *61*, 1361779. [CrossRef] [PubMed]

8. Winkel-Shirley, B. Flavonoid biosynthesis. A colorful model for genetics, biochemistry, cell biology, and biotechnology. *Plant Physiol.* **2001**, *126*, 485–493. [CrossRef]

9. Li, D.; Wang, P.; Luo, Y.; Zhao, M.; Chen, F. Health benefits of anthocyanins and molecular mechanisms: Update from recent decade. *Crit. Rev. Food Sci. Nutr.* **2017**, *57*, 1729–1741. [CrossRef]

10. Smeriglio, A.; Barreca, D.; Bellocco, E.; Trombetta, D. Chemistry, Pharmacology and Health Benefits of Anthocyanins. *Phytother. Res.* **2016**, *30*, 1265–1286. [CrossRef] [PubMed]

11. Tsuda, T.; Ueno, Y.; Aoki, H.; Koda, T.; Horio, F.; Takahashi, N.; Kawada, T.; Osawa, T. Anthocyanin enhances adipocytokine secretion and adipocyte-specific gene expression in isolated rat adipocytes. *Biochem. Biophys. Res. Commun.* **2004**, *316*, 149–157. [CrossRef]

12. Ullah, R.; Khan, M.; Shah, S.A.; Saeed, K.; Kim, M.O. Natural Antioxidant Anthocyanins—A Hidden Therapeutic Candidate in Metabolic Disorders with Major Focus in Neurodegeneration. *Nutrients* **2019**, *11*, 1195. [CrossRef] [PubMed]

13. Riaz, M.; Zia Ul Haq, M.; Saad, B. *Anthocyanins and Human Health: Biomolecular and Therapeutic Aspects*; Springer International Publishing: Madison, WI, USA, 2016; p. 138. [CrossRef]

14. Ficco, D.B.; De Simone, V.; Colecchia, S.A.; Pecorella, I.; Platani, C.; Nigro, F.; Finocchiaro, F.; Papa, R.; De Vita, P. Genetic variability in anthocyanin composition and nutritional properties of blue, purple, and red bread (Triticum aestivum L.) and durum (Triticum turgidum L. ssp. turgidum convar. durum) wheats. *J. Agric. Food Chem.* **2014**, *62*, 8686–8695. [CrossRef] [PubMed]

15. Zhu, F. Anthocyanins in cereals: Composition and health effects. *Food Res. Int.* **2018**, *109*, 232–249. [CrossRef] [PubMed]

16. Gordeeva, E.I.; Shoeva, O.Y.; Khlestkina, E.K. Marker-assisted development of bread wheat near-isogenic lines carrying various combinations of purple pericarp (Pp) alleles. *Euphytica* **2015**, *203*, 469–476. [CrossRef]

17. Morris, C.F.; McLean, D.; Engleson, J.A.; Fuerst, E.P.; Burgos, F.; Coburn, E. Some observations on the granivorous feeding behavior preferences of the house mouse (Mus musculus L.). *Mammalia* **2012**, *76*, 209–218. [CrossRef]

18. Beloshapka, A.N.; Buff, P.R.; Fahey, G.C.; Swanson, K.S. Compositional Analysis of Whole Grains, Processed Grains, Grain Co-Products, and Other Carbohydrate Sources with Applicability to Pet Animal Nutrition. *Foods* **2016**, *5*, 23. [CrossRef]

19. Morgounov, A.; Karaduman, Y.; Akin, B.; Aydogan, S.; Baenziger, P.S.; Bhatta, M.; Chudinov, V.; Dreisigacker, S.; Govindan, V.; Güler, S.; et al. Yield and quality in purple-grained wheat isogenic lines. *Agronomy* **2020**, *10*, 86. [CrossRef]

20. Choi, J.Y.; Cho, E.J.; Lee, H.S.; Lee, J.M.; Yoon, Y.H.; Lee, S. Tartary buckwheat improves cognition and memory function in an in vivo amyloid-beta-induced Alzheimer model. *Food Chem. Toxicol.* **2013**, *53*, 105–111. [CrossRef]

21. Lee, A.Y.; Choi, J.M.; Lee, Y.A.; Shin, S.H.; Cho, E.J. Beneficial effect of black rice (Oryza sativa L. var. japonica) extract on amyloid beta-induced cognitive dysfunction in a mouse model. *Exp. Med.* **2020**, *20*, 64. [CrossRef]

22. Park, S.H.; Kim, J.H.; Bae, S.S.; Hong, K.W.; Lee, D.S.; Leem, J.Y.; Choi, B.T.; Shin, H.K. Protective effect of the phosphodiesterase III inhibitor cilostazol on amyloid beta-induced cognitive deficits associated with decreased amyloid beta accumulation. *Biochem. Biophys. Res. Commun.* **2011**, *408*, 602–608. [CrossRef] [PubMed]

23. Paxinos, G.; Franklin, K.B.J. *Paxinos and Franklin's the Mouse Brain in Stereotaxic Coordinates*, 4th ed.; Elsevier: Amsterdam, The Netherlands; Academic Press: Boston, MI, USA, 2013; p. 360.

24. Pupyshev, A.B.; Tikhonova, M.A.; Akopyan, A.A.; Tenditnik, M.V.; Dubrovina, N.I.; Korolenko, T.A. Therapeutic activation of autophagy by combined treatment with rapamycin and trehalose in a mouse MPTP-induced model of Parkinson's disease. *Pharm. Biochem. Behav.* **2019**, *177*, 1–11. [CrossRef] [PubMed]

25. Deacon, R.M.; Rawlins, J.N. T-maze alternation in the rodent. *Nat. Protoc.* **2006**, *1*, 7–12. [CrossRef] [PubMed]

26. Paul, C.M.; Magda, G.; Abel, S. Spatial memory: Theoretical basis and comparative review on experimental methods in rodents. *Behav. Brain Res.* **2009**, *203*, 151–164. [CrossRef] [PubMed]

27. Dudchenko, P.A. An overview of the tasks used to test working memory in rodents. *Neurosci. Biobehav. Rev.* **2004**, *28*, 699–709. [CrossRef] [PubMed]

28. Lipina, T.V.; Prasad, T.; Yokomaku, D.; Luo, L.; Connor, S.A.; Kawabe, H.; Wang, Y.T.; Brose, N.; Roder, J.C.; Craig, A.M. Cognitive Deficits in Calsyntenin-2-deficient Mice Associated with Reduced GABAergic Transmission. *Neuropsychopharmacology* **2016**, *41*, 802–810. [CrossRef] [PubMed]

29. Tikhonova, M.A.; Ho, S.C.; Akopyan, A.A.; Kolosova, N.G.; Weng, J.C.; Meng, W.Y.; Lin, C.L.; Amstislavskaya, T.G.; Ho, Y.J. Neuroprotective effects of ceftriaxone treatment on cognitive and neuronal deficits in a rat model of accelerated senescence. *Behav. Brain Res.* **2017**, *330*, 8–16. [CrossRef]

30. Garelick, M.G.; Storm, D.R. The relationship between memory retrieval and memory extinction. *Proc. Natl. Acad. Sci. USA* **2005**, *102*, 9091–9092. [CrossRef]

31. Williamson, G.; Manach, C. Bioavailability and bioefficacy of polyphenols in humans. II. Review of 93 intervention studies. *Am. J. Clin. Nutr.* **2005**, *81*, 243S–255S. [CrossRef]

32. Czank, C.; Cassidy, A.; Zhang, Q.; Morrison, D.J.; Preston, T.; Kroon, P.A.; Botting, N.P.; Kay, C.D. Human metabolism and elimination of the anthocyanin, cyanidin-3-glucoside: A (13)C-tracer study. *Am. J. Clin. Nutr.* **2013**, *97*, 995–1003. [CrossRef]

33. Celli, G.B.; Ghanem, A.; Brooks, M.S. A theoretical physiologically based pharmacokinetic approach for modeling the fate of anthocyanins in vivo. *Crit. Rev. Food Sci. Nutr.* **2017**, *57*, 3197–3207. [CrossRef] [PubMed]

34. Sandoval-Ramirez, B.A.; Catalan, U.; Fernandez-Castillejo, S.; Rubio, L.; Macia, A.; Sola, R. Anthocyanin Tissue Bioavailability in Animals: Possible Implications for Human Health. A Systematic Review. *J. Agric. Food Chem.* **2018**, *66*, 11531–11543. [CrossRef] [PubMed]

35. Seeram, N.P.; Adams, L.S.; Hardy, M.L.; Heber, D. Total cranberry extract versus its phytochemical constituents: Antiproliferative and synergistic effects against human tumor cell lines. *J. Agric. Food Chem.* **2004**, *52*, 2512–2517. [CrossRef] [PubMed]

36. Liu, R.H. Health benefits of fruit and vegetables are from additive and synergistic combinations of phytochemicals. *Am. J. Clin. Nutr.* **2003**, *78*, 517S–520S. [CrossRef] [PubMed]

37. Joseph, J.A.; Shukitt-Hale, B.; Denisova, N.A.; Bielinski, D.; Martin, A.; McEwen, J.J.; Bickford, P.C. Reversals of age-related declines in neuronal signal transduction, cognitive, and motor behavioral deficits with blueberry, spinach, or strawberry dietary supplementation. *J. Neurosci.* **1999**, *19*, 8114–8121. [CrossRef] [PubMed]

38. Kent, K.; Charlton, K.; Roodenrys, S.; Batterham, M.; Potter, J.; Traynor, V.; Gilbert, H.; Morgan, O.; Richards, R. Consumption of anthocyanin-rich cherry juice for 12 weeks improves memory and cognition in older adults with mild-to-moderate dementia. *Eur. J. Nutr.* **2017**, *56*, 333–341. [CrossRef]

39. Shih, P.H.; Chan, Y.C.; Liao, J.W.; Wang, M.F.; Yen, G.C. Antioxidant and cognitive promotion effects of anthocyanin-rich mulberry (Morus atropurpurea L.) on senescence-accelerated mice and prevention of Alzheimer's disease. *J. Nutr. Biochem.* **2010**, *21*, 598–605. [CrossRef]

40. Strathearn, K.E.; Yousef, G.G.; Grace, M.H.; Roy, S.L.; Tambe, M.A.; Ferruzzi, M.G.; Wu, Q.L.; Simon, J.E.; Lila, M.A.; Rochet, J.C. Neuroprotective effects of anthocyanin- and proanthocyanidin-rich extracts in cellular models of Parkinsons disease. *Brain Res.* **2014**, *1555*, 60–77. [CrossRef]

41. Ramos, P.; Herrera, R.; Moya-León, M.A. Anthocyanins: Food Sources and Benefits to Consumer's Health. In *Handbook of Anthocyanins: Food Sources, Chemical Applications and Health Benefits*; Warner, L.M., Ed.; Nova Science Publishers Inc.: New York, NY, USA, 2014; pp. 363–384.

42. Strygina, K.V.; Khlestkina, E.K. Anthocyanins synthesis in potato (Solanum tuberosum L.): Genetic markers for smart breeding. *Sel'skokhozyaistvennaya Biol. Agric. Biol.* **2017**, *52*, 37–49. [CrossRef]

43. Bartl, P.; Albreht, A.; Skrt, M.; Tremlova, B.; Ostadalova, M.; Smejkal, K.; Vovk, I.; Ulrih, N.P. Anthocyanins in purple and blue wheat grains and in resulting bread: Quantity, composition, and thermal stability. *Int. J. Food Sci. Nutr.* **2015**, *66*, 514–519. [CrossRef]

44. Khlestkina, E.K.; Usenko, N.I.; Gordeeva, E.I.; Stabrovskaya, O.I.; Sharfunova, I.B.; Otmakhova, Y.S. Evaluation of wheat products with high flavonoid content: Justification of importance of marker-assisted development and production of flavonoid-rich wheat cultivars. *Vavilovskii Zhurnal Genet. I Sel. (Vavilov J. Genet. Breed.)* **2017**, *21*, 545–553. [CrossRef]

45. Ma, D.; Zhang, J.; Li, Y.; Wang, C. Quality of noodles made from colour-grained wheat. *Czech. J. Food Sci.* **2018**, *36*, 314–320. [CrossRef]

46. Pasqualone, A.; Bianco, A.M.; Paradiso, V.M.; Summo, C.; Gambacorta, G.; Caponio, F.; Blanco, A. Production and characterization of functional biscuits obtained from purple wheat. *Food Chem.* **2015**, *180*, 64–70. [CrossRef]

47. Usenko, N.I.; Khlestkina, E.K.; Asavasanti, S.; Gordeeva, E.I.; Yudina, R.S.; Otmakhova, Y.S. Possibilities of enriching food products with anthocyanins by using new forms of cereals. *Foods Raw Mater.* **2018**, *6*, 128–135. [CrossRef]

48. Ghosh, D.; Konishi, T. Anthocyanins and anthocyanin-rich extracts: Role in diabetes and eye function. *Asia Pac. J. Clin. Nutr.* **2007**, *16*, 200–208. [PubMed]

49. Rozanska, D.; Regulska-Ilow, B. The significance of anthocyanins in the prevention and treatment of type 2 diabetes. *Adv. Clin. Exp. Med.* **2018**, *27*, 135–142. [CrossRef]

50. Farrell, K.F.; Krishnamachari, S.; Villanueva, E.; Lou, H.; Alerte, T.N.; Peet, E.; Drolet, R.E.; Perez, R.G. Non-motor parkinsonian pathology in aging A53T alpha-synuclein mice is associated with progressive synucleinopathy and altered enzymatic function. *J. Neurochem.* **2014**, *128*, 536–546. [CrossRef]

51. Paumier, K.L.; Sukoff Rizzo, S.J.; Berger, Z.; Chen, Y.; Gonzales, C.; Kaftan, E.; Li, L.; Lotarski, S.; Monaghan, M.; Shen, W.; et al. Behavioral characterization of A53T mice reveals early and late stage deficits related to Parkinson's disease. *PLoS ONE* **2013**, *8*, e70274. [CrossRef]

52. Unger, E.L.; Eve, D.J.; Perez, X.A.; Reichenbach, D.K.; Xu, Y.; Lee, M.K.; Andrews, A.M. Locomotor hyperactivity and alterations in dopamine neurotransmission are associated with overexpression of A53T mutant human alpha-synuclein in mice. *Neurobiol. Dis.* **2006**, *21*, 431–443. [CrossRef] [PubMed]

53. Selkoe, D.J.; Hardy, J. The amyloid hypothesis of Alzheimer's disease at 25 years. *EMBO Mol. Med.* **2016**, *8*, 595–608. [CrossRef]

54. Haass, C.; Selkoe, D.J. Soluble protein oligomers in neurodegeneration: Lessons from the Alzheimer's amyloid beta-peptide. *Nat. Rev. Mol. Cell Biol.* **2007**, *8*, 101–112. [CrossRef] [PubMed]

55. Walsh, D.M.; Selkoe, D.J. A beta oligomers-a decade of discovery. *J. Neurochem.* **2007**, *101*, 1172–1184. [CrossRef] [PubMed]

56. Mroczko, B.; Groblewska, M.; Litman-Zawadzka, A.; Kornhuber, J.; Lewczuk, P. Amyloid beta oligomers (AbetaOs) in Alzheimer's disease. *J. Neural Transm.* **2018**, *125*, 177–191. [CrossRef]

57. Pike, C.J.; Walencewicz-Wasserman, A.J.; Kosmoski, J.; Cribbs, D.H.; Glabe, C.G.; Cotman, C.W. Structure-activity analyses of beta-amyloid peptides: Contributions of the beta 25-35 region to aggregation and neurotoxicity. *J. Neurochem.* **1995**, *64*, 253–265. [CrossRef] [PubMed]

58. Yankner, B.A.; Duffy, L.K.; Kirschner, D.A. Neurotrophic and neurotoxic effects of amyloid beta protein: Reversal by tachykinin neuropeptides. *Science* **1990**, *250*, 279–282. [CrossRef] [PubMed]

59. El Bitar, F.; Meunier, J.; Villard, V.; Almeras, M.; Krishnan, K.; Covey, D.F.; Maurice, T.; Akwa, Y. Neuroprotection by the synthetic neurosteroid enantiomers ent-PREGS and ent-DHEAS against Abeta(2)(5)(-)(3)(5) peptide-induced toxicity in vitro and in vivo in mice. *Psychopharmacology* **2014**, *231*, 3293–3312. [CrossRef]

60. El-Shiekh, R.A.; Ashour, R.M.; Abd El-Haleim, E.A.; Ahmed, K.A.; Abdel-Sattar, E. Hibiscus sabdariffa L. A potent natural neuroprotective agent for the prevention of streptozotocin-induced Alzheimer's disease in mice. *Biomed. Pharm.* **2020**, *128*, 110303. [CrossRef]

61. Li, J.; Zhao, R.; Jiang, Y.; Xu, Y.; Zhao, H.; Lyu, X.; Wu, T. Bilberry anthocyanins improve neuroinflammation and cognitive dysfunction in APP/PSEN1 mice via the CD33/TREM2/TYROBP signaling pathway in microglia. *Food Funct.* **2020**, *11*, 1572–1584. [CrossRef]

62. Rocha, E.M.; De Miranda, B.; Sanders, L.H. Alpha-synuclein: Pathology, mitochondrial dysfunction and neuroinflammation in Parkinson's disease. *Neurobiol. Dis.* **2018**, *109*, 249–257. [CrossRef]

63. Jagmag, S.A.; Tripathi, N.; Shukla, S.D.; Maiti, S.; Khurana, S. Evaluation of Models of Parkinson's Disease. *Front. Neurosci.* **2015**, *9*, 503. [CrossRef]

64. Oaks, A.W.; Frankfurt, M.; Finkelstein, D.I.; Sidhu, A. Age-dependent effects of A53T alpha-synuclein on behavior and dopaminergic function. *PLoS ONE* **2013**, *8*, e60378. [CrossRef] [PubMed]

65. Kinoshita, K.; Tada, Y.; Muroi, Y.; Unno, T.; Ishii, T. Selective loss of dopaminergic neurons in the substantia nigra pars compacta after systemic administration of MPTP facilitates extinction learning. *Life Sci.* **2015**, *137*, 28–36. [CrossRef] [PubMed]

66. Kinoshita, K.I.; Muroi, Y.; Unno, T.; Ishii, T. Rolipram improves facilitation of contextual fear extinction in the 1-methyl-4-phenyl-1,2,3,6-tetrahydropyridine-induced mouse model of Parkinson's disease. *J. Pharm. Sci.* **2017**, *134*, 55–58. [CrossRef] [PubMed]

67. Hornedo-Ortega, R.; Alvarez-Fernandez, M.A.; Cerezo, A.B.; Richard, T.; Troncoso, A.M.A.; Garcia-Parrilla, M.A.C. Protocatechuic Acid: Inhibition of Fibril Formation, Destabilization of Preformed Fibrils of Amyloid-beta and alpha-Synuclein, and Neuroprotection. *J. Agric. Food Chem.* **2016**, *64*, 7722–7732. [CrossRef] [PubMed]

68. Pogacnik, L.; Pirc, K.; Palmela, I.; Skrt, M.; Kim, K.S.; Brites, D.; Brito, M.A.; Ulrih, N.P.; Silva, R.F. Potential for brain accessibility and analysis of stability of selected flavonoids in relation to neuroprotection in vitro. *Brain Res.* **2016**, *1651*, 17–26. [CrossRef]

69. Tang, Y.; Le, W. Differential Roles of M1 and M2 Microglia in Neurodegenerative Diseases. *Mol. Neurobiol.* **2016**, *53*, 1181–1194. [CrossRef]

70. Meireles, M.; Marques, C.; Norberto, S.; Santos, P.; Fernandes, I.; Mateus, N.; Faria, A.; Calhau, C. Anthocyanin effects on microglia M1/M2 phenotype: Consequence on neuronal fractalkine expression. *Behav. Brain Res.* **2016**, *305*, 223–228. [CrossRef]

71. Park, H.J.; Oh, S.H.; Kim, H.N.; Jung, Y.J.; Lee, P.H. Mesenchymal stem cells enhance alpha-synuclein clearance via M2 microglia polarization in experimental and human parkinsonian disorder. *Acta Neuropathol.* **2016**, *132*, 685–701. [CrossRef]

Publisher's Note: MDPI stays neutral with regard to jurisdictional claims in published maps and institutional affiliations.

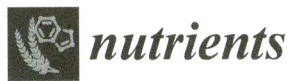

Review

Ketogenic Diet: A Dietary Modification as an Anxiolytic Approach?

Adam Włodarczyk * , **Wiesław Jerzy Cubała** and **Aleksandra Wielewicka**

Department of Psychiatry, Faculty of Medicine, Medical University of Gdańsk, 80-952 Gdańsk, Poland;
cubala@gumed.edu.pl (W.J.C.); wielewicka.aleksandra@gmail.com (A.W.)
* Correspondence: aswlodarczyk@gumed.edu.pl

Received: 1 November 2020; Accepted: 10 December 2020; Published: 14 December 2020

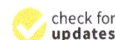

Abstract: Anxiety disorders comprise persistent, disabling conditions that are distributed across the globe, and are associated with the high medical and socioeconomic burden of the disease. Within the array of biopsychosocial treatment modalities—including monoaminergic antidepressants, benzodiazepines, and CBT—there is an unmet need for the effective treatment of anxiety disorders resulting in full remission and recovery. Nutritional intervention may be hypothesized as a promising treatment strategy; in particular, it facilitates relapse prevention. Low-carbohydrate high-fat diets (LCHF) may provide a rewarding outcome for some anxiety disorders; more research is needed before this regimen can be recommended to patients on a daily basis, but the evidence mentioned in this paper should encourage researchers and clinicians to consider LCHF as a piece of advice somewhere between psychotherapy and pharmacology, or as an add-on to those two.

Keywords: GABA; ketogenic diet; low-carbohydrate; anxiety; ketosis; gut microbiota; nutritional psychiatry; mental health; nutrition

1. Introduction

Anxiety disorders comprise a group of persistent, disabling conditions that are distributed across the globe, and are associated with a high burden of the disease being a great cost in the course of healthcare expenses, due to commonly ruling one out from social, professional, and/or educational duties [1–7].

Although intensive research on genetics, neuroimaging, blood-testing, and neurochemical markers has been carried out, the studies failed to determine the anxiety biomarkers, as the majority of them showed solitary findings which sometimes were neither replicable, nor consistent with each other [8].

The array of treatment modalities is still limited in efficacy with regard to remission, prognosis, and relapse prevention. There is an unmet need for novel strategies in the treatment of anxiety disorders, including treatments that fall outside of pharmacotherapy and psychosocial intervention.

1.1. Neurotransmission and Gut-Microbiota Interplay in Anxiety

1.1.1. Monoamines

Within the exploration of the possible biological causes of anxiety, there is evidence on serotonergic and noradrenergic transmission defects in the mechanism of anxiety; there is a need to explore more treatment options to treat these disorders, and a diet regimen could be one of them. The monoaminergic hypothesis led to the development of selective and nonselective inhibitors of serotonin transporters and/or norepinephrine, with the aim of monoaminergic transmission augmentation [9–11]. There is a strong correlation between enhanced noradrenergic activity and fear and anxiety. Additionally, the neurons of the chief noradrenergic projection center in the central nervous system, the locus coeruleus, are hyperactive during anxiety, and the excitation of this part of the brain is related to symptoms such as stress and anxiety responses [9]. Furthermore, pharmacotherapeutic confirmation points towards the involvement of the serotonergic system in the brain [9].

1.1.2. Hypothalamic-Pituitary-Adrenal Axis, Divalent Ions, Inflammation, and Reactive Oxygen Species in Anxiety

Another factor is the disturbance of the hypothalamic–pituitary–adrenal axis (HPA), which is seen to have elevated cortisol levels. However, hypocortisolism has also been noted [12]. Factors such as the divalent ions of zinc or magnesium (the digestion of which is controlled partly by the human microbiota [13]) may exert effects on the progression of the cortical brain-derived neurotrophic factor (zinc and magnesium), N-methyl-D-aspartate (NMDA) antagonists' mechanisms of action, and neuromodulation. The mechanism of action also highlights the linkage between anxiety and some divalent ion deficiencies [14,15]. Inflammation and oxidative stress are also being linked to the anxiety process. The former was consistently found to affect anxiety-related brain regions, i.e., the anterior cingulate cortex, amygdala, and insula, which may result from cytokine effects on monoamines and glutamate. Increased inflammatory cytokines are, in turn, associated with increased oxidative stress, and the generation of reactive oxygen species (ROS) and reactive nitrogen species. The latter could be linked with obsessive-compulsive disorder and panic disorders' etiologies, which show statistically-significant levels of some antioxidant enzymes and malondialdehyde [16–18].

1.1.3. Excess Glutamate

With regard to glutamate, its relationship to anxiety has also already been established. This chief excitatory neurotransmitter in the human brain was found to play a vital role in anxiety. The mechanism consists of NMDA receptor complex activation, which requires both glutamate (which could be depleted by the LCHF diet, as described below) and its co-agonist, glycine. D-cycloserine, for instance, being a partial agonist—at the glycine recognition site—of the glutamatergic NMDA receptor, can act as a cognitive enhancer to augment exposure strategies during the cognitive-behavioral therapy of anxiety disorders [19,20].

1.1.4. GABA Deficiency

Additionally, the main inhibitory gamma-aminobutyric acid (GABA) dysfunctions have been discussed in studies as being responsible for mood fluctuations in affective disorders and the psychopathology of fear (the acquisition, storage, and extinction of fear memory); this has not only been proven theoretically but also practically, by the rapid reduction of symptomatology, anxiety, and sleep disorders when allosteric modulators of GABA were given [21–23]. In patients with General Anxiety Disorder (GAD), the number of GABA type A (GABA-A) receptors is reduced in the temporal lobe [24]; patients with panic disorders also have reduced GABA-A receptor numbers in the parietal, temporal and frontal cortices, the left hippocampus, and the precuneus [25]. Likewise, GABA is responsible for the inhibition of cortisol excretion in stress, and corticotropin-releasing hormone excretion, which also supports the hypothesis that, when altered, GABA could intensify the risk of depression and/or anxiety [23]. Persistent Selective Serotonin Reuptake Inhibitor (SSRIs) intake enhances the cortical GABA concentrations observed in both patients and healthy controls, and are compatible with the antidepressant drug-induced potentiation of GABA release as a mechanism underlying antidepressant effects. Similarly to SSRIs, tricyclic antidepressants that increase the concentration of noradrenaline and serotonin take part in GABAergic transmission modulation. The noradrenergic neuration of GABAergic interneurons increases the GABAergic transmission in the frontal, sensorimotor, and entorhinal cortices; parts of the hippocampus; and the basolateral amygdala. Additionally, significant decreases in the left temporal pole GABA-A receptors were found in a PET study with female GAD patients. Studies have shown that infusions of GABA or GABA-A receptor agonists into the amygdala lessened the measures of anxiety in several animal subjects, while infusions of GABA antagonists managed to show anxiogenic properties [26]. The role of GABA has long been observed as being central to the regulation of anxiety, and this neurotransmitter system is the target of benzodiazepines (and related drugs) used to treat anxiety disorders effectively [27].

1.1.5. Gut Microbiota

Furthermore, the intestinal microbiota have various functions in the organism, including the synthesis of certain bacteria groups that replenish the absorption of ions, calcium and iron, and the transformation of fatty acids, stimulating the development of the immune system and protective functions [13]. The relationship between the development of depression, the immune response, and bowel function is currently explained by the phenomenon of 'leaky gut syndrome'. The research revealed that 'tight junctions'—connections between the cells of the intestinal epithelium—deteriorate under stress, which in turn leads to the translocation of intestinal bacteria through the intestinal barrier into the circulatory system [28].

To summarize, at present, antidepressants augment monoaminergic transmission and also strengthen GABA transmission, the lowered concentration of which is frequently observed in anxiety disorders [9,23].

Among monoaminergic drugs, cognitive-behavioral therapy, or occasional benzodiazepine use, there is a lot to be discovered in the nutrition regimen regarding decreasing anxiety symptoms. The aim of this mini-review is to bring together the existing knowledge of the ways in which certain types of food components affect anxiety.

1.2. Low Carbohydrate Diets and Their Hypothesized Impact on Anxiety Treatment

1.2.1. Low-Carbohydrate Diets

Dietary modification as a treatment intervention modality has been widely discussed since the 19th century [29–31]. A very low-carb diet (up to ca. 50 g carbohydrates per day [32]), the LCHF-ketogenic diet (KD), was the typical treatment for diabetes mellitus (DM) throughout the 19th century [33,34]. A dietary regimen that provided ketosis was found in the treatment amended by the physicians of ancient Greece, including for epilepsy, by altering their patients' diet, mostly by the 'complete abstinence of food and drink' [35].

Diets with low amounts of carbohydrate consumption (low-carb) seem promising both for weight mass optimization among mentally ill patients and for their possible anxiolytic effect. A diet is characterised as being low-carb high-fat (LCHF) when fat comprises >70% of the daily calorie consumption, with sugars being 5–15%, and the rest of the calories being supported by proteins [32].

Although there are various types of LCHF diets, like the Atkins diet, modified Atkins diet, low-glycemic index treatment diet, and the medium-chain triglyceride (MCT) KD [36–38], we will focus on the biological aspect of the mechanism of ketosis. As has previously been said, a very low-carb KD and starvation have something in common, and the process is called ketosis. The difference between physiological ketosis and pathological ketoacidosis (which is seen in DM type 1 or prolonged starvation) is a major limiting factor in the production of ketones [39]. Ketosis, the state of the overproduction of acetoacetate, D-3-hydroxybutyrate, and acetone (called collectively 'the ketone bodies') by the liver, takes place when carbohydrates are removed from the diet (or during starvation). Ketosis seems to only 'imitate' starvation, being different from it, as the daily caloric intake stays on a normal, or even higher, level. The restriction of carbohydrates to under 50 g induces glycogen depletion and ketone production due to the mobilization of fat stored in the adipose tissue, which is the main mechanism associated with a decrease in body weight. Very low-carbohydrate diets and mild low-carbohydrate diets (the latter is commonly defined as carbohydrate consumption up to 130 g per day) differ in the type of body mass loss. In the review by Hashimoto et al. 2016, very low-carb diets were associated with a decrease in fat mass, but mild low-carb diets were not associated with a decrease in fat mass, although both were associated with bodyweight decrease [40]. Furthermore, the Prospective Urban

Rural Epidemiology (PURE) study [41] showed that high carbohydrate consumption (over 60% of daily calories) was linked with an adverse impact on total mortality and non-cardiovascular disease mortality. On the other hand, higher fat consumption was associated with a lower risk of total mortality, non-cardiovascular disease mortality, and stroke [41].

The direct and indirect influence on the central nervous system of KD can be observed in the increasing of the cerebral blood flow, and the decreasing the mammalian target of rapamycin (mTOR) [42] by the increase of the level of endothelial nitric oxide synthase protein expression, but also passively (indirectly). The indirect, 'passive', effects on the central nervous system are supposed to be mediated by microbiota through an increase of short-chain fatty acids and a decrease of GABA [43]. Bacteria such as *Akkermansia muciniphila* and *Lactobacillus* are known as short-chain fatty acid producers [44]. It is known that the KD induces anorexigenic effects: decreased adenosine monophosphate-activated protein (AMP) phosphorylation, and an increase of post-meal free fatty acids. KD has also appetite stimulant (orexigenic) abilities: it increases the brain's GABA concentrations of AMP, and decreases reactive oxygen species (ROS) [45].

In a study on the KD mechanism in epilepsy treatment—by Calderon et al.—in which rodents were set on a two weeks KD trial, the ketone levels in their urine were measured along with GABA, glutamate levels, and weight. Not only did the rats on KD gain weight by only about 1.2 g, whilst the control group gained 20.8 g, but the levels of their neurotransmitters changed significantly in favor of GABA. In probes of microdialysate, the glutamate levels declined non-significantly between KD (3.5 ± 0.6 μM) and the control group (5.18 ± 0.73 μM) ($p = 0.08$), while the GABA levels were significantly higher (47 ± 8 nM) in rats kept in the KD group compared to the control rats (26 ± 3 nM) ($p \leq 0.03$) [45]. This mechanism of KD could be supportive of anxiety disorder treatments.

1.2.2. Gut Microbiota and the Steroid Pathway in the Potentiation of GABA Transmission in Low-Carbohydrate Diets

Furthermore, GABA can be synthesized by the gut microbiota residents: Lactobacilli and Bifidobacteria (Lactobacillus brevis, Bifidobacterium dentium, Bifidobacterium adolescentis, and Bifidobacterium infantis). Lactobacillus rhamnosus has been proven for its therapeutical potential in modulating the expression of central GABA receptors, mediating depression and anxiety-like behaviors [46], which links the possible anxiolytic outcome effect with the gut microbiome. It was suggested that the LCHF diet, and—in general—the inhibition of glycolysis in the brain, could reduce neuronal excitability through the potentiation of GABA transmission via the steroid pathway [47,48]. Forte et al. [47] reported a novel mechanism for the reduction of network hyperexcitability by the inhibition of glycolysis, which involves the potentiation of the shunting inhibition in excitatory neurons, in which a glucose analogue—2-deoxy-D-glucose—potentiates the extra-synaptic tonic GABAergic current through the activation of neurosteroidogenesis. There seems to exist a linkage with the gut–brain axis, neurosteroids, and GABA-A interplay, while neuronal GABA-A receptors are one of the prime molecular targets of neurosteroids [49]. As some gut microbiota residents could be called 'manufacturers of GABA', the gut microbiota diversity seems to influence positively the circulating steroid levels, in particular, that of allopregnanolone. Prebiotic consumption could improve frequently co-existing anxiety disorder symptoms through the promotion of undisturbed non-rapid eye movement (NREM) sleep and stress-related REM sleep rebound, and the prevention of stress-induced reductions in gut microbial alpha diversity [49,50].

Increasingly, low-carb diets are being used to treat behavioral and mood disorders such as attention deficit disorder, for which diets that are low in sugar and high in fatty acids are recommended [51]. Still, little is known about KD and gut microbiota dependence with regard to mental health. Mostly, the evidence found focuses on the effect of KD on the gut microbiota of children with either epilepsy [43,52–54] or autism [55]. Only some articles focus on adult patients, but most focus on subjects with significant comorbidities; such literature is to be found on sclerosis multiplex, in which KD restores the impaired gut microbiome in patients with sclerosis multiplex [56]. Similar data can be found on professional athletes; in a study by Murtaza et al. [57], the researchers found statistically significant differences in some bacteria species between the stool microbiota profiles of those athletes consuming the LCHF diet compared with their baseline measurements. Moreover, tests performed on mice suggest a beneficial role of KD for gut microbiota [43,58]. As a ketogenic diet modifies the gut microbiome, the preservation of proper gut health through the implementation of fermented food (i.e., yogurt, water and milk kefir, kimchi, fermented vegetables) or pre/probiotics consumption (which does not interfere with the assumptions of KD) seem important. It is possible that taking probiotics could help prevent composition disorders of the gut microbiota as a consequence of chronic stress, and the depletion of inflammation and the increasing of serotonin biosynthesis probiotics could be an element of anxiety disorder relapse prevention.

1.2.3. Anti-Inflammatory Effect of the Ketogenic Diet and Fatty Acids

It is hypothesized that a ketogenic diet may reduce inflammation [59]. Compared with glucose metabolism, the metabolism of ketone bodies produces fewer ROS, which contribute to inflammation. Ketolytic metabolism produces fewer free radicals and ROS, affecting the mitochondrial Q coenzyme pair and the cytoplasmic glutathione couple [59,60].

Some research indicates the benefit in the outcome of anxiety when the consumption of particular fats in the diet is increased, i.e., the essential polyunsaturated fatty acids (EPUFAs), also called vitamin F, and omega-3 fatty acids. The clinician-advised dosing of the two omega-3 fatty acids—eicosapentaenoic acid (EPA) and docosahexaenoic acid (DHA)—is at least 1.5–2.5 g daily consumption [61,62]. The American Psychiatric Association guidelines support omega-3 consumption for the mentally ill, through the consumption of at least 1 g of EPA and DHA daily, which is in-line with the guidelines of the American Heart Association [63]. DHA plays a role in the brain's cellular structure construction, because as much as 20% of the brain is composed of it. All omega-3 formulations exhibit anti-inflammatory activity and help to maintain brain cells' stability, with linkages to neurotransmitters' (serotonin, dopamine) proper functioning [64]. Nowadays, with higher depression morbidity in society, studies are showing that omega-3 fatty acids are eaten rarely and in lower doses than in the past decades [64,65]. The proposed mechanisms of action are presented in Figure 1.

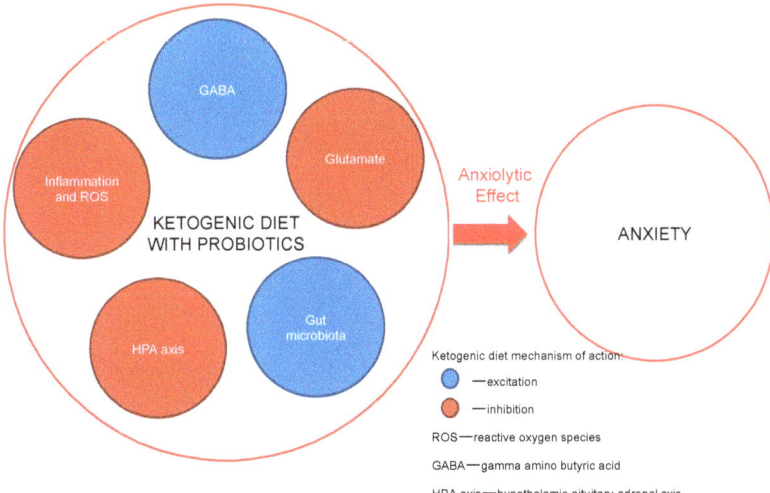

Figure 1. Ketogenic diet mechanisms of action.

1.2.4. The 'Ketogenic Menu'

The 'clean keto' version of KD is mostly based on 'healthy' macronutrients, such as low-processed food, i.e., fat sources such as free-range egg yolks, and polyunsaturated fatty acids such as olive, canola, and grapeseed oil, oily fish, and nuts. As for proteins, fish, meat, cheese, egg whites (mostly high-fat protein sources) are recommended, and carbohydrates are limited to mostly unprocessed, low glycemic index carbohydrates (which are 'smuggled' through green vegetable consumption, brown rice, etc.). A professional dietician's guidance is advised. The previously-mentioned divalent ions linked to anxiety can also be supplied in the LCHF menu, i.e., through zinc-rich foods such as oysters (which are low-carbohydrate meals) and other seafood, etc. Magnesium can be found mostly in green leafy vegetables, while selenium is found in seafood, poultry, fish, and eggs, which all are favorable choices in LCHF diets [35].

A study on over 121,000 participants concluded that high stress and high neuroticism levels were associated with poorer diet quality; however, poor diet quality did not predict emotional or mental health problems [66]. Although the data suggest that enhancing diet quality may not hold promise in preventing mental disorders, patients may benefit from a specific type of nutrition regimen whilst they are mentally ill [67,68]. These findings could help establish the right dietary regimen to enhance the GABAergic transmission and support the gut–brain axis.

2. Conclusions

Although there is a growing body of literature that links nutrition to mood, little can be found on the proposed biological mechanisms of action of certain micro- and macronutrients on neurotransmission, leaving studies with, mainly, epidemiological data [69,70]. There is also evidence with regard to the gut–brain axis, in which some species of bacteria have the ability to generate the neuroendocrine hormones and/or neuroactive compounds involved in a key aspect of neurotransmission [46], which may be responsible for the anxiolytic effect. There is also the vital fact that metabolic acidosis—which is a potentially life-threatening condition that can appear due to ketoacidosis caused by starvation, diabetes, lactate acidosis, alcohol ingestion, or renal failure—is also represented by ketone bodies in the urine and blood, but it differs in those levels of in the blood and urine (due to the lower blood pH in ketoacidosis than in physiological ketosis) [71].

The findings rationalize the need for more detailed, longitudinal research on the ways in which diet and microbiome interactions may be better understood and managed in order to optimize the reduction of anxiety for the benefit of the patients. LCHF diets, in some anxiety disorders, may provide a rewarding outcome, but more research is needed before this regimen can be recommended to patients on a daily basis; however, the evidence mentioned in this paper should encourage psychiatrists to recommend LCHF diets as advice somewhere between psychotherapy and pharmacology, or as an add-on to those two. In our mind, the LCHF diet is a promising, well-accepted diet regimen which has an impact on anxiety disorders, supporting mainly long-term relapse prevention strategies, in combination with the already-approved strategies.

Author Contributions: Study conception and design: A.W. (Adam Włodarczyk); acquisition of data: A.W. (Adam Włodarczyk) and A.W. (Aleksandra Wielewicka); analysis and interpretation of data: A.W. (Adam Włodarczyk) and W.J.C.; drafting of the manuscript: A.W. (Adam Włodarczyk) and A.W. (Aleksandra Wielewicka); critical revision: W.J.C. All authors have read and agreed to the published version of the manuscript.

Funding: The work was completed as a part of grant no. 02-0039/07/221 from the Medical University of Gdańsk, Poland.

Conflicts of Interest: Adam Włodarczyk has received research support from Actavis, Eli Lilly, Minerva Neurosciences, Sunovion Pharmaceuticals, KCR, Janssen, Otsuka, Apodemus, Cortexyme, and Acadia. Wiesław Jerzy Cubała has received research support from Actavis, Alkermes, Allergan, Angelini, Auspex, Biogen, Bristol-Myers Squibb, Cephalon, Eli Lilly, Ferrier, Forest Laboratories, Gedeon Richter, GW Pharmaceuticals, Janssen, KCR, Lundbeck, Orion, Otsuka, Sanofi, and Servier; he has served on speakers' bureaus for Adamed, Angelini, AstraZeneca, Bristol-Myers Squibb, Celon, GlaxoSmithKline, Janssen, Krka, Lekam, Lundbeck,

Novartis, Orion, Pfizer, Polfa Tarchomin, Sanofi, Servier, and Zentiva; and he has served as a consultant for GW Pharmaceuticals, Janssen, KCR, Quintiles, and Roche. Aleksandra Wielewicka: n/a.

References

1. Bandelow, B.; Michaelis, S. Epidemiology of anxiety disorders in the 21st century. *Dialogues Clin. Neurosci.* **2015**, *17*, 327–335. [PubMed]
2. World Health Organization. *ICD-10: International Statistical Classification of Diseases and Related Health Problems: Tenth Revision*, 2nd ed.; World Health Organization: Geneva, Switzerland, 2004; Available online: https://apps.who.int/iris/handle/10665/42980 (accessed on 20 September 2020).
3. Kessler, R.C.; Petukhova, M.; Sampson, N.A.; Zaslavsky, A.M.; Wittchen, H.-U. Twelve-month and lifetime prevalence and lifetime morbid risk of anxiety and mood disorders in the United States. *Int. J. Methods Psychiatry Res.* **2012**, *21*, 169–184. [CrossRef] [PubMed]
4. Leon, A.C.; Portera, L.; Weissman, M.M. The social costs of anxiety disorders. *Br. J. Psychiatry Suppl.* **1995**, 19–22. [CrossRef] [PubMed]
5. Baxter, A.J.; Vos, T.; Scott, K.M.; Ferrari, A.J.; Whiteford, H.A. The global burden of anxiety disorders in 2010. *Psychol. Med.* **2014**, *44*, 2363–2374. [CrossRef]
6. Stein, D.J.; Scott, K.M.; de Jonge, P.; Kessler, R.C. Epidemiology of anxiety disorders: From surveys to nosology and back. *Dialogues Clin. Neurosci.* **2017**, *19*, 127–136. [CrossRef] [PubMed]
7. Andlin-Sobocki, P.; Wittchen, H.U. Cost of anxiety disorders in Europe. *Eur. J. Neurol.* **2005**, *12*, 39–44. [CrossRef] [PubMed]
8. Maron, E.; Nutt, D. Biological markers of generalized anxiety disorder. *Dialogues Clin. Neurosci.* **2017**, *19*, 147–158. [CrossRef] [PubMed]
9. Montoya, A.; Bruins, R.; 1 Katzman, M.A.; Blier, P. The noradrenergic paradox: Implications in the management of depression and anxiety. *Neuropsychiatr. Dis. Treat.* **2016**, *12*, 541–557. [CrossRef] [PubMed]
10. Rickels, K.; Mangano, R.; Khan, A. A double-blind, placebo-controlled study of a flexible dose of venlafaxine ER in adult outpatients with generalized social anxiety disorder. *J. Clin. Psychopharmacol.* **2004**, *24*, 488–496. [CrossRef]
11. Rickels, K.; Zaninelli, R.; McCafferty, J.; Bellew, K.; Iyengar, M.; Sheehan, D. Paroxetine treatment of generalized anxiety disorder: A double-blind, placebo-controlled study. *Am. J. Psychiatry* **2003**, *160*, 749–756. [CrossRef]
12. Jakuszkowiak-Wojten, K.; Landowski, J.; Wiglusz, M.S.; Cubała, W.J. Cortisol as an indicator of hypothalmic-pitituary-adrenal axis dysregulation in patients with panic disorder: A literature review. *Psychiatr. Danub.* **2015**, *27*, S445–S451. [PubMed]
13. Singewald, N.; Sinner, C.; Hetzenauer, A.; Sartori, S.B.; Murck, H. Magnesium deficient diet alter depression-and anxiety-related behavior in mice—Influence of desipramine and Hypericum perforatum extract. *Neuropharmacology* **2004**, *47*, 1189–1197. [CrossRef] [PubMed]
14. Hermann, A. Probiotics supplementation in prophylaxis and treatment of depressive and anxiety disorders - a review of current research. *Psychiatr. Pol.* **2019**, *53*, 459–473. [CrossRef] [PubMed]
15. Jacka, F.N.; Overland, S.; Stewart, R.; Tell, G.S.; Bjelland, I.; Mykletun, A. Association between magnesium intake and depression and anxiety in community-dwelling adults: The Hordaland Health Study. *Aust. N. Z. J. Psychiatry* **2009**, *43*, 45–52. [CrossRef] [PubMed]
16. Kuloglu, M.; Atmaca, M.; Tezcan, E.; Ustundag, B.; Bulut, S. Antioxidant enzyme and malondialdehyde levels in patients with panic disorder. *Neuropsychobiology* **2002**, *46*, 186–189. [CrossRef]
17. Kuloglu, M.; Atmaca, M.; Tezcan, E.; Gecici, O.; Tunckol, H.; Ustundag, B. Antioxidant enzyme activities and malondialdehyde levels in patients with obsessive-compulsive disorder. *Neuropsychobiology* **2002**, *46*, 27–32. [CrossRef]
18. Hassan, W.; Silva, C.E.; Mohammadzai, I.U.; da Rocha, J.B.; Landeira-Fernandez, J. Association of oxidative stress to the genesis of anxiety: Implications for possible therapeutic interventions. *Curr. Neuropharmacol.* **2014**, *12*, 120–139. [CrossRef]
19. Hofmann, S.G. Cognitive processes during fear acquisition and extinction in animals and humans: Implications for exposure therapy of anxiety disorders. *Clin. Psychol. Rev.* **2008**, *28*, 199–210. [CrossRef]

20. Hofmann, S.G.; Sawyer, A.T.; Asnaani, A. ᴅ-cycloserine as an augmentation strategy for cognitive behavioral therapy of anxiety disorders: An update. *Curr. Pharm. Des.* **2012**, *18*, 5659–5662. [CrossRef]
21. Möhler, H. The GABA system in anxiety and depression and its therapeutic potential. *Neuropharmacology* **2012**, *62*, 42–53. [CrossRef]
22. Pehrson, A.L.; Sanchez, C. Altered γ-aminobutyric acid neurotransmission in major depressive disorder: A critical review of the supporting evidence and the influence of serotonergic antidepressants. *Drug Des. Dev. Ther.* **2015**, *9*, 603–624. [CrossRef] [PubMed]
23. Kalueff, A.V.; Nutt, D.J. Role of GABA in anxiety and depression. *Depress. Anxiety* **2007**, *24*, 495–517. [CrossRef] [PubMed]
24. Gross, C.; Hen, R. The developmental origins of anxiety. *Nat. Rev. Neurosci.* **2004**, *5*, 545–552. [CrossRef] [PubMed]
25. Fatemi, S.H.; Folsom, T.D. GABA receptor subunit distribution and FMRP-mGluR5 signaling abnormalities in the cerebellum of subjects with schizophrenia, mood disorders, and autism. *Schizophr. Res.* **2015**, *167*, 42–56. [CrossRef] [PubMed]
26. Nuss, P. Anxiety disorders and GABA neurotransmission: A disturbance of modulation. *Neuropsychiatr. Dis. Treat.* **2015**, *11*, 165–175. [CrossRef] [PubMed]
27. Lydiard, R.B. The role of GABA in anxiety disorders. *J. Clin. Psychiatry* **2003**, *64*, 21–27.
28. Desbonnet, L.; Garrett, L.; Clarke, G.; Kiely, B.; Cryan, J.F.; Dinan, T.G. Effects of the probiotic Bifidobacterium infantis in the maternal separation model of depression. *Neuroscience* **2010**, *170*, 1179–1188. [CrossRef]
29. Banting, W. Letter on Corpulence Addressed to the Public. *Obes. Res.* **1993**, *1*, 153–163. [CrossRef]
30. Johnstone, A.M.; Horgan, G.W.; Murison, S.D.; Bremner, D.M.; Lobley, G.E. Effects of a high-protein ketogenic diet on hunger, appetite, and weight loss in obese men feeding ad libitum. *Am. J. Clin. Nutr.* **2008**, *87*, 44–55. [CrossRef]
31. Paoli, A.; Bosco, G.; Camporesi, E.M.; Mangar, D. Ketosis, ketogenic diet and food intake control: A complex relationship. *Front. Psychol.* **2015**, *2*, 27. [CrossRef]
32. Ludwig, D.S. The Ketogenic Diet: Evidence for Optimism but High-Quality Research Needed. *J. Nutr.* **2020**, *150*, 1354–1359. [CrossRef] [PubMed]
33. Einhorn, M. *Lectures on Dietetics*; Saunders: Philadelphia, PA, USA, 1922.
34. Morgan, W. *Diabetes Mellitus: Its History, Chemistry, Anatomy, Pathology, Physiology, and Treatment. Illustrated with Woodcuts, and Cases Successfully Treated*; Homoeopathic Publishing Company: London, UK, 1877.
35. Hippocrates. *Epidemics 2*; Smith, W.D., Ed.; Harvard University Press: Cambridge, MA, USA, 1994; Volume 7, p. 46.
36. Atkins, R.C. *Dr. Atkins' New Diet Revolution*; M. Evans & Company: New York, NY, USA, 2002.
37. Rezaei, S.; Harsini, S.; Kavoosi, M.; Badv, R.S.; Mahmoudi, M. Efficacy of low glycemic index treatment in epileptic patients: A systematic review. *Acta Neurol. Belg.* **2018**, *118*, 339–349. [CrossRef] [PubMed]
38. Liu, Y.-M.; Wang, H.-S. Medium-chain triglyceride ketogenic diet, an effective treatment for drug-resistant epilepsy and a comparison with other ketogenic diets. *Biomed. J.* **2013**, *36*, 9–15. [CrossRef] [PubMed]
39. Krebs, H.A. The regulation of the release of ketone bodies by the liver. *Adv. Enzyme Regul.* **1966**, *4*, 339–354. [CrossRef]
40. Hashimoto, Y.; Fukuda, T.; Oyabu, C.; Tanaka, M.; Asano, M.; Yamazaki, M.; Fukui, M. Impact of low-carbohydrate diet on body composition: Meta-analysis of randomized controlled studies. *Obes. Rev.* **2016**, *17*, 499–509. [CrossRef] [PubMed]
41. Dehghan, M.; Mente, A.; Zhang, X.; Swaminathan, S.; Li, W.; Mohan, V.; Iqbal, R.; Kumar, R.; Wentzel-Viljoen, E.; Rosengren, A.; et al. Associations of fats and carbohydrate intake with cardiovascular disease and mortality in 18 countries from five continents (PURE): A prospective cohort study. *Lancet* **2017**, *390*, 2050–2062. [CrossRef]
42. Włodarczyk, A.; Wiglusz, M.S.; Cubała, W.J. Ketogenic diet for schizophrenia: Nutritional approach to antipsychotic treatment. *Med. Hypotheses* **2018**, *118*, 74–77. [CrossRef]
43. Olson, C.A.; Vuong, H.E.; Yano, J.M.; Liang, Q.Y.; Nusbaum, D.J.; Hsiao, E.Y. The gut microbiota mediates the anti-seizure effects of the ketogenic diet. *Cell* **2018**, *174*, 497. [CrossRef]
44. Rodríguez-Carrio, J.; Salazar, N.; Margolles, A.; González, S.; Gueimonde, M.; de Los Reyes-Gavilán, C.G.; Suárez, A. Free Fatty Acids Profiles Are Related to Gut Microbiota Signatures and Short-Chain Fatty Acids. *Front. Immunol.* **2017**, *8*, 823. [CrossRef]

45. Calderón, N.; Betancourt, L.; Hernández, L.; Rada, P. A ketogenic diet modifies glutamate, gamma-aminobutyric acid and agmatine levels in the hippocampus of rats: A microdialysis study. *Neurosci. Lett.* **2017**, *642*, 158–162. [CrossRef]

46. Paoli, A.; Mancin, L.; Bianco, A.; Thomas, E.; Mota, J.F.; Piccini, F. Ketogenic Diet and Microbiota: Friends or Enemies? *Genes* **2019**, *10*, 534. [CrossRef] [PubMed]

47. Forte, N.; Medrihan, L.; Cappetti, B.; Baldelli, P.; Benfenati, F. 2-Deoxy-D-glucose enhances tonic inhibition through the neurosteroid-mediated activation of extrasynaptic GABA$_A$ receptors. *Epilepsia* **2016**, *57*, 1987–2000. [CrossRef] [PubMed]

48. Hartman, A.L.; Gasior, M.; Vining, E.P.; Rogawski, M.A. The neuropharmacology of the ketogenic diet. *Pediatr. Neurol.* **2007**, *36*, 281–292. [CrossRef] [PubMed]

49. Carver, C.M.; Reddy, D.S. Neurosteroid interactions with synaptic and extrasynaptic GABAA receptors: Regulation of subunit plasticity, phasic and tonic inhibition, and neuronal network excitability. *Psychopharmacology* **2013**, *230*, 151–188. [CrossRef] [PubMed]

50. Thompson, R.S.; Vargas, F.; Dorrestein, P.C.; Chichlowski, M.; Berg, B.M.; Fleshner, M. Dietary prebiotics alter novel microbial dependent fecal metabolites that improve sleep. *Sci. Rep.* **2020**, *10*. [CrossRef] [PubMed]

51. Millichap, J.G.; Yee, M.M. The diet factor in attention-deficit/hyperactivity disorder. *Pediatrics* **2012**, *129*, 330–337. [CrossRef] [PubMed]

52. Lindefeldt, M.; Eng, A.; Darban, H.; Bjerkner, A.; Zetterstrom, C.K.; Allander, T.; Andersson, B.; Borenstein, E.; Dahlin, M.; Prast-Nielsen, S. The ketogenic diet influences taxonomic and functional composition of the gut microbiota in children with severe epilepsy. *NPJ Biofilms Microbiomes* **2019**, *5*. [CrossRef]

53. Zhang, Y.; Zhou, S.; Zhou, Y.; Yu, L.; Zhang, L.; Wang, Y. Altered gut microbiome composition in children with refractory epilepsy after ketogenic diet. *Epilepsy Res.* **2018**, *145*, 163–168. [CrossRef]

54. Xie, G.; Zhou, Q.; Qiu, C.Z.; Dai, W.K.; Wang, H.P.; Li, Y.H.; Liao, J.X.; Lu, X.G.; Lin, S.F.; Ye, J.H.; et al. Ketogenic diet poses a significant effect on imbalanced gut microbiota in infants with refractory epilepsy. *World J. Gastroenterol.* **2017**, *23*, 6164–6171. [CrossRef]

55. Newell, C.; Bomhof, M.R.; Reimer, R.A.; Hittel, D.S.; Rho, J.M.; Shearer, J. Ketogenic diet modifies the gut microbiota in a murine model of autism spectrum disorder. *Mol. Autism* **2016**, *7*, 37. [CrossRef]

56. Swidsinski, A.; Dorffel, Y.; Loening-Baucke, V.; Gille, C.; Goktas, O.; Reisshauer, A.; Neuhaus, J.; Weylandt, K.H.; Guschin, A.; Bock, M. Reduced mass and diversity of the colonic microbiome in patients with multiple sclerosis and their improvement with ketogenic diet. *Front. Microbiol.* **2017**, *8*, 1141. [CrossRef] [PubMed]

57. Murtaza, N.; Burke, L.M.; Vlahovich, N.; Charlesson, B.; O'Neill, H.; Ross, M.L.; Campbell, K.L.; Krause, L.; Morrison, M. The effects of dietary pattern during intensified training on stool microbiota of elite race walkers. *Nutrients* **2019**, *11*, 261. [CrossRef] [PubMed]

58. Ma, D.; Wang, A.C.; Parikh, I.; Green, S.J.; Hoffman, J.D.; Chlipala, G.; Murphy, M.P.; Sokola, B.S.; Bauer, B.; Hartz, A.M.S.; et al. Ketogenic diet enhances neurovascular function with altered gut microbiome in young healthy mice. *Sci. Rep.* **2018**, *8*, 6670. [CrossRef] [PubMed]

59. Sullivan, P.G.; Rippy, N.A.; Dorenbos, K.; Conception, R.C.; Agarwal, A.K.; Rho, J.M. The ketogenic diet increases mitochondrial uncoupling protein levels and activity. *Ann Neurol.* **2004**, *55*, 576–580. [CrossRef] [PubMed]

60. Veech, R.L. The therapeutic implications of ketone bodies: The effects of ketone bodies in pathological conditions: Ketosis, ketogenic diet, redox states, insulin resistance, and mitochondrial metabolism. *Prostaglandins Leukot. Essent. Fatty Acids* **2004**, *70*, 309–319. [CrossRef] [PubMed]

61. Lakhan, S.E.; Vieira, K.F. Nutritional therapies for mental disorders. *Nutr. J.* **2008**, *7*, 2. [CrossRef] [PubMed]

62. Lim, S.Y.; Kim, E.J.; Kim, A.; Lee, H.J.; Choi, H.J.; Yang, S.J. Nutritional factors affecting mental health. *Clin. Nutr. Res.* **2016**, *5*, 143–152. [CrossRef]

63. Freeman, M.P.; Hibbeln, J.R.; Wisner, K.L.; Davis, J.M.; Mischoulon, D.; Peet, M.; Keck, P.E.; Marangell, L.B., Jr.; Richardson, A.J.; Lake, J.; et al. Omega-3 fatty acids: Evidence basis for treatment and future research in psychiatry. *J. Clin. Psychiatry* **2006**, *67*, 1954–1967. [CrossRef]

64. Martinez-Cengotitabengoa, M.; González-Pinto, A. Nutritional supplements in depressive disorders. *Actas Esp. Psiquiatr.* **2017**, *45*, 8–15.

65. Bodnar, L.M.; Wisner, K.L. Nutrition and Depression: Implications for Improving Mental Health Among Childbearing-Aged Women. *Biol. Psychiatry* **2005**, *58*, 679–685. [CrossRef]

66. Schweren, L.J.S.; Larsson, H.; Vinke, P.C.; Li, L.; Kvalvik, L.G.; Arias-Vasquez, A.; Haavik, J.; Hartman, C.A. Diet quality, stress and common mental health problems: A cohort study of 121,008 adults. *Clin. Nutr.* **2020**. [CrossRef] [PubMed]

67. Murphy, M.; Mercer, J.G. Diet-Regulated Anxiety. *Int. J. Endocrinol.* **2013**, *2013*, 701967. [CrossRef] [PubMed]

68. Bot, M.; Brouwer, I.A.; Roca, M.; Kohls, E.; Penninx, B.W.J.H.; Watkins, E.; van Grootheest, G.; Cabout, M.; Hegerl, U.; Gili, M.; et al. Effect of Multinutrient Supplementation and Food-Related Behavioral Activation Therapy on Prevention of Major Depressive Disorder Among Overweight or Obese Adults with Subsyndromal Depressive Symptoms. The MooDFOOD Randomized Clinical Trial. *JAMA* **2019**, *321*, 858–868. [CrossRef] [PubMed]

69. Jacka, F.N.; Pasco, J.A.; Mykletun, A.; Williams, L.J.; Hodge, A.M.; O'Reilly, S.L.; Nicholson, G.C.; Kotowicz, M.A.; Berk, M. Association of Western and traditional diets with depression and anxiety in women. *Am. J. Psychiatry* **2010**, *167*, 305–311. [CrossRef] [PubMed]

70. Davison, K.M.; Kaplan, B.J. Food intake and blood cholesterol levels of community-based adults with mood disorders. *Davison Kaplan BMC Psychiatry* **2012**, *12*. [CrossRef] [PubMed]

71. Von Geijer, L.; Ekelund, M. Ketoacidosis associated with low-carbohydrate diet in a non-diabetic lactating woman: A case report. *J. Med. Case Rep.* **2015**, *9*, 224. [CrossRef] [PubMed]

Publisher's Note: MDPI stays neutral with regard to jurisdictional claims in published maps and institutional affiliations.

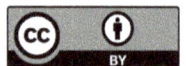

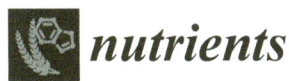

Article

Influence of Dietary Habits and Mediterranean Diet Adherence on Sleep Quality during Pregnancy. The GESTAFIT Project

Marta Flor-Alemany [1,2,3], Teresa Nestares [1,2,*], Inmaculada Alemany-Arrebola [4],
Nuria Marín-Jiménez [3,5], Milkana Borges-Cosic [3,5] and Virginia A. Aparicio [1,3]

[1] Department of Physiology, University of Granada, 18071 Granada, Spain; floralemany@ugr.es (M.F.-A.);
    virginiaparicio@ugr.es (V.A.A.)
[2] Institute of Nutrition and Food Technology (INYTA), Biomedical Research Centre (CIBM),
    University of Granada, 18016 Granada, Spain
[3] Sport and Health University Research Institute (IMUDS), 18007 Granada, Spain;
    nuriaproyecto@gmail.com (N.M.-J.); milkanaa@hotmail.com (M.B.-C.)
[4] Department of Developmental and Educational Psychology, Faculty of Education and Sports Sciences,
    University of Granada, 52005 Melilla, Spain; alemany@ugr.es
[5] Department of Physical Education and Sport, Faculty of Sport Sciences, University of Granada,
    18071 Granada, Spain
*   Correspondence: nestares@ugr.es; Tel.: +34-696989989

Received: 15 October 2020; Accepted: 17 November 2020; Published: 20 November 2020

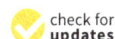

Abstract: We examined the association of the dietary habits and the Mediterranean diet (MD) adherence with sleep quality during pregnancy. A food frequency questionnaire and the Mediterranean Food Pattern were employed to assess dietary habits and MD adherence, respectively. Sleep quality was assessed with the Pittsburgh Sleep Quality Index (PSQI) global score ($n = 150$; mean age 32.9 ± 4.6 years). A higher consumption of fruits was associated with better sleep quality at the 16th gestational week (g.w.; $p < 0.05$). A greater olive oil consumption and a higher MD adherence were associated with better sleep quality at the 16th and 34th g.w. (all, $p < 0.05$). Contrarily, a higher red meat and subproducts consumption was associated with worse sleep quality at the 34th g.w. ($p < 0.05$). The group with the highest adherence to the MD (Tertile 3) showed better sleep quality than the group with the lowest adherence (Tertile 1) at the 16th and 34th g.w. (both, $p < 0.05$). A higher adherence to the MD, a greater intake of fruits and olive oil and a lower intake of red meat and subproducts were associated with better sleep quality along the pregnancy course, especially among sedentary women.

Keywords: dietary pattern; gestation; diet; sleep quality; Pittsburgh sleep quality index

1. Introduction

Sleep disturbances are common complaints during pregnancy, with recent studies suggesting that almost 50% of expectant mothers experience poor sleep quality, with rates close to 75% by the third trimester of pregnancy [1–3]. Assessments of sleep quality during pregnancy might be clinically relevant given the evidence that poor sleep quality is linked with an array of adverse health outcomes including inflammation, metabolic syndrome and type 2 diabetes [1,4–6]. Moreover, recent hypotheses suggest that poor sleep quality is associated with negative birth outcomes such as increased odds of preterm birth, caesarean section, shorter length of gestation and longer labor [1,6,7], whereas good sleep quality is associated with a better Apgar score among neonates and birth weight [8].

Considering the impact of sleep-related habits on adverse health outcomes, it is crucial to investigate and identify potential dietary determinants of sleep quality during pregnancy [9]. Among the many factors studied that could exert an influence on sleep quality, diet seems to have an impact on both sleep quality and its related health outcomes [4]. Indeed, sleep and diet are strongly interrelated, with recent studies [4,10–12] suggesting a bi-directional association: poor sleep quality may negatively affect dietary habits by reducing overall diet quality and increasing appetite and caloric intake [11], while at the same time food choices might influence sleep quality [12]. With this in mind, poorer dietary patterns, such as those characterized by a high fat and sugar content, have been linked to worse sleep quality in all age groups [13–15]. On the contrary, cross-sectional studies [9,11,16] have shown that diets with a high intake of fruits and vegetables and a lower intake of saturated fatty acids, such as the Mediterranean diet (MD), might be beneficial for sleep quality in the adult population. Although these observations helped to establish a sleep–diet relation, little is known about how the MD adherence and its components may be linked to measures of sleep quality in pregnant women. Therefore, the aim of the present study was to explore the association of dietary habits and the MD adherence with sleep quality during pregnancy.

2. Materials and Methods

2.1. Study Design and Participants

The present cross-sectional study forms part of the GESTAFIT project, where a novel exercise intervention was conducted [17]. The entire methodology of the project, the inclusion–exclusion criteria and the sample size calculation to detect clinically meaningful changes in the intervention program have been published elsewhere [17]. The required sample size was only determined for the primary outcome (maternal weight gains and maternal/neonatal glycemic profile) of the GESTAFIT project. A total of 159 Spanish pregnant women (32.9 ± 4.6 years old) enrolled in this study in three waves (from November 2015 to March 2017), for feasibility reasons. The participants were recruited between the 11th to 13th gestational weeks (g.w.) at the "San Cecilio" University Hospital (Granada, Spain) during their first gynecologist checkup. This study was approved by the Ethics Committee on Clinical Research of Granada, Regional Government of Andalusia, Spain (code: GESFIT-0448-N-15). The procedures described in the manuscript have been carried out in accordance with the Code of Ethics of the World Medical Association (Declaration of Helsinki). From the 159 pregnant women recruited, this cross-sectional study included 150 women (mean age 32.9 ± 4.6 years) at the 16th g.w. who had valid data in the food frequency questionnaire and the Pittsburgh Sleep Quality Index (PSQI; Figure 1). From the 150 pregnant women, 32 had missing data in the food frequency questionnaire and/or the PSQI global score at the 34th g.w. As a result, a total of 118 pregnant women were included for the present analyses at the 34th g.w.

2.2. Sociodemographic Characteristics

The evaluation procedures were carried out at the 16th and 34th g.w. at the Sport and Health University Research Institute (iMUDS). The assessments were conducted in a single day. At the 16th g.w., data regarding sociodemographic and lifestyle characteristics (i.e., age; educational, marital and working status; number of children; smoking habit and physical or psychological disease diagnosis) were collected through an initial survey (anamnesis).

2.3. Maternal Anthropometry and Body Composition

Pre-pregnancy body weight was self-reported. Body weight and height were measured using a scale (InBody R20; Biospace, Seoul, Korea) and a stadiometer (Seca 22, Hamburg, Germany), respectively. Those measurements were employed to calculate pre-gestational body mass index and body mass index at the 16th gestational week as weight (kg) divided by squared height (m^2).

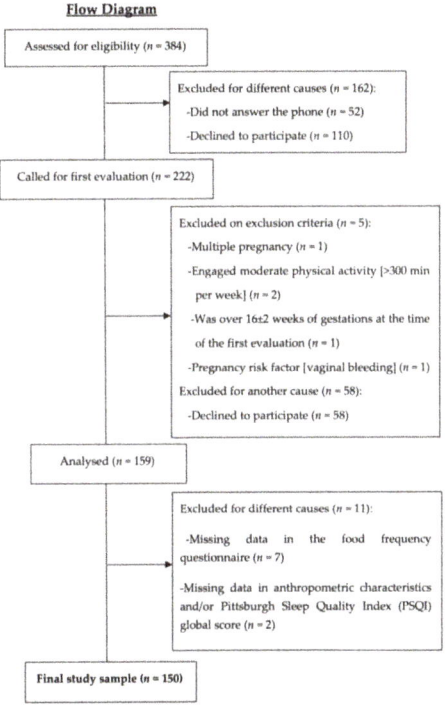

Figure 1. Flow diagram of the study participants.

2.4. Dietary Assessment

Dietary habits were collected by using the food frequency questionnaire designed by Mataix et al. [18]. The same trained nutritionist administered the questionnaires to pregnant women at the 16th and 34th g.w.

The Mediterranean Food Pattern (MFP; a Mediterranean adherence score) was constructed with the data obtained from the food frequency questionnaire [18]. We employed this dietary index because it was previously associated with lower cardiometabolic risk along the pregnancy course in this study sample (submitted data). The MFP was calculated based on previously published literature [19]. It consists of eight elements (olive oil, fiber, fruits, vegetables, fish, cereals, meat and alcohol) ranging from 5 to 40. Notwithstanding, alcohol consumption was not considered when calculating the total score. Thus, the maximum score ranges from 4 to 35, where higher scores indicate greater MD adherence.

2.5. Sleep Quality

The Spanish version of the PSQI [20] was employed to assess sleep quality, since the PSQI has been shown to have a good construct validity among pregnant women [21]. The PSQI is a self-rated questionnaire that measures sleep quality from the previous month, comprising 19 questions divided into seven categories: subjective sleep quality, sleep latency, sleep duration, sleep disturbances, sleep efficiency, use of sleep medication and daytime dysfunction. Each component scores from 0 to 3, with a total score that ranges from 0 to 21 with lower values indicating better sleep quality [20]. The suggested cutoff is 5 points differentiating "good" from "bad" sleepers [20].

2.6. Statistical Analyses

Descriptive statistics (mean (standard deviation) for quantitative variables, and number of women (%) for categorical variables) were employed to describe participants' sociodemographic characteristics. The distribution of the data was examined for all the study variables, and the PSQI global score showed a skewed distribution that could not be normalized after several transformations (e.g., logarithmic transformations). Subsequently, we performed Spearman's correlation analysis between the dietary habits, the MFP score and the PSQI global score at the 16th and 34th g.w. Differences between dietary habits, MFP and PSQI global score by the g.w. (16th g.w. versus 34th g.w.) were tested using the Wilcoxon nonparametric test. The PSQI global score was compared across tertiles using the Kruskal–Wallis test. Post-hoc multiple comparisons with Bonferroni's correction were applied to examine pairwise differences between groups (e.g., Tertile 1 vs. Tertile 3). In order to avoid the discrepancies noted in the literature among the large range of cutoff points for the different tools employed to assess dietary patterns during pregnancy, the MFP was also dichotomized using the 50th percentile with participants being categorized as having low or high adherence, as performed in previous studies [22,23] (Figure S1). Subsequently, the PSQI global score was compared between these dietary indices groups by using the Mann–Whitney U nonparametric test. We performed additional analyses to further explore whether several factors including pre-gestational BMI and the concurrent physical exercise program, which was carried out in the GESTAFIT project [17], exerted an influence on the studied associations. Spearman's correlations were employed to assess the association between the dietary habits, the MFP and the PSQI global score at the 16th and 34th g.w. according to pre-gestational BMI categories and exercise intervention (intervention or control). All analyses were performed using the Statistical Package for Social Sciences (IBM SPSS Statistics for Windows, version 22.0, Armonk, NY, USA); the level of significance was set at $p < 0.05$.

3. Results

Sociodemographic characteristics of the participants are shown in Table 1.

Spearman's correlation analysis assessing the association of dietary habits and the MD adherence with the PSQI global score at the 16th and 34th g.w. is shown in Table 2. At the 16th g.w., a higher consumption of fruits, olive oil and a higher MD adherence were associated with a lower PSQI global score (i.e., better sleep quality; $p = 0.008$, $p = 0.048$ and $p = 0.039$, respectively). In addition, a higher red meat and subproducts consumption was associated with a higher PSQI global score with borderline significance (i.e., worse sleep quality; $p = 0.078$). At the 34th g.w., a higher consumption of olive oil and a higher MD adherence were associated with a lower PSQI global score ($p = 0.038$ and $p = 0.001$, respectively). A higher red meat and subproducts consumption was associated with a greater PSQI global score ($p = 0.032$).

The PSQI global score at the 16th and 34th g.w. by tertiles of the MFP is shown in Figure 2. Pairwise comparisons showed that the group with the highest score (Tertile 3) in the MFP had a lower PSQI global score than the group with the lowest score (Tertile 1) at the 16th g.w. and 34th g.w. ($p = 0.038$ and $p = 0.005$, respectively).

The PSQI global score at the 16th and 34th g.w. according to the 50th percentile of the MFP [19] is shown in Figure S1. The group with the highest score (above the 50th percentile) in the MFP [19] had a lower PSQI global score than the group with the lowest score (below the 50th percentile) at the 16th and 34th g.w. ($p = 0.008$ and $p = 0.005$, respectively).

Differences between the dietary habits, the MFP and the PSQI global score by g.w. (16th g.w. versus 34th g.w.) are shown in Table S1. Regarding dietary habits, pregnant women at the 34th g.w. had higher intake of fruits, vegetables and whole dairy products ($p = 0.010$, $p = 0.014$ and $p = 0.044$, respectively). No differences were found regarding MFP adherence ($p > 0.05$). In addition, pregnant women at the 34th g.w. had a higher PSQI global score ($p < 0.001$).

Table 1. Descriptive characteristics of the study participants ($n = 150$).

Variable	Mean (SD)
Age (years)	32.9 (4.6)
Pre-gestational body mass index categorization ($n = 136$)	
Normal weight (n %)	87 (64.0)
Overweight (n %)	34 (25.0)
Obese (n %)	11 (11.0)
16th gestational week	
Body mass index (kg/m^2; $n = 148$)	24.9 (4.1)
Pittsburgh Sleep Quality Index global score (0–21)	6.01 (3.2)
Poor sleep quality (n %)	72 (48.0)
Mediterranean Food Pattern (4–35)	20.6 (5.1)
34th gestational week ($n = 118$)	
Pittsburgh Sleep Quality Index global score (0–21)	8.83 (3.76)
Poor sleep quality (n %)	89 (75.4)
Mediterranean Food Pattern (4–35)	21.1 (5.4)
Educational Status	n (%)
Non-university studies	62 (41.3)
University studies	88 (58.7)
Marital status	
Single/divorced	62 (41.3)
Married	88 (58.7)
Working status	
Not working (unemployed/homework/student/sick leave)	48 (32.0)
Part-time employment/full-time employment	102 (68.0)
Number of children	
0	90 (60.0)
1 or more	60 (40.0)
Smoking status ((yes, n (%))	13 (8.7)
Physical or psychological disease diagnosis ((yes, n (%))	61 (40.7)

Values shown as mean (SD) unless otherwise indicated. SD—standard deviation.

Table 2. Association between the Mediterranean Food Pattern and the Mediterranean diet components with the Pittsburgh Sleep Quality Index global score at the 16th gestational week ($n = 150$) and 34th gestational week ($n = 118$).

Food Groups	PSQI Global Score [a] (16th Gestational Week)	PSQI Global Score [a] (34th Gestational Week)
Whole-grain cereals (s/week)	−0.056	−0.158
Potatoes (s/week)	−0.012	0.099
Fruits (s/day)	−0.216 **	−0.126
Vegetables (s/day)	−0.025	−0.089
Pulses (s/week)	0.112	0.043
Fish (s/week)	0.032	−0.087
Red meat and subproducts (s/week)	0.144	0.198 *
Poultry (s/week)	0.064	0.101
Whole dairy products (s/week)	0.012	−0.094
Olive oil (s/week)	−0.162 *	−0.192 *
Nuts (s/week)	−0.096	−0.160
Sweets (s/week)	0.048	0.138
Mediterranean Food Pattern (4–35)	−0.169 *	−0.301 **

[a] A higher score means worse sleep quality. PSQI—Pittsburgh Sleep Quality Index; s—servings. * $p < 0.05$; ** $p < 0.01$.

The association between the dietary habits, the MFP and the PSQI global score at the 16th and 34th g.w. according to pre-pregnancy BMI categories and the exercise intervention (intervention or control) are shown in Tables S2 and S3. In the control group, a higher consumption of fruits was associated with better sleep quality at the 16th g.w. ($p < 0.01$). Olive oil and a higher MFP were associated with better sleep quality at the 16th and 34th g.w. (all, $p < 0.05$). All the previous associations were not significant in the intervention group ($p > 0.05$). Regarding pre-pregnancy BMI categories, a higher intake of fruits and olive oil were associated with better sleep quality at the 16th g.w. in normal-weight pregnant women and overweight/obese participants, respectively (both, $p < 0.05$). At the 34th g.w. a higher intake of olive oil and MD adherence were associated with better sleep quality among normal-weight participants (both, $p < 0.05$). A higher MD adherence was associated with better sleep quality in overweight/obese participants at the 34th g.w. ($p < 0.05$).

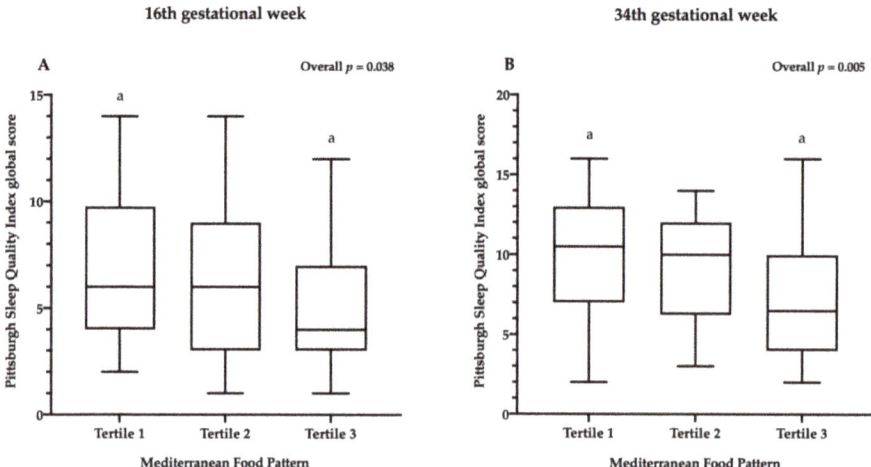

Figure 2. Pittsburgh Sleep Quality Index global score by tertiles of Mediterranean Food Pattern adherence. Box plots demonstrating median, upper and lower quartiles and the minimum and maximum Pittsburgh Sleep Quality Index global scores at the 16th ($n = 150$) and 34th ($n = 118$) gestational weeks. a—indicates a significant difference ($p < 0.05$) between groups. Pairwise comparisons were performed with Bonferroni's adjustment. (**A**) Pittsburgh Sleep Quality Index global score by the Mediterranean Food Pattern tertiles at the 16th gestational week. (**B**) Pittsburgh Sleep Quality Index global score by the Mediterranean Food Pattern tertiles at the 34th gestational week.

Differences between the PSQI global score by exercise intervention (control versus intervention) are shown in Table S4. No differences between groups were found regarding the PSQI global score by exercise intervention ($p > 0.05$).

4. Discussion

The main finding of the present study is that a greater adherence to the MD was associated with better sleep quality during both the 16th and 34th g.w., especially among sedentary pregnant women. In addition, a greater consumption of fruits and olive oil and a lower intake of red meat and subproducts (i.e., beef, pork, viscera and cold meat products) were associated with better sleep quality along gestation. Moreover, pregnant women with the highest adherence to the Mediterranean dietary pattern (Tertile 3) showed better sleep quality than the groups with the lowest scores (Tertile 1) during both the 16th and 34th g.w.

Sleep quality is often compromised in pregnant women and aggravated over the course of pregnancy [24]. A recent study [25] reported that 47% of pregnant women had poor sleep quality (as measured by the PSQI) between the 12th and 20th g.w., similar to our results for the 16th g.w. (48%). Moreover, sleep quality significantly decreased from second to third trimester, with 75% of pregnant women reporting poor sleep quality at the 34th g.w., which is in agreement with a previous study that showed that 75–83% of pregnant women had poor sleep quality in the third trimester of pregnancy (7–8 months) [3].

Comparing the early second trimester with the third trimester, we observed a significantly higher intake of fruits, vegetables and dairy products in the third trimester, as previously reported [26]. It is possible that participants might have increased their fruit, vegetable and dairy product intakes due to nutritional advice, which usually promotes fruit, vegetable and dairy consumption in order to meet the nutritional requirements of pregnancy [27]. However, our results showed that adherence to the Mediterranean diet remained unchanged across pregnancy. This finding suggests that food behavior of our sample did not change during gestation, which concurs with previous studies [28,29]. Moreover, during early gestation, food intake can be often affected by nausea and vomiting, physiological phenomena linked to hormonal changes during this period [30]. However, women recruited in this study were all past the 13th week of gestation, which could partially explain the lack of differences between food habits between different gestational stages.

It has been established that poor sleep quality negatively affects dietary habits by reducing overall diet quality and increasing appetite and caloric intake [11]. Notwithstanding, recent data also suggest a bi-directional association by which food choices might positively influence sleep quality [12]. Recent studies [9,11] showed an association between the adherence to the Mediterranean dietary pattern and sleep quality, suggesting that plant-rich diets might be beneficial for sleep in the adult population. However, evidence in pregnant women is scarce. A study conducted by Chang et al. [31] on overweight and obese pregnant women showed direct associations between sleep disturbances and dietary fat intake and also between shorter time taken to fall asleep and a higher fruit and vegetable intake. Nonetheless, neither diet quality nor dietary patterns were included in these studies. In agreement with our findings, a more recent study [24] showed that better sleep quality was associated with greater diet quality and a greater adherence to a dietary pattern based on fruits, vegetables and rice. In the present study sample, a higher MD (a diet high in fruits, vegetables and fiber and low in saturated fatty acids) adherence was associated with better sleep quality over the course of pregnancy.

Further, participants with the highest MD adherence (Tertile 3) had better sleep quality during the pregnancy course than the groups with the lowest scores (Tertile 1). This concurs with a previous study in a non-pregnant adult population in which individuals with a greater adherence to the Mediterranean dietary pattern presented overall better sleep quality compared to those with less adherence [9]. Moreover, if such an eating pattern influences sleep during pregnancy, it is not clear which specific component or components of the Mediterranean dietary pattern would exert a stronger influence. To further explore this issue, we also studied the different food groups that comprise the Mediterranean dietary pattern, finding that a higher intake of fruits and olive oil and a lower intake of red meat and subproducts were associated with better sleep quality during pregnancy. A previous study [9] checked if any of the MD components alone could explain the association of the MD score with better sleep quality, suggesting that olive oil consumption itself might play an independent role in sleep quality, which is highly in agreement with our results. Regarding fruits, it has been suggested that the odds of meeting or exceeding the sleep recommendations (i.e., 7–9 h per day for adults aged 18–64 years old) increase by 12% in pregnant women for every additional fruit serving consumed [32]. Similarly, a study conducted in women within 5 years of childbirth found that women with longer sleep duration (≥ 9 h) had poorer overall diet quality, a lower intake of fruits and a higher intake of calories from solid fats and added sugar, compared to women with an adequate sleep duration (7–8 h) [33]. Evidence also suggests that diets rich in fats and carbohydrates, with a tendency to include snacks between meals, are associated with poorer sleep quality and fewer sleeping hours in the general population [13,14,34]. The MFP, which was employed to calculate the MD adherence, does not directly assess sugary food intake. For this reason, the sweets variable (including soft drinks, preserved juices, biscuits, baked goods and chocolate) was additionally calculated, as it represents an important component of unhealthy dietary habits. Sweets intake in this study sample was slightly greater than one serving per day, an amount that is within the recommended intake of sugary foods (< 3 servings/day) accordingly to the final nutritional objectives for Spanish population [35]. This result could be due to the limitation of the items of the food frequency questionnaire itself or to underreporting but could also be derived from the wish of the mothers to follow healthier dietary patterns during pregnancy, avoiding highly processed foods. Moreover, the observed lower sugary food intake in this group could also explain why no correlations were found between them and the PSQI global score.

In this study sample, a higher intake of red meat and subproducts were associated with poorer sleep quality along gestation. Similarly, a study conducted by Lana et al. [36] suggested that a high protein intake derived from meat (white or red meat) was associated with poor sleep quality in the non-pregnant adult population. The detrimental effect of red meat and subproducts on sleep quality might be exerted through the protein content of meat as previously stated [36]. The effects of protein on sleep quality could be related to two amino acids (tryptophan and tyrosine) and their capacity to synthesize melatonin, serotonin and dopamine (involved in the sleep–wake cycle) [36]. It has been suggested that a high consumption of protein could reduce the blood circulation ratio of tryptophan/tyrosine, which could result in a lower synthesis of brain sleep inductors and consequently a deterioration of sleep parameters, which is in agreement with our findings [36–38]. Other food groups that are naturally rich in protein and were tested in this study (e.g., dairy, poultry) did not show significant results between them and the PSQI global score. Due to the fact that red meat and subproducts intake was the most consumed group of meat, this finding might overlap the potential influence of other sources of animal protein.

Previous literature showed that BMI and exercise were associated with sleep quality [39–41]. We further studied how these variables affected the association between MD adherence and sleep quality. We found that a higher intake of fruits and olive oil (at the 16th g.w.) and a higher consumption of olive oil and a higher MD adherence (at the 34th g.w.) were associated with better sleep quality independently of pre-pregnancy BMI categories. Regarding the exercise intervention, we found that in the control group a higher consumption of fruits, olive oil and a higher MD adherence were associated with better sleep quality along the pregnancy course. Nevertheless, all of the previous associations disappeared in the intervention group, suggesting that the diet was more effective in improving sleep quality in the control sedentary group. This might be partially explained by the effect that the exercise training could have had by itself regardless of maternal diet. Previous studies [42,43] have reported that after a period of 8–10 weeks of concurrent training, sleep quality improved, suggesting that the improvements could lead to a state of the melatonin hormone being secreted by the allergic pineal glands, which has a hypnotizing effect with central body temperature. Anabolic activity is also stronger during sleep, whereas the catabolic activity is more intense during vigilance. Therefore, for a possible balance of energy, the body consumes more energy to relax, and the body tends to increase sleep duration.

It has been suggested that the high isoflavone and tryptophan content of plant-based diets (e.g., Mediterranean diets) may be the mechanism by which plant foods enhance sleep quality [11]. Interestingly, in a subsample of participants from the PREDIMED study, participants in the two Mediterranean diet groups showed an increment in tryptophan concentrations, and this was related to lower non-stroke outcomes [44]. The authors suggested that changes in tryptophan may be involved in the cardioprotective effects of the Mediterranean diet [44]. Sleep and sleep-related metabolite derivatives of tryptophan, melatonin and serotonin were not measured in this study. Nevertheless, given our understanding of tryptophan metabolism, sleep improvements may have further played a role in this result [11].

When considering the results of the present study, some limitations ought to be kept in mind. Firstly, the cross-sectional design of the study provides information without a clear cause–effect identification. As a result, we cannot determine whether a healthier diet affects sleep quality or, on the contrary, sleep features lead to unhealthy dietary behaviors. Secondly, since we employed a food frequency questionnaire in order to assess dietary habits, we are aware of its recall bias and its lower accuracy when compared to a 24 h food diary. Nonetheless, the food frequency questionnaire (which is widely employed in nutritional epidemiology) was conducted by the same trained nutritionist along the pregnancy course. Importantly, both sleep quality and the dietary adherence were self-reported.

While PSQI is a widely employed tool validated in pregnant population [21], it is not as valid as an objective measure of sleep such as polysomnography.

5. Conclusions

The present study provides some evidence linking the Mediterranean dietary pattern to better sleep quality during pregnancy, especially among sedentary women. Specifically, a higher intake of fruits and olive oil, a lower intake of red meat and subproducts and a greater adherence to the Mediterranean dietary pattern are associated with better sleep quality along the pregnancy course. Given the limited number of studies available, further research is warranted to explore the impact of maternal healthy dietary habits on sleep quality during pregnancy and investigate causality and its mechanisms. Intervention studies are warranted to explore whether plant-based diets (e.g., the Mediterranean dietary pattern) might positively influence sleep quality during gestation.

Supplementary Materials: The following are available online at http://www.mdpi.com/2072-6643/12/11/3569/s1, Figure S1. Pittsburgh Sleep Quality Index global score by Mediterranean Food Pattern adherence; Table S1. Differences in the dietary habits, the Mediterranean Food Pattern and the Pittsburgh Sleep Quality Index global score of pregnant women by gestational week (16th versus 34th gestational weeks) (*n* = 117); Table S2. Association between Mediterranean Food Pattern and Mediterranean diet components with the Pittsburgh Sleep Quality Index global score at the 16th gestational week and 34th gestational week according to pre-pregnancy body mass index categorization; Table S3. Association between Mediterranean Food Pattern and Mediterranean diet components with the Pittsburgh Sleep Quality Index global score at the 16th gestation week and 34th gestational week for the control group and the intervention groups; Table S4. Differences in the Pittsburgh Sleep Quality Index global score of pregnant women at the 34th gestational week by exercise intervention (control versus intervention).

Author Contributions: Conceptualization, M.F.-A. and V.A.A.; methodology, M.F.-A. and V.A.A.; validation, M.F.-A.; T.N.; V.A.A.; N.M.-J.; M.B.-C. and I.A.-A.; formal analysis, M.F.-A. and I.A.-A.; investigation, M.F.-A.; N.M.-J. and M.B.-C.; resources, T.N. and V.A.A.; data curation, M.F.-A. and I.A.-A.; writing—original draft preparation, M.F.-A. and V.A.A.; writing—review and editing, M.F.-A.; T.N.; V.A.A.; N.M.-J.; M.B.-C. and I.A.-A.; project administration, V.A.A.; funding acquisition, T.N. and V.A.A. All authors have read and agreed to the published version of the manuscript.

Funding: This study was partially funded by the Regional Ministry of Health of the Junta de Andalucía (PI-0395-2016) and the Research and Knowledge Transfer Fund (PPIT) 2016, Excellence Actions Programme: Scientific Units of Excellence (UCEES), and the Regional Ministry of Economy, Knowledge, Enterprises and University, European Regional Development Funds (ref. SOMM17/6107/UGR). MFA was additionally funded by the Spanish Ministry of Education, Culture and Sports (Grant number FPU17/03715). This study is included in the thesis of MFA enrolled in the Doctoral Program in Nutrition and Food Sciences of the University of Granada.

Acknowledgments: We are grateful to Ana Yara Postigo-Fuentes for her assistance with the English language.

Conflicts of Interest: The authors declare no conflict of interest.

References

1. Okun, M.L.; Schetter, C.D.; Glynn, L.M. Poor sleep quality is associated with preterm birth. *Sleep* **2011**, *34*, 1493–1498. [CrossRef]
2. Sedov, I.D.; Cameron, E.E.; Madigan, S.; Tomfohr-Madsen, L.M. Sleep quality during pregnancy: A meta-analysis. *Sleep Med. Rev.* **2018**, *38*, 168–176. [CrossRef] [PubMed]
3. Mindell, J.A.; Cook, R.A.; Nikolovski, J. Sleep patterns and sleep disturbances across pregnancy. *Sleep Med.* **2015**, *16*, 483–488. [CrossRef] [PubMed]
4. Jansen, E.C.; Dunietz, G.L.; Tsimpanouli, M.-E.; Guyer, H.M.; Shannon, C.; Hershner, S.D.; O'Brien, L.M.; Baylin, A. Sleep, Diet, and Cardiometabolic Health Investigations: A Systematic Review of Analytic Strategies. *Curr. Nutr. Rep.* **2018**, *7*, 235–258. [CrossRef] [PubMed]
5. Jennings, J.R.; Muldoon, M.F.; Hall, M.; Buysse, D.J.; Manuck, S.B. Self-reported sleep quality is associated with the metabolic syndrome. *Sleep* **2007**, *30*, 219–223. [CrossRef] [PubMed]
6. Blair, L.M.; Porter, K.; Leblebicioglu, B.; Christian, L.M. Poor Sleep Quality and Associated Inflammation Predict Preterm Birth: Heightened Risk among African Americans. *Sleep* **2015**, *38*, 1259–1267. [CrossRef]
7. Naghi, I.; Keypour, F.; Ahari, S.B.; Tavalai, S.A.; Khak, M. Sleep disturbance in late pregnancy and type and duration of labour. *J. Obstet. Gynaecol.* **2011**, *31*, 489–491. [CrossRef]

8.   Zafarghandi, N.; Hadavand, S.; Davati, A.; Mohseni, S.M.; Kimiaiimoghadam, F.; Torkestani, F. The effects of sleep quality and duration in late pregnancy on labor and fetal outcome. *J. Matern. Neonatal Med.* **2012**, *25*, 535–537. [CrossRef]

9.   Godos, J.; Ferri, R.; Caraci, F.; Cosentino, F.I.I.; Castellano, S.; Galvano, F.; Grosso, G. Adherence to the Mediterranean Diet is Associated with Better Sleep Quality in Italian Adults. *Nutrients* **2019**, *11*, 976. [CrossRef]

10. St-Onge, M.-P.; Zuraikat, F.M. Reciprocal Roles of Sleep and Diet in Cardiovascular Health: A Review of Recent Evidence and a Potential Mechanism. *Curr. Atheroscler. Rep.* **2019**, *21*, 11. [CrossRef]

11. St-Onge, M.-P.; Crawford, A.; Aggarwal, B. Plant-based diets: Reducing cardiovascular risk by improving sleep quality? *Curr. Sleep Med. Rep.* **2018**, *4*, 74–78. [CrossRef] [PubMed]

12. St-Onge, M.-P.; Roberts, A.; Shechter, A.; Choudhury, A.R. Fiber and Saturated Fat Are Associated with Sleep Arousals and Slow Wave Sleep. *J. Clin. Sleep Med. Jcsm Off. Publ. Am. Acad. Sleep Med.* **2016**, *12*, 19–24. [CrossRef] [PubMed]

13. Peuhkuri, K.; Sihvola, N.; Korpela, R. Diet promotes sleep duration and quality. *Nutr. Res.* **2012**, *32*, 309–319. [CrossRef] [PubMed]

14. Chaput, J.-P. Sleep patterns, diet quality and energy balance. *Physiol. Behav.* **2014**, *134*, 86–91. [CrossRef]

15. St-Onge, M.-P.; Mikic, A.; Pietrolungo, C.E. Effects of Diet on Sleep Quality. *Adv. Nutr.* **2016**, *7*, 938–949. [CrossRef] [PubMed]

16. Campanini, M.Z.; Guallar-Castillón, P.; Rodríguez-Artalejo, F.; Lopez-Garcia, E. Mediterranean Diet and Changes in Sleep Duration and Indicators of Sleep Quality in Older Adults. *Sleep* **2017**, *40*. [CrossRef]

17. Aparicio, V.A.; Ocon, O.; Padilla-Vinuesa, C.; Soriano-Maldonado, A.; Romero-Gallardo, L.; Borges-Cosic, M.; Coll-Risco, I.; Ruiz-Cabello, P.; Acosta-Manzano, P.; Estevez-Lopez, F.; et al. Effects of supervised aerobic and strength training in overweight and grade I obese pregnant women on maternal and foetal health markers: The GESTAFIT randomized controlled trial. *Bmc Pregnancy Childbirth* **2016**, *16*, 290. [CrossRef]

18. Mataix, J.L.; Martinez de Victoria, E.; Montellano, M.A.; Lopez, M.; Aranda, P.L. *Valoración del estado nutricional de la comunidad autónoma de Andalucía*; Consejería de Salud de la Junta de Andalucía: Sevilla, Spain, 2000.

19. Martinez-Gonzalez, M.A.; Fernandez-Jarne, E.; Serrano-Martinez, M.; Marti, A.; Martinez, J.A.; Martin-Moreno, J.M. Mediterranean diet and reduction in the risk of a first acute myocardial infarction: An operational healthy dietary score. *Eur. J. Nutr.* **2002**, *41*, 153–160. [CrossRef]

20. Buysse, D.J.; Reynolds, C.F., 3rd; Monk, T.H.; Berman, S.R.; Kupfer, D.J. The Pittsburgh Sleep Quality Index: A new instrument for psychiatric practice and research. *Psychiatry Res.* **1989**, *28*, 193–213. [CrossRef]

21. Zhong, Q.Y.; Gelaye, B.; Sánchez, S.E.; Williams, M.A. Psychometric Properties of the Pittsburgh Sleep Quality Index (PSQI) in a Cohort of Peruvian Pregnant Women. *J. Clin. Sleep Med.* **2020**, *11*, 869–877. [CrossRef]

22. Papazian, T.; Serhal, A.; Hout, H.; Younes, H.; Tayeh, G.A.; Azouri, J.; Moussa Lteif, F.H.; Kesrouani, A.; Khabbaz, L.R. Discrepancies among different tools evaluating Mediterranean diet adherence during pregnancy, correlated to maternal anthropometric, dietary and biochemical characteristics. *Clin. Nutr.* **2019**, *38*, 1398–1405. [CrossRef] [PubMed]

23. Aoun, C.; Papazian, T.; Helou, K.; El Osta, N.; Khabbaz, L.R. Comparison of five international indices of adherence to the Mediterranean diet among healthy adults: Similarities and differences. *Nutr. Res. Pract.* **2019**, *13*, 333–343. [CrossRef] [PubMed]

24. van Lee, L.; Chia, A.-R.; Loy, S.L.; Colega, M.; Tham, E.K.H.; Cai, S.; Yap, F.; Godfrey, K.M.; Teoh, O.H.; Goh, D.; et al. Sleep and Dietary Patterns in Pregnancy: Findings from the GUSTO Cohort. *Int. J. Environ. Res. Public Health* **2017**, *14*, 1409. [CrossRef] [PubMed]

25. Conlon, R.P.K.; Wang, B.; Germeroth, L.J.; Cheng, Y.; Buysse, D.J.; Levine, M.D. Demographic, Pregnancy-Related, and Health-Related Factors in Association with Changes in Sleep Among Pregnant Women with Overweight or Obesity. *Int. J. Behav. Med.* **2020**. [CrossRef] [PubMed]

26. Chen, L.-W.; Low, Y.L.; Fok, D.; Han, W.M.; Chong, Y.S.; Gluckman, P.; Godfrey, K.; Kwek, K.; Saw, S.-M.; Soh, S.E.; et al. Dietary changes during pregnancy and the postpartum period in Singaporean Chinese, Malay and Indian women: The GUSTO birth cohort study. *Public Health Nutr.* **2014**, *17*, 1930–1938. [CrossRef] [PubMed]

27. Fowles, E.R. What's a Pregnant Woman to Eat? A Review of Current USDA Dietary Guidelines and MyPyramid. *J. Perinat. Educ.* **2006**, *15*, 28–33. [CrossRef] [PubMed]

28. Gesteiro, E.; Bastida, S.; Rodriguez Bernal, B.; Sanchez-Muniz, F.J. Adherence to Mediterranean diet during pregnancy and serum lipid, lipoprotein and homocysteine concentrations at birth. *Eur. J. Nutr.* **2015**, *54*, 1191–1199. [CrossRef]

29. Jardí, C.; Aparicio, E.; Bedmar, C.; Aranda, N.; Abajo, S.; March, G.; Basora, J.; Arija, V.; the ECLIPSES Study Group. Food Consumption during Pregnancy and Post-Partum. ECLIPSES Study. *Nutrients* **2019**, *11*, 2447.

30. Spadafranca, A.; Bulfoni, C.; Liguori, I.; Mastricci, L.; Bertoli, S.; Battezzati, A.; Ferrazzi, E. Adherence to Mediterranean Diet and Prevention of Excessive Weight Gain during Pregnancy: Study in a Cohort of Normal Weight Caucasian Women. *Res. Heal. Sci.* **2016**, 2. [CrossRef]

31. Chang, M.-W.; Brown, R.; Nitzke, S.; Smith, B.; Eghtedary, K. Stress, sleep, depression and dietary intakes among low-income overweight and obese pregnant women. *Matern. Child Health J.* **2015**, *19*, 1047–1059. [CrossRef]

32. Duke, C.H.; Williamson, J.A.; Snook, K.R.; Finch, K.C.; Sullivan, K.L. Association Between Fruit and Vegetable Consumption and Sleep Quantity in Pregnant Women. *Matern. Child Health J.* **2017**, *21*, 966–973. [CrossRef] [PubMed]

33. Xiao, R.S.; Moore Simas, T.A.; Pagoto, S.L.; Person, S.D.; Rosal, M.C.; Waring, M.E. Sleep Duration and Diet Quality Among Women Within 5 Years of Childbirth in the United States: A Cross-Sectional Study. *Matern. Child. Health J.* **2016**, *20*, 1869–1877. [CrossRef]

34. Dashti, H.S.; Scheer, F.A.; Jacques, P.F.; Lamon-Fava, S.; Ordovás, J.M. Short sleep duration and dietary intake: Epidemiologic evidence, mechanisms, and health implications. *Adv. Nutr.* **2015**, *6*, 648–659. [CrossRef] [PubMed]

35. Aranceta, J.; Serra-Majem, L.; Arija Val, V.; Gil Hernández, Á.; Martínez de Vitoria, E.; Ortega Anta, R.; Peña Quintana, L.; Pérez Rodrigo, C.; Quiles Izquierdo, J.; Salas i Salvadó, J.; et al. Objetivos nutricionales para la población española. *Rev. Esp. Nutr. Comunitaria* **2011**, *17*, 178–199.

36. Lana, A.; Struijk, E.A.; Arias-Fernandez, L.; Graciani, A.; Mesas, A.E.; Rodriguez-Artalejo, F.; Lopez-Garcia, E. Habitual Meat Consumption and Changes in Sleep Duration and Quality in Older Adults. *Aging Dis.* **2019**, *10*, 267–277. [CrossRef]

37. Wurtman, R.J.; Wurtman, J.J.; Regan, M.M.; McDermott, J.M.; Tsay, R.H.; Breu, J.J. Effects of normal meals rich in carbohydrates or proteins on plasma tryptophan and tyrosine ratios. *Am. J. Clin. Nutr.* **2003**, *77*, 128–132. [CrossRef] [PubMed]

38. Lindseth, G.; Murray, A. Dietary Macronutrients and Sleep. *West. J. Nurs. Res.* **2016**, *38*, 938–958. [CrossRef]

39. Kovacevic, A.; Mavros, Y.; Heisz, J.J.; Fiatarone Singh, M.A. The effect of resistance exercise on sleep: A systematic review of randomized controlled trials. *Sleep Med. Rev.* **2018**, *39*, 52–68. [CrossRef]

40. Kelley, G.A.; Kelley, K.S. Exercise and sleep. A systematic review of previous meta-analyses. *J. Evid. Based Med.* **2017**, *10*, 26–36. [CrossRef]

41. Rice, J.R.; Larrabure-Torrealva, G.T.; Luque Fernandez, M.A.; Grande, M.; Motta, V.; Barrios, Y.V.; Sanchez, S.; Gelaye, B.; Williams, M.A. High risk for obstructive sleep apnea and other sleep disorders among overweight and obese pregnant women. *Bmc Pregnancy Childbirth* **2015**, *15*, 1–8. [CrossRef]

42. Monazzami, A.; Momenpour, R.; Alipoor, E.; Yari, K.; Payandeh, M. The Effects of Concurrent Training on the Body Composition, Quality of Life, and Sleep Quality of Postmenopausal Women with Breast Cancer. *J. Kermanshah Univ. Med. Sci.* **2020**, *24*, 101186. [CrossRef]

43. Pooranfar, S.; Shakoor, E.; Shafahi, M.; Salesi, M.; Karimi, M.; Roozbeh, J.; Hasheminasab, M. The effect of exercise training on quality and quantity of sleep and lipid profile in renal transplant patients: A randomized clinical trial. *Int. J. Organ Transplant. Med.* **2014**, *5*, 157–165. [PubMed]

44. Yu, E.; Ruiz-Canela, M.; Guasch-Ferré, M.; Zheng, Y.; Toledo, E.; Clish, C.B.; Salas-Salvadó, J.; Liang, L.; Wang, D.D.; Corella, D.; et al. Increases in Plasma Tryptophan Are Inversely Associated with Incident Cardiovascular Disease in the Prevención con Dieta Mediterránea (PREDIMED) Study. *J. Nutr.* **2017**, *147*, 314–322. [CrossRef] [PubMed]

Publisher's Note: MDPI stays neutral with regard to jurisdictional claims in published maps and institutional affiliations.

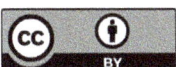

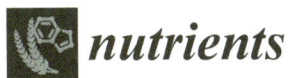

Article

The Relationship between Food Security Status and Sleep Disturbance among Adults: A Cross-Sectional Study in an Indonesian Population

Emyr Reisha Isaura [1,2,3], Yang-Ching Chen [2,4,5], Hsiu-Yueh Su [2,6,*]
and Shwu-Huey Yang [2,7,8,*]

1 Department of Nutrition, Faculty of Public Health, Airlangga University, Surabaya, East Java 60115, Indonesia; emyr.reisha@fkm.unair.ac.id
2 School of Nutrition and Health Sciences, College of Nutrition, Taipei Medical University, Taipei 11031, Taiwan; melisa26@gmail.com
3 Research Group of Food Safety and Food Security, Faculty of Public Health, Airlangga University, Surabaya, East Java 60115, Indonesia
4 Department of Family Medicine, School of Medicine, College of Medicine, Taipei Medical University, Taipei 11031, Taiwan
5 Department of Family Medicine, Taipei Medical University Hospital, Taipei 11031, Taiwan
6 Department of Dietetics, Taipei Medical University Hospital, Taipei 11031, Taiwan
7 Nutrition Research Center, Taipei Medical University Hospital, Taipei 11031, Taiwan
8 Research Center of Geriatric Nutrition, College of Nutrition, Taipei Medical University, Taipei 11031, Taiwan
* Correspondence: hysu@h.tmu.edu.tw (H.-Y.S.); sherry@tmu.edu.tw (S.-H.Y.);
Tel.: +886-2-2737-2181 (ext. 3001) (H.-Y.S.); +886-2-2736-1661 (ext. 6568) (S.-H.Y.)

Received: 10 September 2020; Accepted: 4 November 2020; Published: 6 November 2020

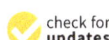

Abstract: Background: The relationship between food insecurity and the experience of sleep disturbance has received little attention among researchers, although food insecurity is associated with poor physical and mental health globally. This study aimed to investigate the relationship between food security status and sleep disturbance among adults 20–64 years old. Methods: The study's population-based sample included 20,212 Indonesian adults who participated in the fifth wave of the Indonesia Family Life Survey (IFLS5) in 2014. Dietary intake data, gathered using a food frequency questionnaire (FFQ), were used to assess the food security status. Sleep disturbance was assessed using the 10-item Patient-Reported Outcomes Measurement Information System (PROMIS) questionnaire. We used multiple linear and logistic regression models to test the study hypothesis. Results: A higher likelihood of experiencing sleep disturbance was recorded in people aged older than 56 years (OR = 1.78, 95% CI: 1.17–2.72, $p = 0.007$), people with depressive symptoms (OR = 3.57, 95% CI: 2.77–4.61, $p < 0.001$), and food-insecure people (OR = 1.32, 95% CI: 1.02–1.70, $p = 0.036$). A lower likelihood of experiencing sleep disturbance was recorded in people with low educational attainment (OR = 0.41, 95% CI: 0.30–0.57, $p < 0.001$). Sleep disturbance was dependent on the food consumption groups and food security status among men ($p = 0.004$). Conclusions: Sleep disturbance may be affected by the food-insecure status of adults, and later, may lead to serious health outcomes.

Keywords: food insecurity; sleep disturbance; adults; cross-sectional study

---

1. Introduction

Food insecurity is a public health problem that exists globally, including in developing countries. Food insecurity is the disruption of dietary patterns or nutrient intake because of a lack of finances and other resources [1]. In the USA, researchers have estimated that food insecurity affects 9–14% of adults aged 24–32 years, and shows higher rates among women and low-income adults [2–4]. Meanwhile, developing countries, such as Indonesia, have reported a high prevalence of food insecurity, with as many as 19.4 million people out of a population of 258.7 million who were unable to meet their dietary requirements [5]. Food-insecure people may encounter anxiety or stress from uncertainty about fulfilling their food requirements or other necessities. The anxiety and stress may lead to depressive symptoms and affect their quality of sleep [6,7]. Poor sleep quality, such as short sleep duration, the presence of sleep disturbance, or difficulty getting to sleep, is associated with the possibility of chronic disease later in life [8–10]. Sleep disturbance is known to be a big problem in developed countries. In the United States, the National Institutes of Health stated that in 2017, about thirty percent of people reported getting less than seven hours of sleep each night [11]. The problem has begun to slide to low-to-middle-income countries, which reported about ten percent of people having severe sleeping problems [12,13]. People with sleep disturbances have reported difficulties with concentrating during the day and feeling restless, anxious, and depressed [14,15]. On the other hand, depressed people may also experience economic difficulties, which leads to food insecurity [16,17]. People with food insecurity are known to be vulnerable and more likely to develop chronic diseases or experience poorer mental health. However, the relationship between food insecurity and sleep disturbance is rather vague. This study's objective was to determine the relationship between food security statuses and sleep disturbance using a nationally representative sample of adults aged 20–64 years in Indonesia.

2. Materials and Methods

2.1. Study Participants and Data Source

This cross-sectional study used the secondary longitudinal data of the fifth wave of the Indonesian Family Life Survey (IFLS5) that was conducted in 2014. The initial survey (IFLS1) was conducted in 1993, representing about 80 percent of the Indonesian population. The IFLS5 datasets were anonymous, included participants of all ages, and were available for researchers who met the criteria based on the RAND Corporation guidelines about the dataset usage [18]. The institutional review board (IRB) review of the IFLS studies went through the sufficient and appropriate review that followed the IRB guidelines and was approved by both the RAND Corporation and Indonesia's Institutions, in particular, the Survey Meter institution for the IFLS5 study [18,19]. The total number of participants for the IFLS5 were 34,464 people, aged from zero to older than 80 years old. The present study included participants who had complete data relating to food, anthropometric characteristics, sociodemographic characteristics, blood pressure, depressive symptoms, and sleep disturbance. We excluded participants who had been diagnosed with cancer, chronic diseases (e.g., diabetes and cardiovascular diseases), had a disability, or who were breastfeeding or pregnant in order to minimize the probability of sampling bias. Therefore, 20,212 participants aged 20–64 years old were included in the present study.

2.2. Assessment of Sleep Disturbance

The assessment of sleep disturbance was based on the guidelines of the Patient-Reported Outcomes Measurement Information System (PROMIS) [20,21]. The IFLS5 used self-reported answers to ten questions based on the PROMIS questionnaire for the assessment of sleep deprivation and sleep quality [18]. Each question on the questionnaire was rated using a one-to-five scale (never, rarely, sometimes, often, and always, respectively). The total score range of the ten questions was then summarized with a range from 10 to 50, which was the so-called total raw score. We used a t-score table to identify the t-score that related to every participant's total raw score and the information was attached to a t-score row based on its value. The t-scores were interpreted as "none to slight" for the participants with scores <55, "mild" for the participants with scores 55.0–59.9, and a combination of "moderate to severe" for the participants with scores >60 [20–22]. For the purposes of this study, we also categorized the data into two groups: participants whose sleep disturbance was "mild or less" or "greater than mild."

2.3. Assessment of Food Security Status

The assessment of food insecurity is associated with a person's lack of secure access to fulfilling their need for a nutritious diet in a sufficient amount to keep an active healthy life, considering both the food frequency and food diversity [23–25]. There are several ways to assess food insecurity at the individual level [26–28]. One of the assessments of the food insecurity concept was developed using the food frequency questionnaire (FFQ). The World Food Programme (WFP) introduced this concept to assess food consumption analysis by producing food consumption scores (FCSs) and cut-off points for food insecurity [24,25]. The FCSs allow data to be categorized into three food consumption groups (FCGs) consisting of poor, borderline, and acceptable groups. Furthermore, the ten food items listed on the IFLS5 food frequency questionnaire were included in the food consumption analysis. The IFLS5 FFQ asked about ten food types that were eaten by the participants during the last seven days before the interview. We then grouped these ten food types into five food groups. The first group was the staple group, consisting of sweet potato. The second group was the protein group, consisting of eggs, fish, and meats. The third group was dairy products. The fourth group was the fruit group, consisting of banana, mango, and papaya. The last group was the vegetable group, consisting of green leafy vegetables and carrots [23–25]. The score for each food group was then summed as the food consumption score in the form of continuous data. The "poor" food consumption group included participants who had an FCS lower than 21. The "borderline" FCG included participants who had food consumption scores that lay between 21 and 35. The "acceptable" FCG included participants who had food consumption scores higher than 35 [24]. The "poor" FGC and "borderline" FGC participants were defined as food-insecure persons [25,29].

2.4. Assessment of Covariates

The covariates of the present study were anthropometric characteristics, blood pressure, physical activity, and sociodemographic measurements. We used the body mass index, and additionally, for the participants aged 40 years and older, the measurements of the waist circumference and the body shape index [30–32] were added. Furthermore, the adult body mass indices (in kg/m^2) adopted the Indonesian cut-off points [33]. The body mass index (BMI) was categorized into "normal weight" for participants with a BMI between 18.5 to 25.0, "overweight" for participants with a BMI between 25.1 to 27.0, and "obese" for participants with a BMI higher than 27.0 [34]. The definition of abdominal obesity used the waist circumference measurement with two cut-off points (for men: >90 cm, for women: >80 cm). Trained nurses performed the anthropometric and blood pressure measurements. For the blood pressure measurements, the participants were in the seated position. Participants were defined as having hypertension if the systolic blood pressure (SBP) was ≥140 mmHg or the diastolic blood pressure (DBP) was ≥90 mmHg, or if they had been diagnosed by paramedics before the interview or were currently consuming blood pressure-lowering medication [32].

Furthermore, physical activity was assessed using the number of days on which respondents had done two types of physical activity (i.e., vigorous and moderate) within the last seven days before the survey. We considered the volume of physical activity (PA) to be a continuous variable in the analysis. Respondents answered the self-reported questionnaires in terms of whether they had engaged in physical activities for at least ten minutes continuously during the last seven days. If the respondents said yes, then they were further asked about the number of days on which they had done each type of physical activity. Eight and four metabolic equivalent of tasks (METs), respectively, were then multiplied by the minutes and days of each type of physical activity to form the physical activity volume (in METs minutes/week) [35]. For example, the vigorous physical activity volume formula was the minutes/day multiplied by days/week of doing vigorous PA multiplied by eight METs.

The sociodemographic variables included smoking habits, educational attainment, living area, and marital status, which were presented as categorical data. The smoking habits of the participants were categorized into never (never had a smoking habit), current smoker (currently has a smoking habit), and former smoker (has stopped a smoking habit). The participants' educational attainment was categorized into low: <12 years of school attainment, and high: ≥12 years of school attainment.

Depressive symptoms were defined using the score of the questionnaire about mental health. The IFLS5 used the ten-item self-reported questionnaire from the Center for Epidemiologic Studies–Depression (CES-D) to assess the mental health of the adult participants. Some prior researchers have used the 10-CES-D questionnaire to assess adults' depressive symptoms [36,37]. The form of the responses to the 10-CES-D questionnaire was based on four scale items: less than one day (rarely or never), one to two days (some days), three to four days (occasionally), and five to seven days (most of the time). The scores of the 10 questions were then added, resulting in a score ranging from ten to forty. Furthermore, the score was rebased so that the lowest score was zero and the highest score was thirty. The highest score identified people with the most symptomatology of depression [38]. The cut-off point for defining a person as having a risk of heightened depressive symptoms was a score higher than or equal to ten [39,40].

2.5. Statistical Analysis

The present study used secondary data from the IFLS5 (2014). The characteristics of participants were presented as a mean and standard deviation for the continuous data and as numbers with percentages for the categorical data. We used one-way ANOVA for the continuous data, with the Bonferroni post hoc test or chi-squared test for the categorical data to compare the values between groups. Furthermore, we used the regression model to assess the relationship between sleep disturbance and depressive symptoms by food consumption group. Furthermore, we also used the sleep disturbance score and CES-D-10 score as continuous data in the linear regression analysis and as categorical data in the logistic regression analysis. To assess the relations of interest, we used a linear and logistic regression model, which was presented using an exponentiated beta coefficient or odds ratio and a 95% confidence interval, respectively. Moreover, this study used three models that accounted for various potential confounders in the multiple logistic regression model. The three models were an unadjusted model, a model with adjustment for age and sex, and a model with a complete adjustment; the complete adjustment was an adjustment for age, sex, educational attainment, marital status, BMI, living area, blood pressure, smoking habit, and physical activity volume. We used a similar sequence of adjustments for potential confounders, which were also used for the linear regression models. Statistical significance was designated as a *p*-value < 0.05. We conducted a multivariate test to identify the characteristics related to sleep disturbance and depressive symptoms, which were analyzed in a separate model. Covariates in these two models included sex, age group, living area, educational attainment, smoking status, blood pressure, physical activity volume, and body mass index. All the analyses were conducted using STATA statistical software (v16.1; StataCorp LP, College Station, TX, USA).

3. Results

This cross-sectional study included 20,212 participants (women = 10,070, men = 10,142) from the IFLS5 dataset (Table 1). The flowchart related to the selection of the participants is shown in Figure S1. The mean age of the participants was 39 (standard deviation (SD): 11) years old. Most of the participants had low educational attainment, were currently or ever married, living in urban areas, and had never had a smoking habit. Additionally, most of the participants aged 40 years and older had abdominal obesity, which was observed in 4494 (51.54%) people. The prevalence of food insecurity in this study was 53.86%, or 10,886 of the total participants. Among the food-insecure participants, women represented as many as 5602 (51.46%) people, low education attainment was found in 6832 (62.76%) people, people who were currently married or had a marriage experience constituted 9707 (89.17%) people, and the number of people who lived in urban areas was 6041 (55.49%). Most of the food-insecure participants, i.e., 6544 (60.11%) people, never had a smoking habit, whereas 3944 (36.23%) people reported that they had quit smoking. We found that 191 (1.75%) food-insecure participants were taking blood-pressure-lowering medication and 61 (0.56%) people were taking cholesterol-lowering medication. Furthermore, 2294 (49.95%) people aged 40 years old and older among the food-insecure groups had abdominal obesity. We found that the number of people with depressive symptoms among the food-insecure group was 3808 (34.98%). Furthermore, 595 (56.67%) of the food-insecure participants were experiencing "mild" sleep disturbance, whereas 168 (62.92%) of the food-insecure participants were experiencing "moderate-to-severe" sleep disturbance. The means of the systolic blood pressures and vigorous physical activity volumes of the food-insecure participants were higher than those in the food-secure group ($p < 0.001$).

Figure 1 shows the prevalence of sleep disturbance by FCG for women and men. Among men, participants reported a "none-to-slight" sleep disturbance level for 94.17% ($n = 4575$) of the acceptable FCG, 93.54% ($n = 3260$) of the borderline FCG, and 92.22% ($n = 1659$) of the poor FCG. Participants reported a "mild" sleep disturbance level for 5.00% ($n = 243$) of the acceptable FCG, 4.99% ($n = 174$) of the borderline FCG, and 6.06% ($n = 109$) of the poor FCG. Furthermore, participants reported a "moderate-to-severe" sleep disturbance level for 0.82% ($n = 40$) of the acceptable FCG, 1.46% ($n = 51$) of the borderline FCG, and 1.72% ($n = 31$) of the poor FCG. The level of sleep disturbance was dependent on the food consumption group or food security status among men ($p = 0.004$).

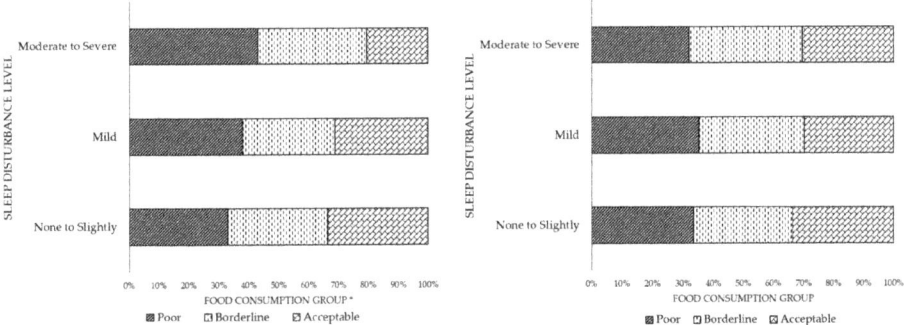

Figure 1. Prevalence of sleep disturbance among men (left) and women (right) by food consumption group. Indonesia Family Life Survey (IFLS) 2014 data were used in the analysis. * Significance: $p < 0.05$.

Among women, participants reported a "none-to-slight" sleep disturbance level for 93.93% ($n = 4197$) of the acceptable FCG, 92.80% ($n = 3370$) of the borderline FCG, and 93.06% ($n = 1825$) of the poor FCG. Participants reported a "mild" sleep disturbance level for 4.74% ($n = 212$) of the acceptable FCG, 5.58% ($n = 203$) of the borderline FCG, and 5.56% ($n = 109$) of the poor FCG. Furthermore, participants reported a "moderate-to-severe" sleep disturbance level for 1.32% ($n = 59$) of the acceptable FCG, 1.62% ($n = 59$) of the borderline FCG, and 1.38% ($n = 27$) of the poor FCG. The level of sleep disturbance was independent of the food consumption group or food security status among women ($p = 0.301$).

Table 2 shows the characteristics related to sleep disturbance, as determined by the regression model. When the confounding variables were taken into account in the multivariate regression model, several characteristics remained independently related to sleep disturbance. A higher likelihood of experiencing sleep disturbance was recorded in participants aged older than 56 years (OR = 1.78, 95% CI: 1.17–2.72, $p = 0.007$), participants with depressive symptoms (OR = 3.57, 95% CI: 2.77–4.61, $p < 0.001$), and food-insecure participants (OR = 1.32, 95% CI: 1.02–1.70, $p = 0.036$). However, a lower likelihood of experiencing sleep disturbance was recorded in participants with low educational attainment (OR = 0.41, 95% CI: 0.30–0.57, $p < 0.001$).

Table 1. The participants' characteristics.

Variable	All	Food-Secure	Food-Insecure	*p*-Value
n	20,212	9326 (46.14)	10,886 (53.86)	
Gender, *n* (%)				<0.001
Women	10,070 (49.82)	4468 (47.91)	5602 (51.46)	
Men	10,142 (50.18)	4858 (52.09)	5284 (48.54)	
Age (years), mean (SD)	39 (11)	39 (11)	38 (11)	0.015
Age Group (years), *n* (%)				0.037
≤35	9050 (44.78)	4088 (43.83)	4962 (45.58)	
36–55	9304 (46.03)	4378 (46.94)	4926 (45.25)	
≥56	1858 (9.19)	860 (9.22)	998 (9.17)	
Educational Attainment, *n* (%)				<0.001
Low (<12 years)	11,037 (54.61)	4205 (45.09)	6832 (62.76)	
High (≥12 years)	9175 (45.39)	5121 (54.91)	4054 (37.24)	
Marital Status, *n* (%)				0.001
Never Married	2328 (11.52)	1149 (12.32)	1179 (10.83)	
Currently or Ever Married	17,884 (88.48)	8177 (87.68)	9707 (89.17)	
Living Areas, *n* (%)				<0.001
Rural	8232 (40.73)	3387 (36.32)	4845 (44.51)	
Urban	11,980 (59.27)	5939 (63.68)	6041 (55.49)	
Smoking Habit, *n* (%)				<0.001
Never	12,148 (60.10)	5604 (60.09)	6544 (60.11)	
Current Smoker	879 (4.35)	481 (5.16)	398 (3.66)	
Former Smoker	7185 (35.55)	3241 (34.75)	3944 (36.23)	
Hypertension Medication User, *n* (%)				0.027
No	19,817 (98.05)	9122 (97.81)	10,695 (98.25)	
Yes	395 (1.95)	204 (2.19)	191 (1.75)	
Cholesterol Medication User, *n* (%)				<0.001
No	20,051 (99.20)	9226 (98.93)	10,825 (99.44)	
Yes	161 (0.80)	100 (1.07)	61 (0.56)	
Abdominal Obesity [a], *n* (%)				0.002
No	4226 (48.46)	1927 (46.69)	2299 (50.05)	
Yes	4494 (51.54)	2200 (53.31)	2294 (49.95)	
Body Mass Index (kg/m^2), mean (SD)	24.28 (4.11)	24.39 (4.06)	24.19 (4.14)	0.001
Body Mass Index Classification [b], *n* (%)				0.013
18.5–25.0	12,664 (57.00)	5749 (61.64)	6915 (63.52)	
25.1–27.0	2923 (13.16)	1407 (15.09)	1516 (13.93)	
>27.0	4625 (20.82)	2170 (23.27)	2455 (22.55)	
Hypertension, *n* (%)				0.542
No	13,689 (67.73)	6296 (67.51)	7393 (67.91)	
Yes	6523 (32.27)	3030 (32.49)	3493 (32.09)	
Sleep Disturbance Level [c], *n* (%)				0.002
None to Slight	18,895 (93.48)	8772 (94.06)	10,123 (92.99)	
Mild	1050 (5.19)	455 (4.88)	595 (5.47)	
Moderate to Severe	267 (1.32)	99 (1.06)	168 (1.54)	
Depressive Symptoms [d], *n* (%)				<0.001
No	12,836 (63.51)	5758 (61.74)	7078 (65.02)	
Yes	7376 (36.49)	3568 (38.26)	3808 (34.98)	
Body Shape Index (m$^{11/6}$ kg$^{-2/3}$), mean (SD)	0.0810 (0.0057)	0.0810 (0.0055)	0.0810 (0.0059)	0.708
Waist Circumference (cm), mean (SD)	85.55 (10.95)	86.19 (10.84)	84.96 (11.03)	<0.001
Systolic Blood Pressures (mmHg), mean (SD)	129.56 (19.76)	129.18 (19.35)	129.89 (20.09)	0.010
Diastolic Blood Pressures (mmHg), mean (SD)	80.04 (11.97)	80.01 (12.01)	80.08 (11.94)	0.667
Food Consumption Score, mean (SD)	34.70 (14.66)	46.70 (10.45)	24.42 (8.75)	<0.001
Moderate PA Volume (METs min/w), mean (SD)	1145.88 (1872.15)	1185.25 (1907.31)	1112.16 (1840.92)	0.943
Vigorous PA Volume (METs min/w), mean (SD)	1190.33 (3136.19)	1093.61 (2950.50)	1273.19 (3284.81)	<0.001
Sleep Disturbance Score, mean (SD)	40.40 (11.51)	40.70 (11.08)	40.14 (11.86)	0.001
CES-D-10 Score, mean (SD)	8.70 (5.00)	9.00 (4.86)	8.45 (5.10)	<0.001

Abbreviations: SD, standard deviation; METs min/w, metabolic equivalent of tasks for minutes per week; CES-D-10, 10 items of the Center for Epidemiological Studies Depression questionnaire; PA, physical activity. Note: The categorical data are presented using *n* (%) and the continuous data are presented using mean (SD). [a] The definition of abdominal obesity for women and men used the waist circumference with cut-off points of >80 cm or >90 cm, respectively. [b] The body mass index used the adult categorization of body mass index for the Indonesian population. [c] The definition of having depressive symptoms used the score of the CES-D-10 with cut-off values ≥10. [d] The sleep disturbance level was defined using the t-score of the Patient-Reported Outcomes Measurement Information System (PROMIS) guidelines of the sleep disturbance questionnaire. Significance was set to *p* < 0.05.

Table 2. Characteristics related to the sleep disturbance level, as determined by the regression model.

Variables	Sleep Disturbance *		
	OR	95% CI	*p*-Value
Gender (Ref: Men)			
Women	1.01	(0.68, 1.48)	0.972
Age (years, Ref: ≤35)			
36–55	1.35	(1.00, 1.82)	0.050
≥56	1.78	(1.17, 2.72)	0.007
Educational attainment (Ref: ≥12 years)			
Low (<12 years)	0.41	(0.30, 0.57)	<0.001
Marital Status (Ref: Never Married)			
Currently or Ever Married	1.49	(0.85, 2.62)	0.165
Living Areas (Ref: Rural)			
Urban	1.01	(0.78, 1.30)	0.949
Smoking Habit (Ref: Never)			
Current Smoker	0.48	(0.20, 1.15)	0.100
Former Smoker	0.81	(0.54, 1.21)	0.297
BMI (kg/m^2, Ref: 18.5–25.0)			
25.1–27.0	0.95	(0.66, 1.37)	0.793
>27.0	0.83	(0.60, 1.15)	0.256
Depressive Symptoms (Ref: No)			
Yes	3.57	(2.77, 4.61)	<0.001
Food Security Status (Ref: Food-Secure)			
Food-Insecure	1.32	(1.02, 1.70)	0.036

Abbreviations: Ref., reference; OR, odds ratio; 95% CI, 95% confidence interval. Note: * Sleep disturbance was categorized into greater than mild or not greater than mild. The models were adjusted for age, gender, body mass index, education attainment, marital status, living area, smoking habits, physical activity volume, blood pressure value, food consumption score, and CES-D-10 score. Statistical significance was set to $p < 0.05$.

Furthermore, Table S1 shows that a higher likelihood of experiencing sleep disturbance after adjusting for age and gender in our study was reported in participants with depressive symptoms (OR = 3.50, 95% CI: 2.72–4.52, $p < 0.001$) and participants with food insecurity (OR = 1.47, 95% CI: 1.15–1.89, $p = 0.002$). On the other hand, a lower likelihood of experiencing sleep disturbance was reported in participants with low educational attainment (OR = 0.38, 95% CI: 0.28–0.51, $p < 0.001$). Furthermore, Table S2 presents the logistic regression between characteristics related to the sleep disturbance level. A higher likelihood of experiencing sleep disturbance among men in our study was reported in participants with depressive symptoms (OR = 3.16, 95% CI: 2.17–4.60, $p < 0.001$) and participants with food insecurity (OR = 1.75, 95% CI: 1.19–2.58, $p = 0.005$). Meanwhile, a higher likelihood of experiencing sleep disturbance among women in our study was reported in participants with depressive symptoms (OR = 3.16, 95% CI: 2.17–4.60, $p < 0.001$) and in participants aged older than 36 years (OR = 1.73–2.54, 95% CI: 1.00–2.72, $p = 0.016$–0.002). On the other hand, a lower likelihood of experiencing sleep disturbance among men in our study was reported in current smoker participants (OR = 0.35, 95% CI: 0.12–0.99, $p = 0.048$) and in participants with low educational attainment (OR = 0.46, 95% CI: 0.30–0.71, $p < 0.001$). Moreover, a lower likelihood of experiencing sleep disturbance among women in our study was reported in participants with low educational attainment (OR = 0.37, 95% CI: 0.22–0.61, $p < 0.001$).

4. Discussion

The present study demonstrates the relationship between food insecurity and sleep disturbance. This study's results show that most of the food-insecure participants were women, people who had marriage experience, people with low educational attainment, and people who lived in urban areas.

In addition, the middle-aged participants (older than 40 years old) were more likely to have abdominal obesity. Furthermore, the means of the systolic blood pressure and vigorous physical activity volume were higher among food-insecure participants compared to food-secure participants. Moreover, participants who were more likely to experience sleep disturbance were aged older than 56 years old, had depressive symptoms, and a food-insecurity status, but this was not the case for the people who had low educational attainment.

Food insecurity is associated with chronic diseases and poor mental health [41–43]. The burden of food insecurity and marriage experience, in particular for women, synergistically contributes to the development of depressive symptoms [44]. A potential explanation may be the stressful decision-making that most food-insecure women have to do related to their financial situation, and women may be more susceptible to harm from life stresses and other environmental factors [4,42,45]. The findings from this study also confirmed previous research that suggests the higher prevalence of food insecurity among women [44,46]. Furthermore, our study results are in line with previous findings showing that most people with low education levels are more likely to encounter food insecurity. One of the possible mechanisms is the contribution of the financial hardship of food-insecure people. The financial hardship of food-insecure people may be affected by the low wage or minimum payment from intensive work. Low-educated people are more likely to do manual labor and to receive a minimum payment, which may affect the difficulty in fulfilling their nutrition requirements through adequate meals [47,48]. Another explanation is that low education may lead to less exposure to nutrition education explaining how to maintain a well-balanced and nutritious diet [49].

Food-insecure people who live in the urban areas may try to keep up with their environment, which includes needs relating to food, or cultural or financial situations [50–52]. People who live in urban areas might also be exposed to more processed food options [53,54]. The problem with processed foods or fast foods is the lack of consumers' ability to control the amount of calories, sodium, fat, and sugar [55]. In particular, for people with inadequate nutrition education, they may prefer to buy the processed foods in a lower price range, which may contain high calories, fat, high sodium, or high sugar, instead of buying well-balanced meals [56]. For food-insecure people, the difficulty of maintaining their nutritional dietary needs may affect their body weight, which leads to being overweight or obese [57]. The findings of the present study support the previous finding that the numbers of food-insecure participants who live in urban areas and who have excess weight were greater than those in the food-secure group. Furthermore, people with food insecurity may encounter sleep disturbance, which is also associated with an increase in systolic blood pressure. The systolic blood pressure may be a result of jobs involving heavy work or of continuous vigorous physical activity [58–60]. A population-based study in a rural area of China found that older age, unemployment, lower-income, disability, and chronic disease comorbidities were significant factors associated with an increased risk of poor sleep quality for both men and women [61]. The significant interactions with race/ethnicity indicate that the relationship between sleep complaints and marital status, income, and employment differs between groups for men, and the relationship with education differs between groups for women [62]. Food insecurity is related to "poor" sleep quality, which may develop from anxiety, stress, or feelings of uncertainty about providing food and other necessities for themselves and their families [6,7].

Moreover, a combination of biological and psychosocial factors is involved in the mechanism of the relationship between food insecurity and poor mental health [9,63]. Meanwhile, the relationship between depression or having depressive symptoms and the experience of sleep disturbance is also known to be closely linked [15]. Food insecurity is related to depressive symptoms [29,64,65], and having depressive symptoms increases the odds of experiencing sleep disturbance in adults [9,14,66]. Another explanation is the compensatory mechanism of leptin, which reduces appetite and increases energy expenditure through the hypothalamic receptors [67,68]. Low leptin levels are associated with increased body mass index, lower quality of sleep, and a higher propensity toward having depressive symptoms [66]. The presence of sleep disturbance is associated with the effect of high levels of ghrelin and low levels of leptin. On the other hand, lower quality of sleep also causes greater neuronal activation in response to food stimuli, which results in increased motivation to seek food to achieve a high-energy intake, particularly by eating energy-dense foods that are high in fat and sugar [66,69]. Food-insecure adults may have diets that are deficient in nutrients, such as folic acid and tryptophan [70,71], which could influence mood and immune functions [72–74], which, in turn, may have an effect on their sleep.

The present study has some limitations. First, the usage of a cross-sectional study limited us from seeing the causal relationship between variables. However, our data were nationally representative for almost a majority of the adult Indonesian population. Second, although we controlled for covariates in the analysis, there remain several sociodemographic factors, such as individual income or house environmental factors that may contribute to sleep disturbance, which we could not include. Third, the sleep disturbance questions in the IFLS survey did not provide more potential sources of sleep disturbance. Thus, we were unable to specifically explain the type of sleep disturbance that the participants experienced (e.g., insomnia, sleep apnea, duration of sleep, and the latency of sleep). The use of self-reported data for sleep disturbance and physical activity variables is likely to suffer from a response bias and may affect the study results [75]. However, the PROMIS self-reported sleep disturbance has been used and validated in former research among adults [20–22]. A possible bidirectional relationship between depressive symptoms and sleep disturbance that we could not test in both directions may also be a limitation of the present work. For the study's purpose, we only focused on the relationship between the exposure (i.e., depressive symptom) and sleep disturbance (as the outcome) because of the general assumption that depression treatment would also resolve the associated symptoms, such as sleep disturbance [76]. Lastly, since we used the food consumption score in the food security assessment, although the outcome investigated may not fully represent food insecurity, this method has been used widely in former studies [29,77,78]. Therefore, the interpretation of the study result must be taken cautiously.

5. Conclusions

In conclusion, the results of this study suggest that sleep disturbance may be affected by food insecurity in adults and may later lead to serious health outcomes. A potential solution that could overcome this problem is to encourage food-insecure people to participate in nutritional education programs that are conducted by health experts that also incorporate advice about the benefits of sleep quality.

Supplementary Materials: The following are available online at http://www.mdpi.com/2072-6643/12/11/3411/s1, Figure S1: Flowchart of the participant sampling process; Table S1: The logistic regression between covariate variables and the outcome; Table S2: The logistic regression between the characteristics related to the sleep disturbance level, stratified by gender; Table S3. The regression test between depressive symptoms and sleep disturbance by food security status.

Author Contributions: E.R.I. and S.-H.Y. conceived and designed the study; E.R.I. and Y.-C.C. performed the data analyses; E.R.I., Y.-C.C., and S.-H.Y. wrote the paper. Y.-C.C., H.-Y.S., and S.-H.Y. provided the supervision. All authors have read and agreed to the published version of the manuscript.

Funding: This research was funded by Taipei Medical University Hospital (109TMU-TMUH-30).

Acknowledgments: E.R.I. was supported by Hibah Riset Mandat Dosen Muda year 2020, Universitas Airlangga.

Conflicts of Interest: The authors declare no conflict of interest.

References

1. Seligman, H.K.; Laraia, B.A.; Kushel, M.B. Food insecurity is associated with chronic disease among low-income NHANES participants. *J. Nutr.* **2010**, *140*, 304–310. [CrossRef] [PubMed]
2. Bruening, M.; van Woerden, I.; Todd, M.; Laska, M.N. Hungry to learn: The prevalence and effects of food insecurity on health behaviors and outcomes over time among a diverse sample of university freshmen. *Int. J. Behav. Nutr. Phys. Act.* **2018**, *15*, 9. [CrossRef] [PubMed]

3. Payne-Sturges, D.C.; Tjaden, A.; Caldeira, K.M.; Vincent, K.B.; Arria, A.M. Student Hunger on Campus: Food Insecurity Among College Students and Implications for Academic Institutions. *Am. J. Health Promot.* **2018**, *32*, 349–354. [CrossRef] [PubMed]

4. Gooding, H.C.; Walls, C.E.; Richmond, T.K. Food insecurity and increased BMI in young adult women. *Obesity* **2012**, *20*, 1896–1901. [CrossRef]

5. World Food Programme. World Food Programme: Indonesia. Available online: https://www.wfp.org/countries/indonesia (accessed on 10 August 2020).

6. Na, M.; Eagleton, S.G.; Jomaa, L.; Lawton, K.; Savage, J.S. Food insecurity is associated with suboptimal sleep quality, but not sleep duration, among low-income Head Start children of pre-school age. *Public Health Nutr.* **2020**, *23*, 701–710. [CrossRef]

7. Ding, M.; Keiley, M.K.; Garza, K.B.; Duffy, P.A.; Zizza, C.A. Food insecurity is associated with poor sleep outcomes among US adults. *J. Nutr.* **2014**, *145*, 615–621. [CrossRef] [PubMed]

8. Arenas, D.J.; Thomas, A.; Wang, J.; DeLisser, H.M. A Systematic Review and Meta-analysis of Depression, Anxiety, and Sleep Disorders in US Adults with Food Insecurity. *J. Gen. Intern. Med.* **2019**, *34*, 2874–2882. [CrossRef]

9. Nagata, J.M.; Palar, K.; Gooding, H.C.; Garber, A.K.; Whittle, H.J.; Bibbins-Domingo, K.; Weiser, S.D. Food Insecurity Is Associated With Poorer Mental Health and Sleep Outcomes in Young Adults. *J. Adolesc. Health* **2019**, *65*, 805–811. [CrossRef]

10. Nutt, D.; Wilson, S.; Paterson, L. Sleep disorders as core symptoms of depression. *Dialogues Clin. Neurosci.* **2008**, *10*, 329.

11. Yong, L.C.; Li, J.; Calvert, G.M. Sleep-related problems in the US working population: Prevalence and association with shiftwork status. *Occup. Environ. Med.* **2017**, *74*, 93–104. [CrossRef]

12. Peltzer, K.; Pengpid, S. Prevalence, social and health correlates of insomnia among persons 15 years and older in Indonesia. *Psychol. Health Med.* **2019**, *24*, 757–768. [CrossRef]

13. Peltzer, K.; Pengpid, S. Sleep duration and health correlates among university students in 26 countries. *Psychol. Health Med.* **2016**, *21*, 208–220. [CrossRef]

14. Dai, H.; Mei, Z.; An, A.; Lu, Y.; Wu, J. Associations of sleep problems with health-risk behaviors and psychological well-being among Canadian adults. *Sleep Health* **2020**. [CrossRef] [PubMed]

15. Hill, T.D.; Ellison, C.; Hale, L. Religious attendance, depressive symptoms, and sleep disturbance in older Mexican Americans. *Mental Health Relig. Cult.* **2020**, *23*, 1–14. [CrossRef]

16. Silverman, J.; Krieger, J.; Kiefer, M.; Hebert, P.; Robinson, J.; Nelson, K. The Relationship Between Food Insecurity and Depression, Diabetes Distress and Medication Adherence Among Low-Income Patients with Poorly-Controlled Diabetes. *J. Gen. Intern. Med.* **2015**, *30*, 1476–1480. [CrossRef]

17. Lent, M.D.; Petrovic, L.E.; Swanson, J.A.; Olson, C.M. Maternal mental health and the persistence of food insecurity in poor rural families. *J. Health Care Poor Underserved* **2009**, *20*, 645–661. [CrossRef]

18. Strauss, J.; Witoelar, F.; Sikoki, B. *The Fifth Wave of the Indonesia Family Life Survey: Overview and Field Report*; RAND: Santa Monica, CA, USA, 2016.

19. Frankenberg, E.; Thomas, D. *The Indonesia Family Life Survey (IFLS): Study Design and Results from Waves 1 and 2. 2000*; DRU2238/1. NIA/NICHD; RAND: Santa Monica, CA, USA, 2000.

20. Buysse, D.J.; Yu, L.; Moul, D.E.; Germain, A.; Stover, A.; Dodds, N.E.; Johnston, K.L.; Shablesky-Cade, M.A.; Pilkonis, P.A. Development and validation of patient-reported outcome measures for sleep disturbance and sleep-related impairments. *Sleep* **2010**, *33*, 781–792. [CrossRef]

21. Yu, L.; Buysse, D.J.; Germain, A.; Moul, D.E.; Stover, A.; Dodds, N.E.; Johnston, K.L.; Pilkonis, P.A. Development of short forms from the PROMIS sleep disturbance and Sleep-Related Impairment item banks. *Behav. Sleep Med.* **2011**, *10*, 6–24. [CrossRef]

22. Sujarwoto, S. Sleep Disturbance in Indonesia: How Much Does Smoking Contribute? *Behav. Sleep Med.* **2019**, 1–14. [CrossRef]

23. United Nations World Food Programme-Food Security Analysis. *Consolidated Approach to Reporting Indicators of Food Security (CARI) Guidelines*; United Nations World Food Programme, Food Security Analysis (VAM): Rome, Italy, 2015.

24. World Food Programme. *Food Consumption Score Nutritional Quality Analysis Guidelines (FCS-N)*; United Nations World Food Programme, Food Security Analysis (VAM): Rome, Italy, 2015.

25. World Food Programme. *Food Consumption Analysis: Calculation and Use of the Food Consumption Score in Food Security Analysis*; World Food Programme: Rome, Italy, 2008.

26. Becker, C.B.; Middlemass, K.M.; Gomez, F.; Martinez-Abrego, A. Eating Disorder Pathology Among Individuals Living With Food Insecurity: A Replication Study. *Clin. Psychol. Sci.* **2019**, *7*, 1144–1158. [CrossRef]

27. Wright, L.; Stallings-Smith, S.; Arikawa, A.Y. Associations between food insecurity and prediabetes in a representative sample of U.S. Adults (NHANES 2005-2014). *Diabetes Res. Clin. Pract.* **2019**, *148*, 130–136. [CrossRef]

28. Laraia, B.A. Food insecurity and chronic disease. *Adv. Nutr.* **2013**, *4*, 203–212. [CrossRef] [PubMed]

29. Isaura, E.R.; Chen, Y.-C.; Adi, A.C.; Fan, H.-Y.; Li, C.-Y.; Yang, S.-H. Association between Depressive Symptoms and Food Insecurity among Indonesian Adults: Results from the 2007–2014 Indonesia Family Life Survey. *Nutrients* **2019**, *11*, 3026. [CrossRef]

30. Krakauer, N.Y.; Krakauer, J.C. Dynamic association of mortality hazard with body shape. *PLoS ONE* **2014**, *9*, e88793. [CrossRef]

31. Krakauer, N.Y.; Krakauer, J.C. A new body shape index predicts mortality hazard independently of body mass index. *PLoS ONE* **2012**, *7*, e39504. [CrossRef]

32. Krakauer, N.Y.; Krakauer, J.C. Untangling Waist Circumference and Hip Circumference from Body Mass Index with a Body Shape Index, Hip Index, and Anthropometric Risk Indicator. *Metab. Syndr. Relat. D* **2018**, *16*, 160–165. [CrossRef]

33. Isaura, E.R.; Chen, Y.C.; Yang, S.H. The Association of Food Consumption Scores, Body Shape Index, and Hypertension in a Seven-Year Follow-Up among Indonesian Adults: A Longitudinal Study. *Int. J. Environ. Res. Public Health* **2018**, *15*, 175. [CrossRef]

34. Departemen Kesehatan Republik Indonesia; Direktorat Jenderal Bina Kesehatan Masyarakat; Direktorat Gizi Masyarakat. *Petunjuk Teknis Pemantauan Status Gizi Orang Dewasa dengan Indeks Massa Tubuh*; Departemen Kesehatan RI: Jakarta, Indonesia, 2003; p. 27.

35. Liu, X.; Zhang, D.; Liu, Y.; Sun, X.; Han, C.; Wang, B.; Ren, Y.; Zhou, J.; Zhao, Y.; Shi, Y.; et al. Dose-Response Association Between Physical Activity and Incident Hypertension: A Systematic Review and Meta-Analysis of Cohort Studies. *Hypertension* **2017**, *69*, 813–820. [CrossRef]

36. Wang, R.; Bishwajit, G.; Zhou, Y.; Wu, X.; Feng, D.; Tang, S.; Chen, Z.; Shaw, I.; Wu, T.; Song, H.; et al. Intensity, frequency, duration, and volume of physical activity and its association with risk of depression in middle- and older-aged Chinese: Evidence from the China Health and Retirement Longitudinal Study, 2015. *PLoS ONE* **2019**, *14*, e0221430. [CrossRef] [PubMed]

37. James, C.; Powell, M.; Seixas, A.; Bateman, A.; Pengpid, S.; Peltzer, K. Exploring the psychometric properties of the CES-D-10 and its practicality in detecting depressive symptomatology in 27 low- and middle-income countries. *Int. J. Psychol.* **2020**, *55*, 435–445. [CrossRef]

38. Kilburn, K.; Prencipe, L.; Hjelm, L.; Peterman, A.; Handa, S.; Palermo, T. Examination of performance of the Center for Epidemiologic Studies Depression Scale Short Form 10 among African youth in poor, rural households. *BMC Psychiatry* **2018**, *18*, 201. [CrossRef] [PubMed]

39. Asante, K.O.; Andoh-Arthur, J. Prevalence and determinants of depressive symptoms among university students in Ghana. *J. Affect. Disord.* **2015**, *171*, 161–166. [CrossRef] [PubMed]

40. Opie, R.S.; Ball, K.; Abbott, G.; Crawford, D.; Teychenne, M.; McNaughton, S.A. Adherence to the Australian dietary guidelines and development of depressive symptoms at 5 years follow-up amongst women in the READI cohort study. *Nutr. J.* **2020**, *19*, 30. [CrossRef]

41. Bergmans, R.S.; Zivin, K.; Mezuk, B. Depression, food insecurity and diabetic morbidity: Evidence from the Health and Retirement Study. *J. Psychosom. Res.* **2019**, *117*, 22–29. [CrossRef]

42. Weigel, M.M.; Armijos, R.X.; Racines, M.; Cevallos, W.; Castro, N.P. Association of Household Food Insecurity with the Mental and Physical Health of Low-Income Urban Ecuadorian Women with Children. *J. Environ. Public Health* **2016**, *2016*, 5256084. [CrossRef]

43. Hanson, K.L.; Olson, C.M. Chronic health conditions and depressive symptoms strongly predict persistent food insecurity among rural low-income families. *J Health Care Poor Underserved* **2012**, *23*, 1174–1188. [CrossRef]

44. Lee, J.W.; Shin, W.K.; Kim, Y. Impact of sex and marital status on the prevalence of perceived depression in association with food insecurity. *PLoS ONE* **2020**, *15*, e0234105. [CrossRef]

45. Harvard Health Publishing. Harvard Mental Health Letter: Women and Depression. Available online: https://www.health.harvard.edu/womens-health/women-and-depression (accessed on 13 August 2020).

46. Maynard, M.; Andrade, L.; Packull-McCormick, S.; Perlman, C.M.; Leos-Toro, C.; Kirkpatrick, S.I. Food Insecurity and Mental Health among Females in High-Income Countries. *Int. J. Environ. Res. Public Health* **2018**, *15*, 1424. [CrossRef]

47. Drewnowski, A. Obesity, diets, and social inequalities. *Nutr. Rev.* **2009**, *67*, S36–S39. [CrossRef]

48. Franklin, B.; Jones, A.; Love, D.; Puckett, S.; Macklin, J.; White-Means, S. Exploring mediators of food insecurity and obesity: A review of recent literature. *J. Community Health* **2012**, *37*, 253–264. [CrossRef]

49. An, R.; Wang, J.; Liu, J.; Shen, J.; Loehmer, E.; McCaffrey, J. A systematic review of food pantry-based interventions in the USA. *Public Health Nutr.* **2019**, *22*, 1704–1716. [CrossRef]

50. Hunt, B.R.; Benjamins, M.R.; Khan, S.; Hirschtick, J.L. Predictors of Food Insecurity in Selected Chicago Community Areas. *J. Nutr. Educ. Behav.* **2019**, *51*, 287–299. [CrossRef]

51. Oh, S.Y.; Hong, M.J. Food insecurity is associated with dietary intake and body size of Korean children from low-income families in urban areas. *Eur. J. Clin. Nutr.* **2003**, *57*, 1598–1604. [CrossRef]

52. Ramsey, R.; Giskes, K.; Turrell, G.; Gallegos, D. Food insecurity among adults residing in disadvantaged urban areas: Potential health and dietary consequences. *Public Health Nutr.* **2012**, *15*, 227–237. [CrossRef] [PubMed]

53. Kaiser, M.L.; Dionne, J.; Carr, J.K. Predictors of Diet-Related Health Outcomes in Food-Secure and Food-Insecure Communities. *Soc. Work Public Health* **2019**, *34*, 214–229. [CrossRef]

54. Vuong, T.N.; Gallegos, D.; Ramsey, R. Household food insecurity, diet, and weight status in a disadvantaged district of Ho Chi Minh City, Vietnam: A cross-sectional study. *BMC Public Health* **2015**, *15*, 232. [CrossRef] [PubMed]

55. Morales, M.E.; Berkowitz, S.A. The Relationship between Food Insecurity, Dietary Patterns, and Obesity. *Curr. Nutr. Rep.* **2016**, *5*, 54–60. [CrossRef] [PubMed]

56. Lee, Y.S.; Kim, T.H. Household food insecurity and breakfast skipping: Their association with depressive symptoms. *Psychiatry Res.* **2019**, *271*, 83–88. [CrossRef]

57. West, C.E.; Goldschmidt, A.B.; Mason, S.M.; Neumark-Sztainer, D. Differences in risk factors for binge eating by socioeconomic status in a community-based sample of adolescents: Findings from Project EAT. *Int. J. Eat. Disord.* **2019**, *52*, 659–668. [CrossRef]

58. Berkowitz, S.A.; Basu, S.; Venkataramani, A.; Reznor, G.; Fleegler, E.W.; Atlas, S.J. Association between access to social service resources and cardiometabolic risk factors: A machine learning and multilevel modeling analysis. *BMJ Open* **2019**, *9*, e025281. [CrossRef]

59. Isaura, E.R.; Chen, Y.C.; Yang, S.H. Pathways from Food Consumption Score to Cardiovascular Disease: A Seven-Year Follow-Up Study of Indonesian Adults. *Int. J. Environ. Res. Public Health* **2018**, *15*, 1567. [CrossRef] [PubMed]

60. Berkowitz, S.A.; Baggett, T.P.; Wexler, D.J.; Huskey, K.W.; Wee, C.C. Food insecurity and metabolic control among U.S. adults with diabetes. *Diabetes Care* **2013**, *36*, 3093–3099. [CrossRef] [PubMed]

61. Wu, W.; Wang, W.; Dong, Z.; Xie, Y.; Gu, Y.; Zhang, Y.; Li, M.; Tan, X. Sleep Quality and Its Associated Factors among Low-Income Adults in a Rural Area of China: A Population-Based Study. *Int. J. Environ. Res. Public Health* **2018**, *15*, 55. [CrossRef]

62. Grandner, M.A.; Patel, N.P.; Gehrman, P.R.; Xie, D.; Sha, D.; Weaver, T.; Gooneratne, N. Who gets the best sleep? Ethnic and socioeconomic factors related to sleep complaints. *Sleep Med.* **2010**, *11*, 470–478. [CrossRef]

63. Nagata, J.M.; Palar, K.; Gooding, H.C.; Garber, A.K.; Bibbins-Domingo, K.; Weiser, S.D. Food Insecurity and Chronic Disease in US Young Adults: Findings from the National Longitudinal Study of Adolescent to Adult Health. *J. Gen. Intern. Med.* **2019**, *34*, 2756–2762. [CrossRef]

64. Kolovos, S.; Zavala, G.A.; Leijen, A.S.; Melgar-Quiñonez, H.; van Tulder, M. Household food insecurity is associated with depressive symptoms: Results from a Mexican population-based survey. *Food Secur.* **2020**, *12*, 1–10. [CrossRef]

65. Whittle, H.J.; Sheira, L.A.; Wolfe, W.R.; Frongillo, E.A.; Palar, K.; Merenstein, D.; Wilson, T.E.; Adedimeji, A.; Weber, K.M.; Adimora, A.A.; et al. Food insecurity is associated with anxiety, stress, and symptoms of posttraumatic stress disorder in a cohort of women with or at risk of HIV in the United States. *J. Nutr.* **2019**, *149*, 1393–1403. [CrossRef]

66. Frank, S.; Gonzalez, K.; Lee-Ang, L.; Young, M.C.; Tamez, M.; Mattei, J. Diet and Sleep Physiology: Public Health and Clinical Implications. *Front. Neurol.* **2017**, *8*, 393. [CrossRef]

67. Lawson, E.A.; Miller, K.K.; Blum, J.I.; Meenaghan, E.; Misra, M.; Eddy, K.T.; Herzog, D.B.; Klibanski, A. Leptin levels are associated with decreased depressive symptoms in women across the weight spectrum, independent of body fat. *Clin. Endocrinol.* **2012**, *76*, 520–525. [CrossRef]

68. Yang, J.L.; Liu, X.; Jiang, H.; Pan, F.; Ho, C.S.; Ho, R.C. The Effects of High-fat-diet Combined with Chronic Unpredictable Mild Stress on Depression-like Behavior and Leptin/LepRb in Male Rats. *Sci. Rep.* **2016**, *6*, 35239. [CrossRef]

69. St-Onge, M.P.; Mikic, A.; Pietrolungo, C.E. Effects of Diet on Sleep Quality. *Adv. Nutr.* **2016**, *7*, 938–949. [CrossRef]

70. Peuhkuri, K.; Sihvola, N.; Korpela, R. Diet promotes sleep duration and quality. *Nutr. Res.* **2012**, *32*, 309–319. [CrossRef]

71. Kirkpatrick, S.I.; Tarasuk, V. Food insecurity is associated with nutrient inadequacies among Canadian adults and adolescents. *J. Nutr.* **2008**, *138*, 604–612. [CrossRef]

72. Benton, D.; Donohoe, R.T. The effects of nutrients on mood. *Public Health Nutr.* **1999**, *2*, 403–409. [CrossRef]

73. Firth, J.; Gangwisch, J.E.; Borisini, A.; Wootton, R.E.; Mayer, E.A. Food and mood: How do diet and nutrition affect mental wellbeing? *BMJ* **2020**, *369*. [CrossRef]

74. Hamer, M.; Dye, L.; Siobhan Mitchell, E.; Laye, S.; Saunders, C.; Boyle, N.; Schuermans, J.; Sijben, J. Examining techniques for measuring the effects of nutrients on mental performance and mood state. *Eur. J. Nutr.* **2016**, *55*, 1991–2000. [CrossRef]

75. Peltzer, K.; Pengpid, S. Loneliness correlates and associations with health variables in the general population in Indonesia. *Int. J. Ment. Health Syst.* **2019**, *13*, 24. [CrossRef]

76. Fang, H.; Tu, S.; Sheng, J.; Shao, A. Depression in sleep disturbance: A review on a bidirectional relationship, mechanisms and treatment. *J. Cell Mol. Med.* **2019**, *23*, 2324–2332. [CrossRef]

77. Wiesmann, D.; Bassett, L.; Benson, T.; Hoddinott, J. *Validation of the World Food Programme s Food Consumption Score and Alternative Indicators of Household Food Security*; International Food Policy Research Institute: Washington, DC, USA, 2009.

78. Marivoet, W.; Becquey, E.; Van Campenhout, B. How well does the Food Consumption Score capture diet quantity, quality and adequacy across regions in the Democratic Republic of the Congo (DRC)? *Food Secur.* **2019**, *11*, 1029–1049. [CrossRef]

Publisher's Note: MDPI stays neutral with regard to jurisdictional claims in published maps and institutional affiliations.

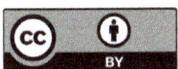

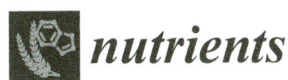

Article

Diet Quality and Health Service Utilization for Depression: A Prospective Investigation of Adults in Alberta's Tomorrow Project

Shelby Marozoff, Paul J. Veugelers, Julia Dabravolskaj, Dean T. Eurich, Ming Ye and Katerina Maximova *

School of Public Health, University of Alberta, Edmonton, AB T6G 1C9, Canada; marozoff@ualberta.ca (S.M.); Paul.Veugelers@ualberta.ca (P.J.V.); dabvravol@ualberta.ca (J.D.); deurich@ualberta.ca (D.T.E.); mye@ualberta.ca (M.Y.)
* Correspondence: katerina.maximova@ualberta.ca; Tel.: +1-780-248-2076

Received: 14 July 2020; Accepted: 11 August 2020; Published: 13 August 2020

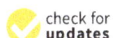

Abstract: Depression is a leading cause of disability and economic burden worldwide. Primary prevention strategies are urgently needed. We examined the association of diet quality with depression in a large provincial cohort of adults. A past year food frequency questionnaire was completed by Alberta's Tomorrow Project (ATP) participants enrolled between 2000–2008 (n = 25,016; average age 50.4 years) and used to calculate Healthy Eating Index-Canada (HEI-C) 2015 scores. The number of physician visits for depression 2000–2015 was obtained via linkage with administrative health records. Negative binomial regression models assessed the relationship between HEI-C 2015 scores and physician visits for depression, adjusting for confounders. Every 10-unit increase in HEI-C 2015 scores was associated with 4.7% fewer physician visits for depression (rate ratio (RR): 0.95; 95% Confidence Interval (CI): 0.92–0.98). This relationship persisted when participants with physician visits for mental illness prior to cohort enrollment were excluded. Higher quality diets were associated with a lower number of physician visits for depression. Results highlight diet may be an important prevention strategy for reducing the burden of health service utilization for depression.

Keywords: diet quality; nutrition; mental health; depression; mood disorders; prevention

1. Introduction

Depression is the leading global cause of disability, affecting over 300 million individuals worldwide [1]. In Canada, the lifetime prevalence of depression is over 11% [2]. Mental illnesses, of which depression represents approximately 42.5% of the burden [3], place a substantial strain on health care systems. In 2011, mental illnesses cost the Canadian economy over $22.6 billion dollars in direct costs, a value which is predicted to increase to $105.6 billion over the following 30 years [4]. About one in seven (14%) Canadians access health care for a mental illness annually [5]. Mental illnesses accounted for 25.5% of all acute care hospital days and diagnoses of mental illness in 2009/10 and were associated with hospital stays over 2.5 times as long as those not involving a mental health diagnosis [6]. Given the large personal, societal, and economic burden of depression, primary prevention strategies are urgently needed.

Diet has recently received attention as a promising intervention target for prevention of depression. Poor quality diets are a leading contributor to the burden of chronic disease in Canada [7,8]. Compliance with dietary recommendations is poor among Canadians, and consumption of beneficial food groups, such as vegetables and fruit, as well as milk and alternatives, has decreased in recent years [7]. While there have been two systematic reviews that synthesized evidence from randomized controlled trials

(RCTs) on the diet-depression relationship [9,10], RCTs included in both reviews focused on dietary interventions in relation to existing depression symptoms (i.e., secondary prevention). To the best of our knowledge, there are no RCTs that examined diet as a potential target for primary prevention of depression. There are several factors that limit the feasibility of the RCT design when it comes to the diet-depression relationship. Complex exposures, such as diet, affect disease risk through multiple systems and pathways, and these effects aggregate over long periods of time [11], thus requiring sufficient follow-up time [12]. This results in additional costs, as well as non-compliance and high dropout rates among participants. Blinding is also problematic (if at all possible) in RCTs of dietary interventions, and these interventions are often examined in high-risk populations (e.g., obese and overweight) rather than the general population.

Given these challenges, evidence from high-quality observational studies is required to understand if diet is a novel intervention target for primary prevention of depression. Emerging evidence from observational studies indicates that this might be true. For example, several systematic reviews and meta-analyses report the link between adherence to high quality, healthy diets with high intakes of vegetables, fruit, whole grains, and healthy fats and reduced consumption of saturated fat, sugar, and red meat (e.g., whether healthy/prudent, Mediterranean, pro-vegetarian, or Tuscan) and as much as 33% lower risk of incident depression [13–17]. While most of the studies appropriately assessed diet quality (as opposed to individual food constituents) using a variety of tools, the assessment of depression has been limited by the use of symptom severity scales rather than other outcome measures, such as healthcare utilization. For example, available observational studies most commonly included symptom severity scales (e.g., Center for Epidemiologic Studies Depression Scale [18], Beck Depression Inventory-II [19], Composite International Diagnostic Interview Short Form [20]), antidepressant use, or self-report of physician diagnoses, with mixed results that vary by age, sex, and diagnosis [14,15]. While symptom severity scales evaluate the presence of mental illness symptoms regardless of whether formal diagnostic criteria are fulfilled, individuals with symptoms of depression and individuals seeking physician-provided mental health care form two separate yet overlapping groups [21], as not all individuals with symptoms of mental illness will seek physician care. There is value in examining whether the association between diet quality and symptoms of depression extends to individuals seeking health care for depression. Filling this gap can contribute to our understanding of the potential for using dietary approaches to reduce the health service utilization burden.

There is an acknowledged need for large prospective investigations that account for a range of relevant confounders, and focus on population-based samples without a previous history of mental health problems [14]. The aim of the present study was to fill this gap and examine the association between diet quality and health service utilization for depression in a large prospective study of community dwelling adults, accounting for a range of relevant confounders.

2. Materials and Methods

From 2000 to 2008, Alberta's Tomorrow Project (ATP) enrolled 29,876 participants into a population-based prospective cohort study of cancer and chronic disease. Participants were considered eligible if they were ages 35–69 years, with no personal history of cancer other than non-melanoma skin cancer, plans to stay in Alberta for at least one year, and able to complete written questionnaires in English [22]. Participants were recruited using random digit dialing mapped to Regional Health Authority boundaries to facilitate balanced recruitment throughout the province. Eligible participants were mailed baseline questionnaires: the Health and Lifestyle Questionnaire (HLQ), the Canadian Diet History Questionnaire (CDHQ-I), and the Past-Year Total Physical Activity Questionnaire (PYTPAQ), which assessed sociodemographic characteristics, diet, and physical activity, respectively [22]. ATP methods have been previously published [22–24]. ATP data were linked to Alberta Health administrative health care databases via Personal Health Numbers and covered the years 2000 to 2015. Over 99% of ATP participants were successfully linked after providing valid Personal Health Numbers and consenting to data linkage [25]. ATP study procedures were approved by the Health Research Ethics Board of Alberta (HREBA)—Cancer Committee (HREBA.CC-17-0461). Ethics approval for the linkage to Alberta Health databases and current analyses was obtained from the University of Alberta Health Research Ethics Board (Pro00058561). All ATP participants provided written consents to participating in ATP and allowing healthcare data linkage and long-term follow-ups at the time of enrolment.

The CDHQ-I, a 124-item past year food frequency questionnaire (FFQ) of foods, beverages, and dietary supplements was based on the Diet History Questionnaire from the U.S. National Cancer Institute [26] and adapted to Canadian food availability, brand names, nutrient composition, and food fortification [23,27]. Responses were analyzed using Diet*Calc (version 1.4.2) software (National Cancer Institute, Bethesda, MD, USA) with a nutrient database adapted for the CDHQ-I to measure each participant's mean daily intake of energy, nutrients, foods, and supplement use. Diet quality was assessed by the Healthy Eating Index Canada (HEI-C) 2015 (Table S1), based on the American Healthy Eating Index (HEI) 2015 scoring criteria [28] and adapted to age- and sex-specific recommendations from Canada's Food Guide (CFG) 2007 [29]. The HEI-C 2015 assesses two major components of diet: adequacy (sufficiency of intake of healthy foods and nutrients (e.g., total fruits, whole fruits, total vegetables, greens and beans, whole grains, dairy, total protein foods, seafood and plant proteins, and fatty acids)) and moderation (excess consumption of unhealthy foods and nutrients (e.g., refined grains, sodium, added sugars, and saturated fats)). Moderation components are reverse-scored to reward the restriction of consumption the unhealthy components. The HEI-C 2015 score ranges 0–100, with higher scores indicating better diet quality and greater adherence to dietary recommendations.

We also calculated the Modified Mediterranean Diet Score (MMDS), which has nine components and total index score ranges from zero to nine, with higher scores indicating greater adherence to the Mediterranean diet [30]. Each of the nine components is scored either zero or one based on the sex-specific median, with the exception of alcohol which is based on set consumption values. The MMDS components are constituents of the traditional Mediterranean diet, which is associated with a number of beneficial chronic disease outcomes [31,32].

Health service utilization for depression was estimated using hospital discharge abstracts, physician claims, and prescription medication data between cohort enrollment (2000–2008) and 2015. International Classification of Diseases (ICD), Ninth and 10th Revision codes from administrative health databases of hospital inpatient datasets and the primary, secondary, and tertiary diagnosis fields from physician claims were used to identify depression. Additionally, Anatomical Therapeutic Chemical Classification (ATC) codes for antidepressants or mood stabilizers from Alberta Blue Cross (ABC) pharmacy claims or Pharmaceutical Information Network (PIN) dispenses were used (see Table S2 for ICD-9/10 and ATC codes). The codes for hospital discharge abstracts, physician claims, and prescription medication data were drawn from a validated algorithm from the Manitoba Centre for Health Policy's Regional Health Authority Indicators Atlas [33,34] to identify health service utilization for depression.

We considered a range of potential confounders. Sociodemographic factors included sex; age; region of residence (urban or rural) determined by postal code; family history of gambling, alcohol, or drug addiction (yes/no); household income (<$30,000, $30,000–59,999, $60,000–99,999, ≥$100,000); highest level of education (high school, some university, post-graduate); marital status (attached or unattached); and employment status (full-time, part-time, other). Lifestyle factors included body weight status (underweight/normal weight, overweight, obese); leisure time moderate-to-vigorous physical activity (MVPA) (rounded quartiles: <70.0 min/week, 70.0–209.9 min/week, 210.0–389.9 min/week, ≥390.0 min/week); smoking status (present, former, never); alcohol intake (g/week); use of supplements (yes/no), specifically vitamin D and other (vitamin A, beta carotene, vitamin E, vitamin C, thiamin, riboflavin, niacin, folic acid, calcium, magnesium, iron, zinc, copper, selenium). The Charlson comorbidity index (0, 1, ≥2 comorbidities) was calculated at baseline, using administrative health records and the ICD-9/10 coding algorithm for administrative healthcare data [35].

Data Analyses

Given the overdispersion ($p < 0.05$) of physician visits for depression, associations between diet quality and health service utilization for depression were calculated using Negative Binomial Regression Models (NBM). The effect of each of the HEI, moderation, adequacy, and MMDS were evaluated sequentially using four separate models. Rate ratios and 95% confidence intervals were derived from unadjusted, parsimonious, and fully adjusted NBMs. Parsimonious models adjusted for covariates commonly identified in the literature: age, sex, annual household income, educational attainment, physical activity, Body Mass Index (BMI), and energy intake. Fully adjusted models included all covariates from the parsimonious models plus rural/urban residence, marital status, family history of addiction, smoking status, disease comorbidities, vitamin D supplement use, other supplement use, and alcohol intake. Missing values for confounding variables were treated as separate covariate categories in the multivariable NBMs, but their estimates are not presented.

Participants were excluded if they had daily caloric intakes (<500 or >5000 kcal) [36], had not completed the three baseline questionnaires (HLQ, PYTPAQ, and CDHQ-I), or had missing dietary data (>10 missing responses on the CDHQ-I). In order to exclude prevalent cases of depression, we excluded participants with one or more physician visits for mental illness (see Table S3 for ICD-9/10 and ATC codes) during four time periods prior to enrollment in the ATP cohort, including three periods of fixed length (six months, one year and two years prior to cohort enrollment ($n = 2597, 5391$ and $12{,}657$, respectively)) and one period of variable length (from October 2000 to cohort enrollment ($n = 7681$)). These "washout" periods were implemented to increase the chance that depression episodes were incident and are recommended for examining chronic, episodic disorders in administrative health databases [37]. Analyses also included models that excluded physician visits for mental illness in the three months following enrollment to account for the possibility of increased health-consciousness immediately following enrollment in the ATP study. All analyses were conducted using STATA statistical software (Stata Corp LP, College Station, Texas, USA. 2007, Release 14). Statistical significance was set at $p < 0.05$.

3. Results

A total of 25,016 participants were available for analysis (Supplementary Materials Figure S1). Excluded participants did not significantly differ from those included in the analytic sample in terms of age, gender, geographic residence, education and presence of comorbidities (data not presented). Baseline characteristics of ATP participants are presented in Table 1. Of 25,016 participants included in analysis, 62.8% were female and 65.7% were overweight or obese. More than one-third (31.1%) of participants had one or more physician visits for depression between enrollment in the ATP cohort and end of follow-up in 2015 (Table 1). Participants' HEI-C 2015 score was, on average, 61.6 ± 11.0 out of 100 (Table 2), while the MMDS score was, on average, 4.3 ± 1.7 out of 10. Overall, 31.1% of participants saw a physician for depression following enrollment.

Table 1. Baseline characteristics of ATP participants ($n = 25{,}016$).

	Number of Physician Visits			
	Total ($n = 25{,}016$)	0 ($n = 17{,}227$)	1–2 ($n = 3881$)	3+ ($n = 3908$)
	% or Mean (SD)	% or Mean (SD)	% or Mean (SD)	% or Mean (SD)
Age (years)	50.39 (9.17)	50.56 (9.21)	50.49 (9.28)	49.50 (8.87)
Sex				
Male	37.18%	42.70%	28.45%	21.52%
Female	62.82%	57.30%	71.55%	78.48%

Table 1. *Cont.*

	Total (n = 25,016)	0 (n = 17,227)	1–2 (n = 3881)	3+ (n = 3908)
	% or Mean (SD)	% or Mean (SD)	% or Mean (SD)	% or Mean (SD)
BMI (kg/m^2)				
Underweight/normal weight (≤24.9)	34.03%	34.14%	35.02%	32.55%
Overweight (25.0–29.9)	39.11%	40.29%	37.64%	35.36%
Obese (≥30.0)	26.63%	25.37%	27.11%	31.70%
Location				
Rural	23.64%	24.50%	22.78%	20.70%
Urban	76.36%	75.50%	77.22%	79.30%
Smoking status				
Never	45.12%	47.75%	41.07%	37.54%
Former	37.73%	36.96%	38.52%	40.32%
Current	17.13%	15.27%	20.41%	22.11%
Household income				
<$30,000	12.71%	10.89%	14.33%	19.14%
$30,000–59,999	26.89%	26.09%	28.06%	29.25%
$60,000–99,999	31.87%	32.58%	30.92%	29.68%
≥$100,000	26.29%	28.22%	24.19%	19.83%
Highest level of education				
High school	27.49%	26.97%	29.27%	28.02%
Some university	46.94%	46.18%	47.46%	49.80%
Post-graduate	25.56%	26.85%	23.27%	22.16%
Charlson comorbidity index				
0	83.24%	85.52%	80.06%	76.33%
1	14.31%	12.56%	16.52%	19.83%
2+	2.45%	1.92%	3.43%	3.84%
Energy intake (Kcal/day)	1826.81 (730.92)	1840.59 (732.73)	1797.23 (719.15)	1795.47 (732.82)

ATP, Alberta's Tomorrow Project; BMI, Body Mass Index; SD, Standard Deviation.

Table 2. Average HEI-C 2015 and component scores of ATP participants (*n* = 25,016).

Category/Component	Possible Range	Mean (SD)
Overall HEI-C 2015	0–100	61.56 (11.02)
Adequacy	0–60	34.93 (8.88)
Total vegetables and fruit	0–10	8.02 (2.28)
Whole fruits	0–5	4.04 (1.40)
Greens and beans	0–5	2.53 (1.65)
Whole grains	0–10	3.64 (2.30)
Dairy	0–10	5.86 (3.14)
Total protein foods	0–5	3.43 (1.26)
Seafood and plant proteins	0–5	2.42 (1.44)
Fatty acids	0–10	4.98 (2.78)
Moderation	0–40	26.64 (6.33)
Refined grains	0–10	5.29 (2.33)
Sodium	0–10	7.08 (3.39)
Added sugars	0–10	7.86 (2.37)
Saturated fats	0–10	6.42 (2.90)

ATP, Alberta's Tomorrow Project; HEI-C 2015, Health Eating Index-Canada 2015; SD, Standard Deviation.

Table 3 presents the estimated reduction in the number of physician visits for depression for every 10-unit increase in HEI-C 2015 and component scores. After adjusting for all covariates, every 10-unit increase in HEI-C 2015 score was associated with 4.68% fewer physician visits for depression (rate ratio (RR): 0.95; 95% Confidence Interval (CI): 0.92–0.98). Dietary adequacy was also negatively associated with physician visits, leading to 8.78% fewer visits for depression (RR: 0.91; 95% CI: 0.87–0.96). For each 1-unit increase in MMDS score, there was a 2.48% reduction in the number of physician visits for depression (RR: 0.98; 95% CI: 0.96–0.99) (Table 3). Results capturing the association of diet quality measured with HEI-C 2015 or MMDS and health service utilization for depression remained robust regardless of the covariates adjusted for in parsimonious and fully adjusted models.

A similar reduction in the number of physician visits for depression associated with 10-unit increases in HEI-C 2015 scores was observed when participants were excluded in different periods prior to cohort enrollment. In fully adjusted models, participants had 5.39% (RR: 0.95; 95% CI: 0.91–0.98), 5.38% (RR: 0.95; 95% CI: 0.91–0.98), and 8.34% (RR: 0.92; 95% CI: 0.88–0.96) fewer physician visits when we excluded visits in the six months, one year, or variable-length period from 2000 to cohort enrollment, respectively (Table 4). However, the results were no longer significant after excluding physician visits for mental health in the two years prior to enrollment. Lastly, after excluding physician visits in the three months after cohort enrollment, every 10-unit increase in HEI-C 2015 score and adequacy component score was associated with 4.68% (RR: 0.95; 95% CI: 0.92–0.98) and 8.78% (RR: 0.91; 95% CI: 0.87–0.96) fewer physician visits for depression, respectively (Table 4).

Table 3. Associations of increases in HEI-C 2015 and MMDS scores with number of physician visits for depression (n = 25,016).

	Unadjusted			Parsimonious [a]			Fully Adjusted [b]		
	RR (95% CI)	(1-RR)%	p-Value	RR (95% CI)	(1-RR)%	p-Value	RR (95% CI)	(1-RR)%	p-Value
HEI-C 2015 [c]	0.96 (0.94, 0.99)	3.68%	0.010	0.95 (0.92, 0.98)	5.12%	0.001	0.95 (0.92, 0.98)	4.68%	0.002
Moderation [c]	0.94 (0.89, 0.99)	6.03%	0.016	0.93 (0.88, 0.99)	6.55%	0.034	0.96 (0.89, 1.02)	4.48%	0.172
Adequacy [c]	0.97 (0.94, 1.01)	2.75%	0.122	0.92 (0.88, 0.96)	8.10%	<0.001	0.91 (0.87, 0.96)	8.78%	<0.001
MMDS [d]	0.94 (0.92, 0.96)	5.76%	<0.001	0.97 (0.95, 0.99)	2.75%	0.004	0.98 (0.96, 0.99)	2.48%	0.010

95% CI, 95% Confidence Interval; HEI-C 2015, Health Eating Index-Canada 2015; MMDS, Modified Mediterranean Diet Score; RR, rate ratio; [a] Adjusted for sex, age, BMI, leisure time moderate-to-vigorous physical activity (MVPA), household income, educational attainment, caloric intake; [b] Adjusted for sex, age, BMI, urban/rural location, family history of addiction, leisure time MVPA, smoking status, household income, educational attainment, marital status, employment status, chronic disease comorbidities, use of vitamin D supplements, use of other supplements, weekly alcohol intake, caloric intake; [c] Per 10-unit increase in score; [d] Per 1-unit increase in score.

Table 4. Associations of increases in HEI-C 2015 and MMDS scores with number of physician visits for depression following exclusions.

	Unadjusted			Parsimonious [a]			Fully Adjusted [b]		
	RR (95% CI)	(1-RR)%	p-Value	RR (95% CI)	(1-RR)%	p-Value	RR (95% CI)	(1-RR)%	p-Value
Six-Month Exclusion Prior to Enrollment (n = 22,419)									
HEI-C 2015 [c]	0.96 (0.93, 1.00)	3.58%	0.125	0.94 (0.91, 0.98)	5.60%	0.001	0.95 (0.91, 0.98)	5.39%	0.002
Moderation [c]	0.94 (0.89, 1.00)	5.85%	0.033	0.92 (0.86, 0.99)	7.69%	0.026	0.93 (0.86, 1.00)	7.00%	0.056
Adequacy [c]	0.97 (0.94, 1.01)	2.53%	0.202	0.92 (0.87, 0.96)	8.36%	0.001	0.91 (0.86, 0.96)	8.98%	0.001
MMDS [d]	0.95 (0.93, 0.97)	5.39%	<0.001	0.97 (0.95, 0.99)	2.61%	0.014	0.98 (0.96, 1.00)	2.31%	0.030
One-Year Exclusion Prior to Enrollment (n = 19,625)									
HEI-C 2015 [c]	0.96 (0.93, 0.99)	4.07%	0.023	0.94 (0.91, 0.98)	5.85%	0.002	0.95 (0.91, 0.98)	5.38%	0.006
Moderation [c]	0.92 (0.86, 0.98)	8.35%	0.006	0.91 (0.84, 0.98)	9.21%	0.017	0.92 (0.84, 1.00)	8.50%	0.039
Adequacy [c]	0.98 (0.94, 1.03)	1.91%	0.395	0.92 (0.87, 0.97)	7.96%	0.004	0.92 (0.86, 0.98)	8.12%	0.006
MMDS [d]	0.94 (0.92, 0.97)	5.58%	<0.001	0.97 (0.95, 0.99)	2.84%	0.017	0.98 (0.95, 1.00)	2.50%	0.036
Two-Year Exclusion Prior to Enrollment (n = 12,359)									
HEI-C 2015 [c]	0.99 (0.94, 1.03)	1.50%	0.537	0.96 (0.91, 1.01)	4.39%	0.088	0.98 (0.93, 1.03)	2.14%	0.426
Moderation [c]	0.94 (0.86, 1.02)	6.12%	0.144	0.89 (0.80, 0.99)	11.03%	0.035	0.94 (0.84, 1.05)	6.05%	0.278
Adequacy [c]	1.01 (0.95, 1.07)	-0.78%	0.796	0.96 (0.89, 1.04)	4.11%	0.290	0.98 (0.90, 1.07)	1.83%	0.660
MMDS [d]	0.96 (0.93, 0.99)	3.94%	0.013	0.98 (0.95, 1.00)	2.27%	0.160	0.98 (0.95, 1.01)	2.06%	0.203

Table 4. *Cont.*

	Unadjusted			Parsimonious [a]			Fully Adjusted [b]		
	RR (95% CI)	(1-RR)%	p-Value	RR (95% CI)	(1-RR)%	p-Value	RR (95% CI)	(1-RR)%	p-Value
Variable-Length Exclusion Prior to Enrollment (n = 17,335)									
HEI-C 2015 [c]	0.92 (0.89, 0.96)	7.61%	<0.001	0.91 (0.87, 0.95)	9.17%	<0.001	0.92 (0.88, 0.96)	8.34%	<0.001
Moderation [c]	0.88 (0.82, 0.94)	11.87%	<0.001	0.87 (0.79, 0.95)	13.45%	0.002	0.87 (0.79, 0.96)	12.85%	0.005
Adequacy [c]	0.94 (0.90, 0.99)	5.74%	0.022	0.87 (0.81, 0.93)	13.04%	<0.001	0.87 (0.81, 0.93)	12.76%	<0.001
MMDS [d]	0.94 (0.92, 0.97)	5.91%	<0.001	0.97 (0.95, 1.00)	2.75%	0.043	0.97 (0.95, 1.00)	2.57%	0.059
Exclusion of Visits Three Months Following Enrollment (n = 25,016)									
HEI-C 2015 [c]	0.96 (0.94, 0.99)	3.75%	0.009	0.95 (0.92, 0.98)	5.08%	0.001	0.95 (0.92, 0.98)	4.68%	0.002
Moderation [c]	0.94 (0.89, 0.99)	6.11%	0.015	0.94 (0.88, 1.00)	6.41%	0.039	0.96 (0.89, 1.02)	4.48%	0.172
Adequacy [c]	0.97 (0.94, 1.01)	2.81%	0.115	0.92 (0.88, 0.96)	8.06%	<0.001	0.91 (0.87, 0.96)	8.78%	<0.001
MMDS [d]	0.94 (0.92, 0.96)	5.82%	<0.001	0.97 (0.95, 0.99)	2.75%	0.004	0.98 (0.96, 0.99)	2.46%	0.011

95% CI, 95% Confidence Interval; HEI-C 2015, Health Eating Index-Canada 2015; MMDS, Modified Mediterranean Diet Score; RR, rate ratio; [a] Adjusted for sex, age, BMI, leisure time MVPA, household income, educational attainment, caloric intake; [b] Adjusted for sex, age, BMI, urban/rural location, family history of addiction, leisure time MVPA, smoking status, household income, educational attainment, marital status, employment status, chronic disease comorbidities, use of vitamin D supplements, use of other supplements, weekly alcohol intake, caloric intake; [c] Per 10-unit increase in score; [d] Per 1-unit increase in score.

4. Discussion

Our study provides evidence that a high-quality diet in adulthood is associated with reduced health service utilization, where every 10-unit increase in diet quality as measured with the HEI-C 2015 was associated with a 4.68% reduction in the number of physician visits for depression. We also observed a similar 2.48% reduction in physician visits for depression for every 1-unit increase in MMDS score, which measures adherence to the Mediterranean diet, high in vegetables, fruit, grains, and legumes, and low in meat and dairy. In addition, our results remained robust when participants with pre-existing physician-diagnosed mental illness were excluded from analyses.

The association between diet quality indices and depression in adults was recently summarized in two systematic reviews. One of the two reviews was limited to 29 prospective studies and found that adherence to high-quality (i.e., healthy/prudent, Mediterranean, pro-vegetarian, or Tuscan) and anti-inflammatory diets was associated with 23% and 19% lower risk of depression, respectively [14]. Another systematic review and meta-analysis of 41 observational studies found that individuals in the highest category of adherence to high-quality and Mediterranean diets had 24% and 33% lower risk of incident depression, respectively, compared to those with lowest adherence [15]. The coefficients from our analyses translate into a difference of up to 17.26% for higher versus lower adherence to the HEI-C 2015 (scores >75 vs. <50) and up to 9.38% for the MMDS (scores >6 vs. <4). These results are of similar magnitude to earlier studies and further corroborate the previously reported associations.

Previous studies often have not accounted for baseline depression status [38–40], with findings pointing to complex and bidirectional relations between diet, other lifestyle behaviors, and mental disorders and depression in particular. Given the chronic and episodic nature of depression, our exclusion of participants using four periods prior to cohort enrollment sought to mitigate the issue of reverse causation. It is compelling that our results remained significant with exclusions of six months (*n* = 22,419), one year (*n* = 19,625), and all visits between 2000 and cohort enrollment (*n* = 17,335). Although our results were no longer significant following exclusion of participants with any physician visits for mental illness in the two years prior to cohort enrollment, this is likely due to additionally excluding all participants enrolled in the first two years of ATP. This resulted in a substantial reduction of study sample (12,359/25,016 or approximately half) and a loss of statistical power. As suggested by Molendijk et al. (2018), the correction for depression status at baseline may negate the cumulative effects of lifestyle behaviors in the years before the study. Our work in children demonstrated that adherence to established recommendations for diet, physical activity, sleep, and sedentary behavior at age 10–11 years was associated with 56% fewer physician visits for mental illness in the subsequent four years [41]. This reduction was of similar magnitude with and without correction for mental illness at baseline, i.e., exclusion of all children with a mental illness diagnosis before the baseline. As less than 10% of children in the sample met this exclusion criteria, the similar magnitude of the association with and without correction for baseline mental illness corroborates the findings from this study, and suggests that the lack of association after excluding participants with physician visits in the two years prior to cohort enrollment may indeed be a statistical power issue.

We found that the adequacy component of the HEI-C 2015 remained significant following adjustment for confounders, but the moderation component did not. This finding is interesting and corroborates existing literature. In a recent meta-analysis, the highest category of adherence to healthy diets was associated with less depressive symptoms; however, adherence to unhealthy dietary patterns and food groups was not associated with incident depressive symptoms [14]. Taken together, these findings suggest that a diet sufficient in beneficial foods and nutrients may be more important than a diet restrictive in foods and nutrients recommended to be consumed in moderation. To our knowledge, other studies that have used versions of the HEI to investigate the relationship between diet quality and mental illness have not examined or reported the components of adequacy or moderation.

Existing studies also relied predominantly on cross-sectional design and often did not include several potential confounding variables, such as obesity, energy intake, baseline socioeconomic status (income, parents' educational level), and medical conditions (e.g., diabetes, food allergies, hypothyroidism) that may be correlated with mood or diet [14,15]. Diet is the product of the interplay among a large number of factors and a lack of consistency in the adjustment for confounders leads to errors in inference and makes comparison across studies difficult [14]. We adjusted for a range of relevant confounders identified in the literature and observed that even after the inclusion of confounders in the models, the results remained robust.

The large sample of the general adult population of Alberta with a diverse range of demographic and behavioral characteristics, followed prospectively for up to 14 years of follow-up and low attrition, the nearly complete linkage with administrative databases, little missing data due to rigorous quality control measures, and the use of multiple measures of diet quality are major strengths. Several limitations warrant consideration. First, although we included a wide range of relevant covariates, the possibility of residual confounding remains. Second, the exposures of interest and confounders, with the exclusion of disease comorbidities, were based on self-report. Nonetheless, the HLQ, CDHQ-I, and PYTPAQ were either composed of existing items used in other studies, adapted from a validated questionnaire, or specifically developed and tested for validity and reliability in this cohort, respectively [22]. Third, since ATP recruited participants when they were already aged 35–69 years, this precludes our ability to observe lifetime incidence of depression. Last, our outcome measure was mental health service utilization, which included participants who had sought out and received physician care for a mental illness. Those who encountered barriers to care or received care outside of the medical system (e.g., psychological counselling through community mental health services) were not included, thus underestimating the burden of depression. Additionally, individuals of higher socioeconomic status may have chosen to seek mental health support through private psychological services, which was also not included. However, if misclassification of outcome did occur, the literature suggests that the result is typically an estimate biased toward the null [42].

5. Conclusions

We observed an inverse relationship between diet quality measured with two different dietary indices and health service utilization for depression, independent of socio-economic status (SES), other lifestyle behaviors, and disease comorbidities. Given that the diet quality of many Canadians is of poor quality and either stagnating or declining [7,8], interventions to improve the diets of Canadians at the population level may have important implications for reducing the health care burden for depression in addition to reducing the established risk for chronic disease.

Supplementary Materials: The following are available online at http://www.mdpi.com/2072-6643/12/8/2437/s1: Figure S1: Flow chart for the inclusion and exclusion of Alberta's Tomorrow Project (ATP) cohort (2000–2008); Table S1: Scoring Criteria for the Healthy Eating Index-Canada 2015; Table S2: ICD 9/10 and ATC Codes Identifying Physician Visits for Depression; Table S3: ICD 9/10 and ATC Codes Identifying Physician Visits for Mental Illness.

Author Contributions: S.M. conceived, designed, and conducted the analysis and drafted the manuscript; K.M. and P.J.V. conceived and designed the analysis, assisted in interpreting the data, and critically reviewed the manuscript; J.D. conducted literature reviews, drafted the manuscript, and critically reviewed the manuscript for important intellectual content; M.Y. and D.T.E. assisted in interpreting the data and critically reviewed the manuscript for important intellectual content. All authors have read and agreed to the published version of the manuscript.

Funding: Alberta's Tomorrow Project is funded by Alberta Health, Alberta Cancer Foundation, Canadian Partnership against Cancer and Health Canada, and substantial in kind funding from Alberta Health Services.

Acknowledgments: Alberta's Tomorrow Project is only possible because of the commitment of its research participants, its staff and its funders: Alberta Health, Alberta Cancer Foundation, Canadian Partnership against Cancer and Health Canada, and substantial in kind funding from Alberta Health Services. The views expressed herein represent the views of the author(s) and not of Alberta's Tomorrow Project or any of its funders. This study is based in part on data provided by Alberta Health. The interpretation and conclusions contained herein are those of the researchers and do not necessarily represent the views of the Government of Alberta. Neither the Government nor Alberta Health express any opinion in relation to this study.

Conflicts of Interest: The authors have no conflicts of interest relevant to this article to disclose.

References

1. World Health Organization. *Depression and Other Common Mental Disorders: Global Health Estimates*; World Health Organization: Geneva, Switzerland, 2017.

2. Pearson, C.; Janz, T.; Ali, J. *Mental and Substance Use Disorders in Canada*; Statistics Canada: Ottawa, ON, Canada, 2013.

3. Whiteford, H.A.; Degenhardt, L.; Rehm, J.; Baxter, A.J.; Ferrari, A.J.; Erskine, H.E.; Charlson, F.J.; Norman, R.E.; Flaxman, A.D.; Johns, N. Global burden of disease attributable to mental and substance use disorders: Findings from the Global Burden of Disease Study 2010. *Lancet* **2013**, *382*, 1575–1586. [CrossRef]

4. Smetanin, P.; Stiff, D.; Briante, C.; Adair, C.; Ahmad, S.; Khan, M. *The Life and Economic Impact of Major Mental Illnesses in Canada: 2011 to 2041*; RiskAnalytica on behalf of the Mental Health Commission of Canada: Toronto, ON, Canada, 2011.

5. Public Health Agency of Canada. *Report from the Canadian Chronic Disease Surveillance System*; Public Health Agency of Canada: Ottawa, ON, Canada, 2015.

6. Johansen, H.; Finès, P. Acute care hospital days and mental diagnoses. *Health Rep.* **2012**, *23*, 61–65.

7. Tugault-Lafleur, C.N.; Black, J.L. Differences in the Quantity and Types of Foods and Beverages Consumed by Canadians between 2004 and 2015. *Nutrients* **2019**, *11*, 526. [CrossRef] [PubMed]

8. Lieffers, J.R.; Ekwaru, J.P.; Ohinmaa, A.; Veugelers, P.J. The economic burden of not meeting food recommendations in Canada: The cost of doing nothing. *PLoS ONE* **2018**, *13*, e0196333. [CrossRef] [PubMed]

9. Firth, J.; Marx, W.; Dash, S.; Carney, R.; Teasdale, S.B.; Solmi, M.; Stubbs, B.; Schuch, F.B.; Carvalho, A.F.; Jacka, F.; et al. The Effects of Dietary Improvement on Symptoms of Depression and Anxiety: A Meta-Analysis of Randomized Controlled Trials. *Psychosom. Med.* **2019**, *81*, 265–280. [CrossRef] [PubMed]

10. Opie, R.S.; O'Neil, A.; Itsiopoulos, C.; Jacka, F.N. The impact of whole-of-diet interventions on depression and anxiety: A systematic review of randomised controlled trials. *Public Health Nutr.* **2015**, *18*, 2074–2093. [CrossRef]

11. Satija, A.; Yu, E.; Willett, W.C.; Hu, F.B. Understanding nutritional epidemiology and its role in policy. *Adv. Nutr.* **2015**, *6*, 5–18. [CrossRef]

12. Satija, A.; Stampfer, M.J.; Rimm, E.B.; Willett, W.; Hu, F.B. Perspective: Are Large, Simple Trials the Solution for Nutrition Research? *Adv. Nutr.* **2018**, *9*, 378–387. [CrossRef]

13. Nicolaou, M.; Colpo, M.; Vermeulen, E.; Elstgeest, L.E.M.; Cabout, M.; Gibson-Smith, D.; Knuppel, A.; Sini, G.; Schoenaker, D.A.; Mishra, G.D. Association of a priori dietary patterns with depressive symptoms: A harmonized meta-analysis of observational studies. *Psychol. Med.* **2019**, 1–12. [CrossRef]

14. Molendijk, M.; Molero, P.; Ortuño Sánchez-Pedreno, F.; Van der Does, W.; Angel Martínez-González, M. Diet quality and depression risk: A systematic review and dose-response meta-analysis of prospective studies. *J. Affect. Disord.* **2018**, *226*, 346–354. [CrossRef]

15. Lassale, C.; Batty, G.D.; Baghdadli, A.; Jacka, F.; Sánchez-Villegas, A.; Kivimäki, M.; Akbaraly, T. Healthy dietary indices and risk of depressive outcomes: A systematic review and meta-analysis of observational studies. *Mol. Psychiatry* **2019**, *24*, 965–986. [CrossRef] [PubMed]

16. Li, Y.; Lv, M.R.; Wei, Y.J.; Sun, L.; Zhang, J.X.; Zhang, H.G.; Li, B. Dietary patterns and depression risk: A meta-analysis. *Psychiatry Res.* **2017**, *253*, 373–382. [CrossRef] [PubMed]

17. Lai, J.S.; Hiles, S.; Bisquera, A.; Hure, A.J.; McEvoy, M.; Attia, J. A systematic review and meta-analysis of dietary patterns and depression in community-dwelling adults. *Am. J. Clin. Nutr.* **2014**, *99*, 181–197. [CrossRef] [PubMed]

18. Radloff, L.S. The CES-D scale: A self-report depression scale for research in the general population. *Appl. Psychol. Meas.* **1977**, *1*, 385–401. [CrossRef]

19. Beck, A.T.; Steer, R.A.; Brown, G.K. *Manual for the Beck Depression Inventory-II*; Psychological Corporation: San Antonio, TX, USA, 1996.

20. World Health Organization. *Composite International Diagnostic Interview–Version 1.1*; World Health Organization: Geneva, Switzerland, 1993.

21. Parslow, R.A.; Jorm, A.F. Who uses mental health services in Australia? An analysis of data from the National Survey of Mental Health and Wellbeing. *Aust. N. Z. J. Psychiatry* **2000**, *34*, 997–1008. [CrossRef]

22. Bryant, H.; Robson, P.J.; Ullman, R.; Friedenreich, C.; Dawe, U. Population-based cohort development in Alberta, Canada: A feasibility study. *Chronic Dis. Can.* **2006**, *27*, 51–59.

23. Csizmadi, I.; Kahle, L.; Ullman, R.; Dawe, U.; Zimmerman, T.P.; Friedenreich, C.M.; Bryant, H.; Subar, A.F. Adaptation and evaluation of the National Cancer Institute's Diet History Questionnaire and nutrient database for Canadian populations. *Public Health Nutr.* **2007**, *10*, 88–96. [CrossRef]

24. Friedenreich, C.M.; Courneya, K.S.; Neilson, H.K.; Matthews, C.E.; Willis, G.; Irwin, M.; Troiano, R.; Ballard-Barbash, R. Reliability and validity of the Past Year Total Physical Activity Questionnaire. *Am. J. Epidemiol.* **2006**, *163*, 959–970. [CrossRef]

25. Ye, M.; Robson, P.J.; Eurich, D.T.; Vena, J.E.; Xu, J.Y.; Johnson, J.A. Cohort Profile: Alberta's Tomorrow Project. *Int. J. Epidemiol.* **2017**, *46*, 1097–1098l. [CrossRef]

26. National Institutes of Health. *Diet History Questionnaire*; National Institutes of Health: Washington, DC, USA, 2007.

27. Subar, A.F.; Midthune, D.; Kulldorff, M.; Brown, C.C.; Thompson, F.E.; Kipnis, V.; Schatzkin, A. Evaluation of alternative approaches to assign nutrient values to food groups in food frequency questionnaires. *Am. J. Epidemiol.* **2000**, *152*, 279–286. [CrossRef]

28. Krebs-Smith, S.M.; Pannucci, T.E.; Subar, A.F.; Kirkpatrick, S.I.; Lerman, J.L.; Tooze, J.A.; Wilson, M.M.; Reedy, J. Update of the Healthy Eating Index: HEI-2015. *J. Acad. Nutr. Diet.* **2018**, *118*, 1591–1602. [CrossRef] [PubMed]

29. Health Canada. *Eating Well with Canada's Food Guide*; Health Canada: Ottawa, ON, Canada, 2007.

30. Trichopoulou, A.; Costacou, T.; Bamia, C.; Trichopoulos, D. Adherence to a Mediterranean diet and survival in a Greek population. *N. Engl. J. Med.* **2003**, *348*, 2599–2608. [CrossRef] [PubMed]

31. Dinu, M.; Pagliai, G.; Casini, A.; Sofi, F. Mediterranean diet and multiple health outcomes: An umbrella review of meta-analyses of observational studies and randomised trials. *Eur. J. Clin. Nutr.* **2018**, *72*, 30–43. [CrossRef] [PubMed]

32. Galbete, C.; Schwingshackl, L.; Schwedhelm, C.; Boeing, H.; Schulze, M.B. Evaluating Mediterranean diet and risk of chronic disease in cohort studies: An umbrella review of meta-analyses. *Eur. J. Epidemiol.* **2018**, *33*, 909–931. [CrossRef] [PubMed]

33. Fransoo, R.; Martens, P.; Burland, E.; The Need to Know Team; Prior, H.; Burchill, C. *Manitoba RHA Indicators Atlas 2009*; Manitoba Centre for Health Policy: Winnipeg, MB, Canada, 2009.

34. Burchill, C.; Burland, E.; Chateau, D.; De Coster, C.; Ekuma, O.; Fransoo, R.; Jebamani, L.; Martens, P.J.; McKeen, N.; Metge, C.; et al. *Patterns of Regional Mental Illness Disorder Diagnoses and Service Use in Manitoba: A Population-Based Study*; Manitoba Centre for Health Policy: Winnipeg, MB, Canada, 2004.

35. Quan, H.; Sundararajan, V.; Halfon, P.; Fong, A.; Burnand, B.; Luthi, J.C.; Saunders, L.D.; Beck, C.A.; Feasby, T.E.; Ghali, W.A. Coding algorithms for defining comorbidities in ICD-9-CM and ICD-10 administrative data. *Med. Care* **2005**, *43*, 1130–1139. [CrossRef] [PubMed]

36. Willett, W. *Nutritional Epidemiology*, 3rd ed.; Oxford University Press: Oxford, UK, 2013.

37. Lewis, J.D.; Bilker, W.B.; Weinstein, R.B.; Strom, B.L. The relationship between time since registration and measured incidence rates in the General Practice Research Database. *Pharmacoepidemiol. Drug Saf.* **2005**, *14*, 443–451. [CrossRef]

38. McMartin, S.E.; Kuhle, S.; Colman, I.; Kirk, S.F.; Veugelers, P.J. Diet quality and mental health in subsequent years among Canadian youth. *Public Health Nutr.* **2012**, *15*, 2253–2258. [CrossRef]

39. Timonen, M.; Horrobin, D.; Jokelainen, J.; Laitinen, J.; Herva, A.; Räsänen, P. Fish consumption and depression: The Northern Finland 1966 birth cohort study. *J. Affect. Disord.* **2004**, *82*, 447–452. [CrossRef]

40. Sánchez-Villegas, A.; Toledo, E.; de Irala, J.; Ruiz-Canela, M.; Pla-Vidal, J.; Martínez-González, M.A. Fast-food and commercial baked goods consumption and the risk of depression. *Public Health Nutr.* **2012**, *15*, 424–432. [CrossRef]

41. Loewen, O.K.; Maximova, K.; Ekwaru, J.P.; Faught, E.L.; Asbridge, M.; Ohinmaa, A.; Veugelers, P.J. Lifestyle Behavior and Mental Health in Early Adolescence. *Pediatrics* **2019**, *143*, e20183307. [CrossRef]

42. Copeland, K.T.; Checkoway, H.; McMichael, A.J.; Holbrook, R.H. Bias due to misclassification in the estimation of relative risk. *Am. J. Epidemiol.* **1977**, *105*, 488–495. [CrossRef] [PubMed]

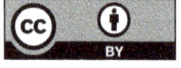

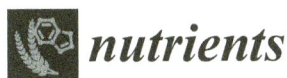

Article

Specific Dietary (Poly)phenols Are Associated with Sleep Quality in a Cohort of Italian Adults

Justyna Godos [1], Raffaele Ferri [1], Sabrina Castellano [2], Donato Angelino [3], Pedro Mena [4], Daniele Del Rio [5,6], Filippo Caraci [1,7], Fabio Galvano [8] and Giuseppe Grosso [8,*]

1   Oasi Research Institute—IRCCS, 94018 Troina, Italy; justyna.godos@gmail.com (J.G.); rferri@oasi.en.it (R.F.); carafil@hotmail.com (F.C.)
2   Department of Educational Sciences, University of Catania, 95124 Catania, Italy; sabrina.castellano@unict.it
3   Faculty of Bioscience and Technology for Food, Agriculture and Environment, University of Teramo, 64100 Teramo, Italy; dangelino@unite.it
4   Human Nutrition Unit, Department of Food and Drugs, University of Parma, 43125 Parma, Italy; pedromiguel.menaparreno@unipr.it
5   School of Advanced Studies on Food and Nutrition, University of Parma, 43125 Parma, Italy; daniele.delrio@unipr.it
6   Department of Veterinary Medicine, University of Parma, 43125 Parma, Italy
7   Department of Drug Sciences, University of Catania, 95125 Catania, Italy
8   Department of Biomedical and Biotechnological Sciences, University of Catania, 95123 Catania, Italy; fgalvano@unict.it
*   Correspondence: giuseppe.grosso@unict.it; Tel.: +39-095-478-1187

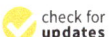

Received: 28 March 2020; Accepted: 24 April 2020; Published: 26 April 2020

Abstract: Background: Diet has been the major focus of attention as a leading risk factor for non-communicable diseases, including mental health disorders. A large body of literature supports the hypothesis that there is a bidirectional association between sleep and diet quality, possibly via the modulation of neuro-inflammation, adult neurogenesis and synaptic and neuronal plasticity. In the present study, the association between dietary total, subclasses of and individual (poly)phenols and sleep quality was explored in a cohort of Italian adults. Methods: The demographic and dietary characteristics of 1936 adults living in southern Italy were analyzed. Food frequency questionnaires (FFQs) were used to assess dietary intake. Data on the (poly)phenol content in foods were retrieved from the Phenol-Explorer database. The Pittsburg Sleep Quality Index was used to measure sleep quality. Multivariate logistic regression analyses were used to test the associations. Results: A significant inverse association between a higher dietary intake of lignans and inadequate sleep quality was found. Additionally, individuals with the highest quartile of hydroxycinnamic acid intake were less likely to have inadequate sleep quality. When individual compounds were taken into consideration, an association with sleep quality was observed for naringenin and apigenin among flavonoids, and for matairesinol among lignans. A secondary analysis was conducted, stratifying the population into normal weight and overweight/obese individuals. The findings in normal weight individuals showed a stronger association between certain classes of, subclasses of and individual compounds and sleep quality. Notably, nearly all individual compounds belonging to the lignan class were inversely associated with inadequate sleep quality. In the overweight/obese individuals, there were no associations between any dietary (poly)phenol class and sleep quality. Conclusions: The results of this study suggest that a higher dietary intake of certain (poly)phenols may be associated with better sleep quality among adult individuals.

Keywords: polyphenol; sleep; mental health; cohort; antioxidant; cognitive; brain; Sicily; population

1. Introduction

Diet has been the focus of major attention as a leading risk factor for non-communicable diseases [1,2]. These estimates are based on convincing evidence that dietary factors may play a role in the risks of cardiovascular diseases and certain cancers [3–8]. A more intriguing hypothesis recently explored is that diet may also influence brain health and mental disorders [9,10]. A large body of literature supports the hypothesis that there is an association between sleeping patterns and diet quality, possibly mediating weight status and obesity-related disorders [11]. Generally, most of the evidence relies on the positive association between sleep quality or duration and diet quality, but relatively recent studies suggest that a bidirectional relationship may exist, with dietary factors influencing sleep features [12]. Several mechanisms have been hypothesized to explain this association, including inflammation, oxidative stress, the gut microbiome, epigenetic modifications and the direct effects of nutrients and non-nutrients on neuroplasticity [13]. Among the healthy dietary patterns suggested for their putative influence on sleep quality, plant-based foods, including vegetables, grains, nuts, seeds, legumes and fruits, have demonstrated to have a mechanistic relationship with better mental health, potentially influencing sleep features [12]. Those foods are rich sources of bioactive compounds that, in the context of a healthy lifestyle, may play a potential role in preventing subclinical low-grade inflammation, a starting point for several chronic non-communicable diseases as well as for impaired sleep quality and duration [14,15]. There is, in fact, evidence that inflammation may mediate a variety of brain disorders involving sleep quality but also stress, depression, dementia and Alzheimer's disease [16]. Thus, it is crucial to understand whether diet may affect the level of inflammation and which compounds should be of major interest.

Dietary (poly)phenols represent a group of compounds present in plant-derived foods that, based on their biochemical structure, may play a pivotal role in radical scavenging and in mediating inflammation processes [17–19]. Several families are commonly consumed when adhering to healthy dietary patterns, including flavonoids (mostly contained in fruits, vegetables, tea and cocoa products), phenolic acids (contained in fruits, coffee, pulses and nuts), stilbenes (mainly contained in wine) and phytoestrogens (including isoflavones and lignans, contained in soy products and legumes). Dietary (poly)phenols have been related to several potential health benefits [20]: recently, they have been hypothesized to also play a role in brain health [21,22]. We previously reported that individuals more adherent to healthy dietary patterns (i.e., the Mediterranean diet) and to a diet with low inflammatory potential were more likely to have higher sleep quality [23,24]. In the present study, we aimed to test whether total, subclasses of and individual (poly)phenols may be candidate molecules associated with sleep quality in a cohort of Italian adults.

2. Materials and Methods

2.1. Study Population

The MEAL study is an observational study aiming to investigate the association between the nutritional and lifestyle habits characterizing the classical Mediterranean area and non-communicable diseases. The baseline data included a sample of 2044 men and women aged 18 or more years old. Individuals were randomly selected in the main districts of the city of Catania, Sicily, Italy. The enrolment and data collection were performed between 2014 and 2015. Details of the study protocol are published elsewhere [25]. All participants were informed about the aims of the study and provided written informed consent. All the study procedures were carried out in accordance with the Declaration of Helsinki (1989) of the World Medical Association. The study protocol has been reviewed and approved by the concerning ethical committee of the Municipal Health Authority (protocol number: 802/23 December 2014).

2.2. Data Collection

Electronic data collection was performed by face-to-face assisted personal interviews, using tablet computers. In order to visualize the response options, participants were provided with a paper copy of the questionnaire. However, final answers were registered directly by the interviewer. The demographic data included gender, age at recruitment, highest educational degree achieved, occupation (specifying the nature of the most important employment during the year before the investigation) or last occupation before retirement, and marital status. Educational status was categorized as (i) low (primary/secondary), (ii) medium (high school), and (iii) high (university). Occupational status was categorized as (i) unemployed, (ii) low (unskilled workers), (iii) medium (partially skilled workers), and (iv) high (skilled workers). Physical activity status was evaluated using International Physical Activity Questionnaires (IPAQ) [26], which demonstrated an acceptable validity for the Italian population (the Cronbach's alpha values were 0.73 and 0.60 for the short and long versions, respectively) [27]: the instrument included a set of questionnaires (five domains) investigating the time spent being physically active in the last 7 days. Based on the IPAQ guidelines, the final score allows categorizing physical activity levels as (i) low, (ii) moderate, and (iii) high. Smoking status was categorized as (i) non-smoker, (ii) ex-smoker, and (iii) current smoker. Alcohol consumption was categorized as (i) none, (ii) moderate drinker (0.1–12 g/d) and (iii) regular drinker (>12 g/d). Anthropometric measurements have been collected following standard procedures [28]. Arterial blood pressure was measured in sitting position and after at least 5 min of rest, at the end of the physical examination. Because of the possibility of differences in blood pressure measurements, the measurements were taken three times at the right arm, relaxed and well supported by a table, with an angle of 45° from the trunk. A mean of the last two measurements was considered for inclusion in the database. Patients were considered hypertensive when their average systolic/diastolic blood pressure levels were higher than or equal to 140/90 mm Hg, they were taking anti-hypertensive medications, or they had previously been diagnosed with hypertension.

2.3. Dietary Assessment

The dietary assessment was performed by the administration of two food frequency questionnaires (FFQ, long and short versions) that had been previously tested for validity and reliability for individuals living in Sicily [29,30]. For the purposes of this study, the data from the most comprehensive FFQ including 110 food items were used. The identification of food intake, energy content and macro- and micro-nutrient intake was performed through comparison with the food composition tables from the Research Center for Foods and Nutrition [31]. The intake of seasonal foods referred to consumption during the period in which the food was available, proportionally adjusted by its intake in one year. The instrument showed a good relative validity (all major food groups with the exception of bread and soft drinks had significant Person's correlation coefficients, over 0.60, and the highest correlation coefficients for coffee ($R = 0.96$ in men and women), tea ($R = 0.79$ in men and 0.80 in women) and alcoholic beverages ($R = 0.83$ in men and 0.88 in women)) and reliability (all major food groups besides bread had significant Person's correlation coefficients, over 0.60, and the highest correlation coefficients for coffee ($R = 0.97$ in men and $R = 0.96$ in women), tea ($R = 0.82$ in men and 0.84 in women) and alcoholic beverages ($R = 0.87$ in men and 0.92 in women)). FFQs with unreliable intakes (<1000 or >6000 kcal/d) were excluded from the analyses ($n = 107$), leaving a total of 1936 individuals included in the analysis.

2.4. Estimation of Polyphenol Intake

The process of the estimation of habitual (poly)phenol intakes has been previously described in detail [32]. Briefly, data on the (poly)phenol content in foods were retrieved from the Phenol-Explorer database (www.phenol-explorer.eu) [33]. A new version of the Phenol-Explorer database containing data on the effects of cooking and food processing on (poly)phenol contents was used whenever possible, in order to apply (poly)phenol-specific retention factors [34]. Foods that contained no (poly)phenols were excluded from the calculation, leaving a total of 75 items included in the analyses. Food weight loss or gain during cooking was corrected using yield factors [35]. Average food consumption was calculated (in g or mL) by following the standard portion sizes used in the study and then converted to 24 h intake. Finally, a search was carried out in the Phenol-Explorer database to retrieve the mean content values for all (poly)phenols contained in the selected foods. Next, (poly)phenol intake from each food was calculated by multiplying the content of each (poly)phenol class by the daily consumption of each food. The total (poly)phenol intake was considered as the sum of all the main classes and subclasses. Finally, (poly)phenol intake was adjusted for total energy intake (kcal/d) using the residual method [36].

2.5. Sleep Quality

The Pittsburg sleep quality index (PSQI) [37] was used to assess participants' sleep quality and disturbances in the past six months, which has also been demonstrated to be a good and reliable tool in the Italian population (the internal consistency was represented by a Cronbach's alpha of 0.835) [38]. It consists of 19 items that are rated on a four-point scale (0–3) and grouped into seven components (sleep quality, sleep latency, sleep duration, habitual sleep efficiency, sleep disturbance, the use of sleeping medications, and daytime dysfunction). The item scores in each component were summed and converted to component scores ranging from 0 (better) to 3 (worse) based on guidelines. The total PSQI score was calculated as the summation of seven component scores, ranging from 0 to 21, where a higher score indicates a worse condition. A score of <5 on for total global PSQI is indicative of adequate sleep quality.

2.6. Statistical Analysis

Frequencies are expressed as absolute numbers and percentages; continuous variables are expressed as means and standard deviations. Individuals were divided into quartiles of dietary (poly)phenol intake and the distributions of background characteristics were compared between the groups. Differences were tested with Chi-square tests for categorical variables, ANOVA for continuous variables distributed normally, and Kruskall–Wallis tests for variables not normally distributed. Energy-adjusted multivariate logistic regression models were used to test the association between the variables of exposure (including total (poly)phenols, their classes, subclasses and individual compounds) and inadequate sleep quality; a multivariate model adjusted for all other background characteristics (body mass index, physical activity, educational status, occupational status, smoking status, alcohol consumption, occurrence of hypertension, diabetes, dyslipidemias, cardiovascular disease, cancer, and menopausal status) was also used to test whether the observed associations were independent from the aforementioned variables. All reported *P*-values were based on two-sided tests and compared to a significance level of 5%. Bonferroni correction was applied and *P*-values meeting the threshold of 0.05 divided by the number of polyphenol quartiles were noted. The SPSS 17 (SPSS Inc., Chicago, IL, USA) software was used for all the statistical calculations.

3. Results

The baseline characteristics of the study population by quartiles of energy-adjusted total (poly)phenol intake are presented in Table 1. The distributions of certain variables, such as age and education level, did not follow linear trends, as individuals in the middle quartiles were significantly older and had lower educational levels than the others. The participants in the highest quartile of total (poly)phenol intake had moderate levels of physical activity and were moderate or regular alcohol drinkers, and they also had a lower prevalence of hypertension, while concerning type 2 diabetes, the distribution was not linear and higher rates were registered in the middle quartiles (Table 1). High total (poly)phenol intake was also correlated with higher total energy intake (Table 1).

Table 1. Background characteristics of participants in the MEAL cohort by quartiles of total (poly)phenol intake (energy-adjusted).

	Total (Poly)phenol Intake				*P*
	Q1	Q2	Q3	Q4	
Age (years), mean (SD)	47.0 (19.3)	48.9 (18.0)	50.1 (16.7)	47.6 (16.4)	0.036
Men, *n* (%)	193 (43.0)	217 (43.4)	195 (39.0)	199 (40.9)	0.472
BMI, mean (SD)	25.9 (4.4)	25.9 (4.8)	25.9 (4.5)	25.5 (4.6)	0.393
Smoking status, *n* (%)					0.598
Current	96 (21.4)	127 (25.4)	130 (26.0)	112 (23.0)	
Former	62 (13.8)	71 (14.2)	75 (15.0)	68 (14.0)	
Never	291 (64.8)	302 (60.4)	295 (59.0)	307 (63.0)	
Educational level, *n* (%)					0.001
Low	147 (32.7)	185 (37.0)	187 (37.4)	178 (36.6)	
Medium	153 (34.1)	180 (36.0)	213 (42.6)	174 (35.7)	
High	149 (33.2)	135 (27.0)	100 (20.0)	135 (27.7)	
Occupational level, *n* (%)					0.046
Unemployed	90 (23.7)	115 (26.7)	131 (28.8)	125 (31.9)	
Low	64 (16.8)	66 (15.3)	74 (16.3)	62 (15.8)	
Medium	87 (22.9)	126 (29.2)	123 (27.0)	104 (26.5)	
High	139 (36.6)	124 (28.8)	127 (27.9)	101 (25.8)	
Physical activity level, *n* (%)					0.010
Low	82 (20.4)	92 (20.4)	69 (19.7)	86 (19.7)	
Medium	192 (47.8)	236 (52.2)	200 (45.8)	228 (52.2)	
High	128 (31.8)	124 (27.4)	168 (38.4)	123 (28.1)	
Alcohol consumption, *n* (%)					<0.001
None	125 (27.8)	118 (23.6)	74 (14.8)	58 (11.9)	
Moderate (0.1–12 g/d)	317 (70.6)	340 (67.9)	306 (61.2)	243 (49.9)	
Regular (>12 g/d)	7 (1.6)	43 (8.6)	120 (24.0)	186 (38.2)	
Health status, *n* (%)					
Hypertension	240 (53.5)	275 (54.9)	261 (52.2)	200 (41.1)	<0.001
Diabetes	21 (4.7)	50 (10.0)	41 (8.2)	34 (7.0)	0.018
Dyslipidemias	69 (15.4)	100 (20.0)	102 (20.4)	85 (17.5)	0.158
Cardiovascular disease	40 (9.1)	36 (7.4)	42 (8.7)	36 (7.6)	0.732
Cancer	17 (3.8)	18 (3.6)	18 (3.6)	25 (5.1)	0.556
Menopausal status (women only), *n* (%)	118 (45.4)	129 (44.6)	146 (46.9)	133 (44.5)	0.926
Total energy intake (kcal/d), mean (SD)	1749.9 (563.4)	1916.2 (552.7)	2062.8 (625.2)	2704.2 (1068.9)	<0.001

A total of 509 individuals (32.4%) reported inadequate sleep quality. No association between total or individual major classes of (poly)phenols and sleep quality was found, with the exception of lignans, for which participants in the third quartile of intake were less likely to have inadequate sleep quality after adjusting for potential confounding factors (OR = 0.62; 95% CI: 0.43, 0.88; Table 2). None of the flavonoid subclasses showed an association with sleep quality. Conversely, individuals with the highest quartile of hydroxycinnamic acid intake were less likely to have inadequate sleep quality (OR = 0.67; 95% CI: 0.46, 0.98; Table 2). When individual compounds were taken into consideration, inverse associations with inadequate sleep quality were observed for naringenin (OR = 0.66; 95% CI: 0.46, 0.95) and apigenin (OR = 0.63; 95% CI: 0.44, 0.90) among flavonoids, and for matairesinol (OR= 0.66; 95% CI: 0.46, 0.96) among lignans (Table 2).

Table 2. Odds ratios (ORs) and 95% confidence intervals (CIs) for the associations between (poly)phenol intake (total, main classes, subclasses and individual compounds) and adequate sleep quality in the MEAL cohort.

	\(Poly)phenol Quartiles, OR (95% CI)				
	Q1	Q2	Q3	Q4	*P* for Trend
Total (poly)phenols	1	1.12 (0.80, 1.58)	0.87 (0.61, 1.25)	1.04 (0.69, 1.55)	0.476
Total flavonoids	1	0.83 (0.58, 1.18)	0.92 (0.64, 1.31)	0.97 (0.66, 1.43)	0.948
Flavanols	1	0.90 (0.63, 1.28)	0.93 (0.66, 1.32)	1.25 (0.89, 1.77)	0.603
Catechins	1	0.81 (0.57, 1.15)	0.96 (0.67, 1.38)	1.05 (0.73, 1.50)	0.255
Flavonols	1	1.07 (0.68, 1.67)	0.90 (0.48, 1.68)	1.32 (0.59, 2.92)	0.645
Quercetin	1	1.44 (0.97, 2.11)	1.51 (1.04, 2.20)	1.33 (0.88, 2.01)	0.368
Kaempferol	1	0.72 (0.50, 1.02)	0.74 (0.53, 1.05)	0.91 (0.59, 1.41)	0.104
Flavanones	1	1.03 (0.72, 1.45)	0.75 (0.53, 1.06)	0.72 (0.50, 1.03)	0.263
Hesperetin	1	0.85 (0.60, 1.21)	0.96 (0.68, 1.36)	0.81 (0.58, 1.15)	0.249
Naringenin	1	0.76 (0.54, 1.08)	0.62 (0.44, 0.89)	0.66 (0.46, 0.95)	0.020
Flavones	1	1.03 (0.72, 1.45)	0.75 (0.53, 1.06)	0.72 (0.50, 1.03)	0.016
Apigenin	1	0.67 (0.46, 0.96)	0.61 (0.41, 0.90)	0.63 (0.44, 0.90)	0.046
Luteolin	1	1.09 (0.77, 1.53)	0.85 (0.60, 1.20)	0.84 (0.56, 1.15)	0.043
Anthocyanins	1	0.91 (0.63, 1.31)	0.97 (0.68, 1.37)	0.86 (0.59, 1.26)	0.459
Isoflavones	1	0.90 (0.64, 1.27)	0.95 (0.68, 1.33)	0.92 (0.65, 1.30)	0.356
Daidzein	1	0.90 (0.64, 1.27)	0.98 (0.70, 1.38)	0.89 (0.62, 1.27)	0.301
Genistein	1	0.90 (0.64, 1.27)	0.93 (0.66, 1.32)	0.93 (0.65, 1.32)	0.263
Biochanin A	1	0.75 (0.51, 1.10)	0.96 (0.66, 1.41)	1.07 (0.72, 1.60)	0.025
Phenolic acids	1	1.32 (0.93, 1.87)	1.31 (0.97, 1.87)	1.16 (0.81, 1.65)	0.457
Hydroxybenzoic acids	1	1.10 (0.80, 1.53)	1.07 (0.74, 1.53)	1.13 (0.79, 1.61)	0.852
Vanillic acid	1	1.00 (0.69, 1.44)	1.34 (0.93, 1.93)	1.27 (0.85, 1.89)	0.624
Hydroxycinnamic acids	1	0.89 (0.63, 1.26)	0.77 (0.51, 1.09)	0.67 (0.46, 0.98)	0.005 [a]
Caffeic acid	1	0.95 (0.67, 1.36)	0.72 (0.50, 1.04)	0.88 (0.54, 1.43)	0.055
Cinnamic acid	1	1.02 (0.73, 1.42)	0.93 (0.65, 1.35)	1.09 (0.77, 1.52)	0.680
Ferulic acid	1	0.71 (0.50, 1.01)	0.94 (0.67, 1.31)	0.77 (0.53, 1.12)	0.299
Stilbenes	1	0.73 (0.50, 1.06)	0.83 (0.56, 1.24)	0.97 (0.60, 1.56)	0.828
Lignans	1	0.85 (0.60, 1.21)	0.62 (0.43, 0.88)	0.78 (0.54, 1.12)	0.051
Lariciresinol	1	0.90 (0.64, 1.27)	0.69 (0.49, 0.98)	0.85 (0.59, 1.22)	0.187
Matairesinol	1	0.72 (0.51, 1.02)	0.67 (0.47, 0.95)	0.66 (0.46, 0.96)	0.017
Pinoresinol	1	0.90 (0.64, 1.27)	0.64 (0.45, 0.92)	0.78 (0.54, 1.12)	0.090
Secoisolariciresinol	1	0.72 (0.51, 1.02)	0.68 (0.48, 0.98)	0.80 (0.55, 1.16)	0.187

Adjusted for total energy intake (continuous), body mass index (continuous), physical activity (low/medium/high), educational status (low/medium/high), occupational status (unemployed/low/medium/high), smoking status (current/former/never), alcohol consumption (none/moderate/regular), occurrence of hypertension, diabetes, dyslipidemias, cardiovascular disease, cancer (yes/no), and menopausal status (women only, yes/no). [a] *P*-value meeting threshold for Bonferroni correction.

A secondary analysis was conducted, stratifying the population into normal weight and overweight/obese individuals. The findings in normal weight individuals showed a stronger association between certain classes, subclasses and individual compounds and sleep quality (Table 3). Notably, nearly all individual compounds belonging to the lignan class (secoisolariciresinol, matairesinol and pinoresinol) were inversely associated with inadequate sleep quality (Table 3).

Table 3. Odds ratios (ORs) and 95% confidence intervals (CIs) for the associations between (poly)phenol intake (total, main classes, subclasses and individual compounds) and adequate sleep quality in normal weight individuals.

	(Poly)phenol Quartiles, OR (95% CI)				
	Q1	Q2	Q3	Q4	P for Trend
Total (poly)phenols	1	0.74 (0.45, 1.21)	0.52 (0.31, 0.89)	0.70 (0.39, 1.25)	0.060
Total flavonoids	1	0.60 (0.36, 1.01)	0.60 (0.36, 1.01)	0.66 (0.38, 1.13)	0.308
Flavanols	1	0.88 (0.44, 1.75)	0.66 (0.25, 1.71)	1.21 (0.39, 3.75)	0.571
Catechins	1	0.76 (0.45, 1.27)	0.84 (0.49, 1.42)	0.94 (0.57, 1.55)	0.869
Flavonols	1	0.86 (0.52, 1.45)	0.78 (0.47, 1.29)	1.03 (0.62, 1.71)	0.914
Quercetin	1	1.24 (0.71, 2.16)	1.55 (0.90, 2.68)	1.17 (0.63, 2.16)	0.827
Kaempferol	1	0.65 (0.39, 1.09)	0.68 (0.42, 1.10)	1.00 (0.53, 1.87)	0.228
Flavanones	1	1.32 (0.78, 2.23)	1.05 (0.61, 1.81)	0.88 (0.50, 1.52)	0.774
Hesperetin	1	1.24 (0.74, 2.09)	0.96 (0.56, 1.65)	0.87 (0.50, 1.50)	0.724
Naringenin	1	0.80 (0.48, 1.32)	0.51 (0.30, 0.85)	0.49 (0.28, 0.85)	0.016
Flavones	1	0.94 (0.56, 1.56)	0.64 (0.38, 1.07)	0.52 (0.30, 0.91)	0.037
Apigenin	1	0.78 (0.45, 1.34)	0.61 (0.34, 1.07)	0.67 (0.40, 1.13)	0.062
Luteolin	1	1.34 (0.82, 2.17)	0.77 (0.47, 1.28)	0.68 (0.39, 1.18)	0.106
Anthocyanins	1	1.04 (0.63, 1.69)	0.73 (0.44, 1.21)	0.59 (0.34, 1.03)	0.033
Isoflavones	1	0.99 (0.59, 1.63)	1.11 (0.66, 1.84)	1.00 (0.61, 1.63)	0.878
Daidzein	1	1.04 (0.63, 1.72)	1.14 (0.68, 1.91)	1.02 (0.62, 1.68)	0.803
Genistein	1	1.06 (0.64, 1.75)	1.02 (0.59, 1.76)	1.09 (0.66, 1.78)	0.992
Biochanin A	1	0.59 (0.33, 1.04)	0.79 (0.46, 1.37)	0.89 (0.49, 1.60)	0.823
Phenolic acids	1	1.22 (0.72, 2.05)	1.18 (0.70, 1.96)	0.79 (0.46, 1.35)	0.538
Hydroxybenzoic acids	1	1.24 (0.76, 2.00)	0.73 (0.42, 1.27)	1.15 (0.67, 1.97)	0.631
Vanillic acid	1	0.93 (0.55, 1.56)	1.18 (0.71, 1.97)	1.31 (0.74, 2.31)	0.816
Hydroxycinnamic acids	1	0.59 (0.36, 0.97)	0.60 (0.37, 0.97)	0.39 (0.22, 0.69)	0.049
Caffeic acid	1	1.22 (0.74, 1.99)	0.49 (0.29, 0.84)	0.86 (0.42, 1.79)	0.044
Cinnamic acid	1	0.84 (0.52, 1.35)	0.88 (0.52, 1.49)	0.73 (0.44, 1.21)	0.481
Ferulic acid	1	0.87 (0.51, 1.47)	0.92 (0.55, 1.54)	0.91 (0.52, 1.60)	0.312
Stilbenes	1	0.57 (0.33, 0.99)	0.79 (0.45, 1.39)	0.95 (0.43, 2.09)	0.553
Lignans	1	0.70 (0.42, 1.15)	0.45 (0.27, 0.77)	0.54 (0.31, 0.94)	0.040
Lariciresinol	1	0.79 (0.48, 1.30)	0.54 (0.32, 0.90)	0.61 (0.36, 1.05)	0.061
Matairesinol	1	0.70 (0.42, 1.16)	0.57 (0.35, 0.95)	0.50 (0.29, 0.87)	0.025
Pinoresinol	1	0.68 (0.41, 1.12)	0.47 (0.27, 0.80)	0.55 (0.32, 0.96)	0.030
Secoisolariciresinol	1	0.54 (0.33, 0.88)	0.54 (0.31, 0.92)	0.51 (0.29, 0.89)	0.047

Adjusted for total energy intake (continuous), body mass index (continuous), physical activity (low/medium/high), educational status (low/medium/high), occupational status (unemployed/low/medium/high), smoking status (current/former/never), alcohol consumption (none/moderate/regular), occurrence of hypertension, diabetes, dyslipidemias, cardiovascular disease, cancer (yes/no), and menopausal status (women only, yes/no).

To the contrary, in the overweight/obese individuals, there were no associations between any dietary (poly)phenol class and sleep quality. Among the individual components, only apigenin was significantly associated with sleep quality (OR = 0.53; 95% CI: 0.31, 0.90) (Table 4).

Table 4. Odds ratios (ORs) and 95% confidence intervals (CIs) for the associations between (poly)phenol intake (total, main classes, subclasses and individual compounds) and adequate sleep quality in overweight/obese individuals.

	(Poly)phenol Quartiles, OR (95% CI)				
	Q1	Q2	Q3	Q4	P for Trend
Total (poly)phenols	1	1.64 (0.98, 2.73)	1.13 (0.82, 2.29)	1.57 (0.86, 2.83)	0.219
Total flavonoids	1	1.24 (0.73, 2.10)	1.50 (0.88, 2.55)	1.69 (0.93, 3.05)	0.075
Flavanols	1	1.37 (0.73, 2.56)	1.10 (0.46, 2.60)	1.37 (0.42, 4.46)	0.982
Catechins	1	0.88 (0.54, 1.43)	1.26 (0.74, 2.12)	1.31 (0.77, 2.24)	0.114
Flavonols	1	0.89 (0.53, 1.48)	1.16 (0.71, 1.91)	1.47 (0.90, 2.40)	0.183
Quercetin	1	1.55 (0.88, 2.73)	1.44 (0.83, 2.49)	1.46 (0.82, 2.60)	0.180
Kaempferol	1	0.90 (0.53, 1.53)	0.97 (0.57, 1.63)	0.93 (0.49, 1.76)	0.918
Flavanones	1	0.61 (0.37, 1.01)	1.00 (0.62, 1.61)	0.82 (0.51, 1.32)	0.847
Hesperetin	1	0.60 (0.36, 1.00)	0.99 (0.62, 1.59)	0.82 (0.51, 1.33)	0.803
Naringenin	1	0.86 (0.51, 1.43)	0.77 (0.46, 1.28)	0.99 (0.59, 1.65)	0.899
Flavones	1	1.00 (0.61, 1.64)	0.81 (0.50, 1.33)	0.89 (0.54, 1.47)	0.195
Apigenin	1	0.56 (0.33, 0.95)	0.61 (0.34, 1.07)	0.53 (0.31, 0.90)	0.555
Luteolin	1	0.80 (0.47, 1.34)	0.79 (0.48, 1.30)	0.88 (0.53, 1.45)	0.208
Anthocyanins	1	0.84 (0.48, 1.48)	1.17 (0.69, 1.97)	1.29 (0.73, 2.27)	0.155
Isoflavones	1	0.87 (0.53, 1.41)	0.96 (0.60, 1.53)	0.91 (0.54, 1.54)	0.349
Daidzein	1	0.81 (0.50, 1.32)	0.97 (0.60, 1.55)	0.84 (0.49, 1.44)	0.269
Genistein	1	0.80 (0.49, 1.30)	0.94 (0.58, 1.52)	0.85 (0.50, 1.43)	0.286
Biochanin A	1	1.02 (0.58, 1.79)	1.27 (0.73, 2.23)	1.45 (0.81, 2.60)	0.024
Phenolic acids	1	1.35 (0.83, 2.20)	1.38 (0.83, 2.28)	1.49 (0.90, 2.45)	0.079
Hydroxybenzoic acids	1	0.94 (0.58, 1.51)	1.41 (0.85, 2.35)	1.06 (0.64, 1.76)	0.308
Vanillic acid	1	1.04 (0.60, 1.80)	1.39 (0.80, 2.39)	1.14 (0.63, 2.04)	0.324
Hydroxycinnamic acids	1	1.28 (0.77, 2.12)	0.86 (0.50, 1.47)	1.03 (0.60, 1.78)	0.260
Caffeic acid	1	0.69 (0.40, 1.20)	0.90 (0.52, 1.52)	0.81 (0.40, 1.62)	0.860
Cinnamic acid	1	1.22 (0.75, 2.00)	0.99 (0.58, 1.69)	1.53 (0.93, 2.51)	0.195
Ferulic acid	1	0.61 (0.37, 1.00)	0.92 (0.58, 1.47)	0.72 (0.42, 1.22)	0.609
Stilbenes	1	0.99 (0.57, 1.69)	0.84 (0.46, 1.53)	0.91 (0.48, 1.72)	0.555
Lignans	1	1.15 (0.69, 1.91)	0.86 (0.52, 1.43)	1.23 (0.73, 2.07)	0.538
Lariciresinol	1	1.09 (0.66, 1.80)	0.90 (0.55, 1.47)	1.30 (0.77, 2.17)	0.396
Matairesinol	1	0.86 (0.52, 1.44)	0.84 (0.50, 1.41)	0.99 (0.58, 1.69)	0.864
Pinoresinol	1	1.13 (0.69, 1.84)	0.84 (0.50, 1.41)	1.11 (0.67, 1.86)	0.520
Secoisolariciresinol	1	1.02 (0.62, 1.70)	0.90 (0.54, 1.51)	1.37 (0.80, 2.33)	0.342

Adjusted for total energy intake (continuous), body mass index (continuous), physical activity (low/medium/high), educational status (low/medium/high), occupational status (unemployed/low/medium/high), smoking status (current/former/never), alcohol consumption (none/moderate/regular), occurrence of hypertension, diabetes, dyslipidemias, cardiovascular disease, cancer (yes/no), and menopausal status (women only, yes/no).

4. Discussion

In this article, we tested whether dietary (poly)phenols were associated with sleep quality in a cohort of Italian adults. Individuals showing a higher intake of some flavonoid subclasses (flavanones and flavones), phenolic acids (such as hydroxycinnamic acids) and lignans were significantly less likely to have inadequate sleep quality. These findings suggest that some classes of (poly)phenol may play a specific role when exploring their relationship with brain and mental health. Interestingly, the associations were more evident when stratifying the cohort by weight status, showing significant results in normal weight individuals, but no confirmed associations for overweight/obese participants.

To date, only one recent study has investigated the relationship between dietary (poly)phenols derived from fruit and vegetables and sleep duration [39]. The study was conducted on 13,958 women with about 4 years of follow-up in the UK Women's Cohort Study: total fruit and vegetable consumption and their estimated content of total polyphenols were directly associated with sleep duration, while individual (poly)phenol classes were not associated with the outcome of interest [39]. Despite no other studies being focused on polyphenols, some studies reported a direct relationship between sleep duration and quality, and fruit and vegetable intake [40,41]. Other studies showed the role of certain polyphenol-rich foods (i.e., black tea and cocoa products) in improving sleep quality [42,43]. Despite there being no other studies specifically conducted on (poly)phenols and sleep quality, there is consistent evidence from the literature suggesting a potential role of dietary (poly)phenols in improving mental health and preventing conditions that are associated with sleep disorders. For instance, some cohort studies showed that individuals with higher intakes of the same flavonoid, hydroxycinnamic and lignan classes found to be significantly associated with better sleep quality in this study were less likely to have depressive symptoms [44,45]. Other studies also showed an inverse association between fruit and vegetable intake and depressive symptoms and perceived stress, despite most of them have been conducted on students [46–49].

From a general mechanistic point of view, (poly)phenol circulating metabolites are able to pass through the blood–brain barrier to various extents, depending on their degree of lipophilicity, with less polar (poly)phenol metabolites capable of greater brain uptake than more polar ones [50,51]. The main potential beneficial effects of dietary (poly)phenols in the central nervous system include the suppression of neuronal apoptosis, modulation of signaling pathways implicated in neuron survival, and stimulation of adult neurogenesis [52–54]. With special regard to specific mechanisms related to sleep features, dietary (poly)phenols have been shown to improve resilience after sleep deprivation [55]; some individual molecules, such as apigenin, are able to reduce locomotor activity, prolong sleep time, increase sleep rate increase and sleep time in combined administration with a GABA(A) receptor agonist, and show synergic effects in potentiating sleep onset in animal models [56–58]. Additionally, derivates of hydroxycinnamic acids have been identified as agonists for both gamma-amino butyric acid (GABA) receptors and act synergistically with 5-hydroxytryptophan (5-HTP), both of which play a role in sleep quality, including having sedative effects on locomotion activity, prolonging sleeping time and shortening sleep latency [59–61].

Dietary (poly)phenols have been shown to decrease systemic inflammation [62] but also exert anti-neuroinflammatory properties and reduce oxidative stress and inflammation-related conditions [63]. Several studies have shown that molecules of interest from our study, including some flavonoids (i.e., apigenin) and hydroxycinnamic acids, improve cell antioxidant activity against oxidative stress in the central nervous system [64,65]. Additionally, lignans have been demonstrated to exert anti-oxidative and anti-inflammatory properties in neurons and protect the blood–brain barrier against inflammatory cells by reducing oxidative stress, inflammation and permeability [66–68]. Dietary (poly)phenols may ameliorate poor endothelial function [69] and help to control blood pressure [70], which, in turn, has been associated with measures of sleep quality together with decreases in the percentage of REM sleep and increases in REM sleep latency [71–73]. Previous epidemiological studies have shown an inverse association between the intake of specific classes of (poly)phenol (in line with the findings shown in the present study)—including flavones and flavanones among flavonoids [74], and hydroxycinnamic acids—and the occurrence of hypertension [75,76]. The mechanisms underlying these relationships are still under investigation; besides, regarding the direct effect of (poly)phenols (especially hydroxycinnamic acids) on low-grade inflammation, which, in turn, may affect endothelial function [77,78], an intriguing hypothesis involves nitric oxide-mediated vasodilation in the brain, which has been shown to facilitate REM sleep [79].

An emerging body of literature investigates the double interexchange of information between the gut microbiota and the brain through a complex system of signals involving neural, endocrine and inflammatory mechanisms [80]. In fact, the gut microbiota has been shown to affect brain and behaviors related to anxiety and depressive symptoms depending on bacterial family ratios, dysbiosis, and subsequent modulation through dietary (poly)phenol intake [81]; the status of the pro- and anti-inflammatory balance in the gut has been demonstrated to have an impact at the systemic level and on the central nervous system [82,83]. Recent studies show that dietary (poly)phenols may play a role in the modulation of gut microbiota metabolism and that variations in the gut microbiota can affect (poly)phenol activity [84]. This hypothesis is particularly valid in light of our results stratified by weight status; in the intestinal microbiota of obese people, a specific increase in the proportion of class Firmicutes to class Bacteroidetes has been shown compared to in normal-weight individuals [85], which may affect (poly)phenol transformation and absorption in the gut [86] and their anti-oxidant effects [87–89]. However, current evidence is still limited, largely based on cell and animal studies, and future studies conducted on humans are needed to identify specific metabotypes associated with activity in the brain.

To the best of our knowledge, this is the first study investigating such a comprehensive group of compounds in order to identify key (poly)phenol molecules of potential interest to improve sleep quality. Moreover, based on our previous results [32], no unique food source is responsible for specific compounds or classes of (poly)phenols; thus, the present analysis is able to detect the potential role of (poly)phenols rather than of the individual foods underlying their consumption. However, the findings presented in this study should be considered in light of some limitations. Firstly, this study provided evidence from a cross-sectional analysis, which cannot exclude reverse causation nor describe a causal relation. Secondly, all methods used to assess food consumption and dietary polyphenol intake provide only estimations, while true intake cannot be estimated without measuring biomarkers or metabolites. Despite the use of the Phenol-Explorer database being validated and widespread, this method cannot take into account molecular transformation or interaction. Moreover, recall bias and unmeasured confounding factors (i.e., jobs requiring night shifts) should be considered as potential limitations. However, these methods are commonly used in the current scientific literature, representing the standard for scientific research until new methods are validated and made available. Thirdly, no other aspects related to sleeping problems or other mental health issues have been considered, while they may be associated with sleep quality. Thus, the potential mediating effect of such intermediary conditions should be taken into account.

5. Conclusions

Our study suggests that a higher dietary intake of certain (poly)phenols may be potentially associated with better sleep quality. However, further epidemiological studies are needed to confirm the presented hypothesis, with a major focus on sleep quality. Several aspects should be further considered in future studies, such as the use of caffeinated beverages or the timing of food and alcohol intake. Future studies should additionally focus on the inter-individual variation in response to the consumption of (poly)phenols and thus investigate the associations not only for their dietary intake but also for the true internal exposure to their metabolites. In this context, attention to the gut microbiota composition should also be paid as differences in microbial species may condition (poly)phenol metabolite formation and bioactivity. Finally, intervention studies will be needed to explore the level of absorption and bioavailability of dietary (poly)phenols and the characterization of biologically available (poly)phenol metabolites responsible for the promotion of resilience against cognitive impairment in response to poor sleep quality.

Author Contributions: Conceptualization, J.G., R.F., F.C., F.G., G.G.; methodology J.G., R.F., F.C., F.G., G.G.; validation, J.G., R.F., S.C., F.C., F.G., G.G.; formal analysis, J.G. and G.G.; investigation, J.G., R.F., F.C., F.G., G.G.; data curation, J.G. and S.C.; writing—original draft preparation, J.G., R.F., F.C., F.G., G.G.; writing—review and editing, J.G., R.F., S.C., D.A., P.M., D.D.R., F.C., F.G., G.G.; supervision, R.F., F.C., F.G., G.G. All authors have read and agreed to the published version of the manuscript.

Funding: This study was partially supported by a fund from the Italian Ministry of Health "Ricerca Corrente" (RC n. 2751594) (Ferri, Caraci and Godos).

Conflicts of Interest: The authors declare no conflict of interest.

References

1. Afshin, A.; Sur, P.J.; Fay, K.A.; Cornaby, L.; Ferrara, G.; Salama, J.S.; Mullany, E.C.; Abate, K.H.; Abbafati, C. Health effects of dietary risks in 195 countries, 1990–2017: A systematic analysis for the Global Burden of Disease Study 2017. *Lancet* **2019**, *393*, 1958–1972. [CrossRef]

2. Stanaway, J.D.; Afshin, A.; Gakidou, E.; Lim, S.S.; Abate, D.; Abate, K.H.; Abbafati, C.; Abbasi, N.; Abbastabar, H.; Abd-Allah, F.; et al. Global, regional, and national comparative risk assessment of 84 behavioural, environmental and occupational, and metabolic risks or clusters of risks for 195 countries and territories, 1990–2017: A systematic analysis for the Global Burden of Disease Study 2017. *Lancet* **2018**, *392*, 1923–1994. [CrossRef]

3. Angelino, D.; Godos, J.; Ghelfi, F.; Tieri, M.; Titta, L.; Lafranconi, A.; Marventano, S.; Alonzo, E.; Gambera, A.; Sciacca, S.; et al. Fruit and vegetable consumption and health outcomes: An umbrella review of observational studies. *Int. J. Food Sci. Nutr.* **2019**, *70*, 652–667. [CrossRef] [PubMed]

4. Godos, J.; Tieri, M.; Ghelfi, F.; Titta, L.; Marventano, S.; Lafranconi, A.; Gambera, A.; Alonzo, E.; Sciacca, S.; Buscemi, S.; et al. Dairy foods and health: An umbrella review of observational studies. *Int. J. Food Sci. Nutr.* **2019**, *71*, 138–151. [CrossRef] [PubMed]

5. Grosso, G.; Godos, J.; Galvano, F.; Giovannucci, E.L. Coffee, Caffeine, and Health Outcomes: An Umbrella Review. *Annu. Rev. Nutr.* **2017**, *37*, 131–156. [CrossRef]

6. Marventano, S.; Godos, J.; Tieri, M.; Ghelfi, F.; Titta, L.; Lafranconi, A.; Gambera, A.; Alonzo, E.; Sciacca, S.; Buscemi, S.; et al. Egg consumption and human health: An umbrella review of observational studies. *Int. J. Food Sci. Nutr.* **2019**, *71*, 325–331. [CrossRef]

7. Tieri, M.; Ghelfi, F.; Vitale, M.; Vetrani, C.; Marventano, S.; Lafranconi, A.; Godos, J.; Titta, L.; Gambera, A.; Alonzo, E.; et al. Whole grain consumption and human health: An umbrella review of observational studies. *Int. J. Food Sci. Nutr.* **2020**, 1–10. [CrossRef]

8. Schwingshackl, L.; Hoffmann, G.; Missbach, B.; Stelmach-Mardas, M.; Boeing, H. An Umbrella Review of Nuts Intake and Risk of Cardiovascualr Disease. *Curr. Pharm. Des.* **2017**, *22*, 1. [CrossRef]

9. Huang, Q.; Liu, H.; Suzuki, K.; Ma, S.; Liu, C. Linking What We Eat to Our Mood: A Review of Diet, Dietary Antioxidants, and Depression. *Antioxidants* **2019**, *8*, 376. [CrossRef]

10. Dominguez, L.J.; Barbagallo, M.; Garcia, M.M.; Godos, J.; Martinez-Gonzalez, M.A. Dietary Patterns and Cognitive Decline: Key features for prevention. *Curr. Pharm. Des.* **2019**, *25*, 2428–2442. [CrossRef]

11. Manna, P.; Jain, S.K. Obesity, Oxidative Stress, Adipose Tissue Dysfunction, and the Associated Health Risks: Causes and Therapeutic Strategies. *Metab. Syndr. Relat. Disord.* **2015**, *13*, 423–444. [CrossRef] [PubMed]

12. St-Onge, M.-P.; Mikic, A.; Pietrolungo, C.E. Effects of Diet on Sleep Quality. *Adv. Nutr.* **2016**, *7*, 938–949. [CrossRef] [PubMed]

13. Godos, J.; Currenti, W.; Angelino, D.; Mena, P.; Castellano, S.; Caraci, F.; Galvano, F.; Del Rio, D.; Ferri, R.; Grosso, G. Diet and mental health: Review of the recent updates on molecular mechanisms. *Antioxidants* **2020**, *9*, 346. [CrossRef]

14. Kanagasabai, T.; Ardern, C.I. Inflammation, Oxidative Stress, and Antioxidants Contribute to Selected Sleep Quality and Cardiometabolic Health Relationships: A Cross-Sectional Study. *Mediat. Inflamm.* **2015**, *2015*, 824589. [CrossRef] [PubMed]

15. Kanagasabai, T.; Ardern, C.I. Contribution of Inflammation, Oxidative Stress, and Antioxidants to the Relationship between Sleep Duration and Cardiometabolic Health. *Sleep* **2015**, *38*, 1905–1912. [CrossRef] [PubMed]

16. Pace-Schott, E.F.; Spencer, R. Sleep-Dependent Memory Consolidation in Healthy Aging and Mild Cognitive Impairment. *Curr. Top. Behav. Neurosci.* **2014**, *25*, 307–330.

17. Del Rio, D.; Rodriguez-Mateos, A.; Spencer, J.P.; Tognolini, M.; Borges, G.; Crozier, A. Dietary (poly)phenolics in human health: Structures, bioavailability, and evidence of protective effects against chronic diseases. *Antioxid. Redox Signal.* **2012**, *18*, 1818–1892. [CrossRef]

18. Mena, P.; Domínguez-Perles, R.; Gironés-Vilaplana, A.; Baenas, N.; García-Viguera, C.; Villaño, D. Flavan-3-ols, anthocyanins, and inflammation. *IUBMB Life* **2014**, *66*, 745–758. [CrossRef]

19. Rodriguez-Mateos, A.; Vauzour, D.; Krueger, C.G.; Shanmuganayagam, D.; Reed, J.; Calani, L.; Mena, P.; Del Rio, D.; Crozier, A. Bioavailability, bioactivity and impact on health of dietary flavonoids and related compounds: An update. *Arch. Toxicol.* **2014**, *88*, 1803–1853. [CrossRef]

20. Fraga, C.G.; Croft, K.D.; Kennedy, D.O.; Tomas-Barberan, F. The effects of polyphenols and other bioactives on human health. *Food Funct.* **2019**, *10*, 514–528. [CrossRef]

21. Gomez-Pinilla, F.; Nguyen, T.T.J. Natural mood foods: The actions of polyphenols against psychiatric and cognitive disorders. *Nutr. Neurosci.* **2012**, *15*, 127–133. [CrossRef] [PubMed]

22. Brickman, A.M.; Khan, U.A.; Provenzano, F.A.; Yeung, L.-K.; Suzuki, W.; Schroeter, H.; Wall, M.; Sloan, R.P.; Small, S.A. Enhancing dentate gyrus function with dietary flavanols improves cognition in older adults. *Nat. Neurosci.* **2014**, *17*, 1798–1803. [CrossRef] [PubMed]

23. Godos, J.; Ferri, R.; Caraci, F.; Cosentino, F.I.I.; Castellano, S.; Galvano, F.; Grosso, G. Adherence to the Mediterranean Diet is Associated with Better Sleep Quality in Italian Adults. *Nutrients* **2019**, *11*, 976. [CrossRef] [PubMed]

24. Godos, J.; Ferri, R.; Caraci, F.; Cosentino, F.I.I.; Castellano, S.; Shivappa, N.; Hébert, J.R.; Galvano, F.; Grosso, G. Dietary Inflammatory Index and Sleep Quality in Southern Italian Adults. *Nutrients* **2019**, *11*, 1324. [CrossRef] [PubMed]

25. Grosso, G.; Marventano, S.; D'Urso, M.; Mistretta, A.; Galvano, F. The Mediterranean healthy eating, ageing, and lifestyle (MEAL) study: Rationale and study design. *Int. J. Food Sci. Nutr.* **2017**, *68*, 577–586. [CrossRef]

26. Craig, C.L.; Marshall, A.; Sjöström, M.; Bauman, A.E.; Booth, M.L.; Ainsworth, B.E.; Pratt, M.; Ekelund, U.; Yngve, A.; Sallis, J.F.; et al. International Physical Activity Questionnaire: 12-Country Reliability and Validity. *Med. Sci. Sports Exerc.* **2003**, *35*, 1381–1395. [CrossRef]

27. Mannocci, A.; Di Thiene, D.; Del Cimmuto, A.; Masala, D.; Boccia, A.; De Vito, E.; La Torre, G. International Physical Activity Questionnaire: Validation and assessment in an Italian sample. *Ital. J. Public Health* **2010**, *7*, 369–376.

28. Mistretta, A.; Marventano, S.; Platania, A.; Godos, J.; Galvano, F.; Grosso, G. Metabolic profile of the Mediterranean healthy Eating, Lifestyle and Aging (MEAL) study cohort. *Mediterr. J. Nutr. Metab.* **2017**, *10*, 131–140. [CrossRef]

29. Buscemi, S.; Rosafio, G.; Vasto, S.; Massenti, F.M.; Grosso, G.; Galvano, F.; Rini, N.; Barile, A.M.; Maniaci, V.; Cosentino, L.; et al. Validation of a food frequency questionnaire for use in Italian adults living in Sicily. *Int. J. Food Sci. Nutr.* **2015**, *66*, 426–438. [CrossRef]

30. Marventano, S.; Mistretta, A.; Platania, A.; Galvano, F.; Grosso, G. Reliability and relative validity of a food frequency questionnaire for Italian adults living in Sicily, Southern Italy. *Int. J. Food Sci. Nutr.* **2016**, *67*, 857–864. [CrossRef]

31. Istituto Nazionale di Ricerca per gli Alimenti e la Nutrizione. *Tabelle di Composizione degli Alimenti*; CREA: Rome, Italy, 2009.

32. Godos, J.; Marventano, S.; Mistretta, A.; Galvano, F.; Grosso, G. Dietary sources of polyphenols in the Mediterranean healthy Eating, Aging and Lifestyle (MEAL) study cohort. *Int. J. Food Sci. Nutr.* **2017**, *68*, 750–756. [CrossRef] [PubMed]

33. Neveu, V.; Pérez-Jiménez, J.; Vos, F.; Crespy, V.; Du Chaffaut, L.; Mennen, L.; Knox, C.; Eisner, R.; Cruz, J.; Wishart, D.; et al. Phenol-Explorer: An online comprehensive database on polyphenol contents in foods. *Database* **2010**, *2010*, bap024. [CrossRef] [PubMed]

34. Rothwell, J.A.; Pérez-Jiménez, J.; Neveu, V.; Medina-Remón, A.; M'Hiri, N.; García-Lobato, P.; Manach, C.; Knox, C.; Eisner, R.; Wishart, D.S.; et al. Phenol-Explorer 3.0: A major update of the Phenol-Explorer database to incorporate data on the effects of food processing on polyphenol content. *Database* **2013**, *2013*, bat070. [CrossRef]

35. Bognar, A. *Tables on Weight Yield of Food and Retention Factors of Food Constituents for the Calculation of Nutrient Composition of Cooked Foods (Dishes)*; Bundesforschungsanstalt für Ernährung: Karlsruhe, Germany, 2002.

36. Willett, W.C. Reproducibility and Validity of Food-Frequency Questionnaires. In *Nutritional Epidemiology*; Oxford University Press (OUP): New York, NY, USA, 1998; pp. 101–147.

37. Buysse, D.J.; Reynolds, C.F.; Monk, T.H.; Berman, S.R.; Kupfer, D.J. The Pittsburgh sleep quality index: A new instrument for psychiatric practice and research. *Psychiatry Res. Neuroimaging* **1989**, *28*, 193–213. [CrossRef]

38. Curcio, G.; Tempesta, D.; Scarlata, S.; Marzano, C.; Moroni, F.; Rossini, P.M.; Ferrara, M.; De Gennaro, L. Validity of the Italian Version of the Pittsburgh Sleep Quality Index (PSQI). *Neurol. Sci.* **2012**, *34*, 511–519. [CrossRef]

39. Noorwali, E.; Hardie, L.J.; Cade, J.E. Fruit and Vegetable Consumption and Their Polyphenol Content Are Inversely Associated with Sleep Duration: Prospective Associations from the UK Women's Cohort Study. *Nutrients* **2018**, *10*, 1803. [CrossRef]

40. Noorwali, E.; Cade, J.E.; Burley, V.J.; Hardie, L.J. The relationship between sleep duration and fruit/vegetable intakes in UK adults: A cross-sectional study from the National Diet and Nutrition Survey. *BMJ Open* **2018**, *8*, e020810. [CrossRef]

41. Jansen, E.C.; She, R.; Rukstalis, M.M.; Alexander, G.L. Sleep Duration and Quality in Relation to Fruit and Vegetable Intake of US Young Adults: A Secondary Analysis. *Int. J. Behav. Med.* **2020**, *2020*, 1–12. [CrossRef]

42. Zhao, W.; Li, Y.; Ma, W.; Ge, Y.; Huang, Y. A study on quality components and sleep-promoting effects of GABA black tea. *Food Funct.* **2015**, *6*, 3393–3398. [CrossRef]

43. Socci, V.; Tempesta, D.; Desideri, G.; De Gennaro, L.; Ferrara, M. Enhancing Human Cognition with Cocoa Flavonoids. *Front. Nutr.* **2017**, *4*. [CrossRef]

44. Godos, J.; Castellano, S.; Ray, S.; Grosso, G.; Galvano, F. Dietary Polyphenol Intake and Depression: Results from the Mediterranean Healthy Eating, Lifestyle and Aging (MEAL) Study. *Molecules* **2018**, *23*, 999. [CrossRef] [PubMed]

45. Chang, S.-C.; Cassidy, A.; Willett, W.C.; Rimm, E.B.; O'Reilly, E.J.; Okereke, O.I. Dietary flavonoid intake and risk of incident depression in midlife and older women. *Am. J. Clin. Nutr.* **2016**, *104*, 704–714. [CrossRef]

46. Mikolajczyk, R.; El Ansari, W.; Maxwell, A.E. Food consumption frequency and perceived stress and depressive symptoms among students in three European countries. *Nutr. J.* **2009**, *8*, 31. [CrossRef] [PubMed]

47. Liu, C.; Xie, B.; Chou, C.-P.; Koprowski, C.; Zhou, D.; Palmer, P.; Sun, P.; Guo, Q.; Duan, L.; Sun, X.; et al. Perceived stress, depression and food consumption frequency in the college students of China seven cities. *Physiol. Behav.* **2007**, *92*, 748–754. [CrossRef]

48. Laugero, K.; Falcon, L.M.; Tucker, K.L. Relationship between perceived stress and dietary and activity patterns in older adults participating in the Boston Puerto Rican Health Study. *Appetite* **2010**, *56*, 194–204. [CrossRef]

49. Errisuriz, V.L.; Pasch, K.E.; Perry, C.L. Perceived stress and dietary choices: The moderating role of stress management. *Eat. Behav.* **2016**, *22*, 211–216. [CrossRef]

50. Youdim, K.A.; Qaiser, M.; Begley, D.J.; Rice-Evans, C.A.; Abbott, N.J. Flavonoid permeability across an in situ model of the blood–brain barrier. *Free Radic. Boil. Med.* **2004**, *36*, 592–604. [CrossRef]

51. Angelino, D.; Carregosa, D.; Domenech-Coca, C.; Savi, M.; Figueira, I.; Brindani, N.; Jang, S.; Lakshman, S.; Molokin, A.; Urban, J.J.F.; et al. 5-(Hydroxyphenyl)-γ-Valerolactone-Sulfate, a Key Microbial Metabolite of Flavan-3-ols, Is Able to Reach the Brain: Evidence from Different in Silico, In Vitro and In Vivo Experimental Models. *Nutrients* **2019**, *11*, 2678. [CrossRef]

52. Dias, G.P.; Cavegn, N.; Nix, A.; Bevilaqua, M.C.D.N.; Stangl, R.; Zainuddin, M.S.A.; Nardi, A.E.; Gardino, P.F.; Thuret, S. The Role of Dietary Polyphenols on Adult Hippocampal Neurogenesis: Molecular Mechanisms and Behavioural Effects on Depression and Anxiety. *Oxidative Med. Cell. Longev.* **2012**, *2012*, 541971. [CrossRef]

53. Moghadam, F.H.; Mesbah-Ardakani, M.; Esfahani, M.H.N. Ferulic Acid exerts concentration-dependent anti-apoptotic and neuronal differentiation-inducing effects in PC12 and mouse neural stem cells. *Eur. J. Pharmacol.* **2018**, *841*, 104–112. [CrossRef]

54. Kurauchi, Y.; Hisatsune, A.; Isohama, Y.; Mishima, S.; Katsuki, H. Caffeic acid phenethyl ester protects nigral dopaminergic neurons via dual mechanisms involving haem oxygenase-1 and brain-derived neurotrophic factor. *Br. J. Pharmacol.* **2012**, *166*, 1151–1168. [CrossRef]

55. Zhao, W.; Wang, J.; Bi, W.; Ferruzzi, M.G.; Yemul, S.; Freire, D.; Mazzola, P.; Ho, L.; Dubner, L.; Pasinetti, G.M. Novel application of brain-targeting polyphenol compounds in sleep deprivation-induced cognitive dysfunction. *Neurochem. Int.* **2015**, *89*, 191–197. [CrossRef]

56. Zanoli, P.; Avallone, R.; Baraldi, M. Behavioral characterisation of the flavonoids apigenin and chrysin. *Fitoterapia* **2000**, *71*, S117–S123. [CrossRef]

57. Kim, J.-W.; Kim, C.-S.; Hu, Z.; Han, J.-Y.; Kim, S.K.; Yoo, S.-K.; Yeo, Y.M.; Chong, M.S.; Lee, K.; Hong, J.T.; et al. Enhancement of pentobarbital-induced sleep by apigenin through chloride ion channel activation. *Arch. Pharmacal Res.* **2012**, *35*, 367–373. [CrossRef]

58. Fernandez, S.P.; Wasowski, C.; Paladini, A.C.; Marder, M. Synergistic interaction between hesperidin, a natural flavonoid, and diazepam. *Eur. J. Pharmacol.* **2005**, *512*, 189–198. [CrossRef]

59. Varin, C.; Rancillac, A.; Geoffroy, H.; Arthaud, S.; Fort, P.; Gallopin, T. Glucose Induces Slow-Wave Sleep by Exciting the Sleep-Promoting Neurons in the Ventrolateral Preoptic Nucleus: A New Link between Sleep and Metabolism. *J. Neurosci.* **2015**, *35*, 9900–9911. [CrossRef]

60. Garrido, J.; Gaspar, A.; Garrido, J.; Miri, R.; Tavakkoli, M.; Pourali, S.; Saso, L.; Borges, F.; Firuzi, O. Alkyl esters of hydroxycinnamic acids with improved antioxidant activity and lipophilicity protect PC12 cells against oxidative stress. *Biochimie* **2012**, *94*, 961–967. [CrossRef]

61. Tu, Y.; Cheng, S.; Sun, H.-T.; Ma, T.-Z.; Zhang, S. Ferulic acid potentiates pentobarbital-induced sleep via the serotonergic system. *Neurosci. Lett.* **2012**, *525*, 95–99. [CrossRef]

62. Ou, Q.; Zheng, Z.; Zhao, Y.; Lin, W. Impact of quercetin on systemic levels of inflammation: A meta-analysis of randomised controlled human trials. *Int. J. Food Sci. Nutr.* **2019**, *71*, 152–163. [CrossRef]

63. Rendeiro, C.; Rhodes, J.S.; Spencer, J.P. The mechanisms of action of flavonoids in the brain: Direct versus indirect effects. *Neurochem. Int.* **2015**, *89*, 126–139. [CrossRef]

64. Rehman, S.U.; Ali, T.; Alam, S.I.; Ullah, R.; Zeb, A.; Lee, K.W.; Rutten, B.P.F.; Kim, M.O. Ferulic Acid Rescues LPS-Induced Neurotoxicity via Modulation of the TLR4 Receptor in the Mouse Hippocampus. *Mol. Neurobiol.* **2018**, *56*, 2774–2790. [CrossRef] [PubMed]

65. Morroni, F.; Sita, G.; Graziosi, A.; Turrini, E.; Fimognari, C.; Tarozzi, A.; Hrelia, P. Neuroprotective Effect of Caffeic Acid Phenethyl Ester in A Mouse Model of Alzheimer's Disease Involves Nrf2/HO-1 Pathway. *Aging Dis.* **2018**, *9*, 605–622. [CrossRef] [PubMed]

66. Jung, H.W.; Mahesh, R.; Lee, J.G.; Lee, S.H.; Kim, Y.S.; Park, Y.-K. Pinoresinol from the fruits of Forsythia koreana inhibits inflammatory responses in LPS-activated microglia. *Neurosci. Lett.* **2010**, *480*, 215–220. [CrossRef]

67. Lee, K.; Kim, S.-H.; Jeong, E.; Park, J.; Kim, S.; Kim, Y.; Sung, S. New Secoisolariciresinol Derivatives fromLindera obtusilobaStems and Their Neuroprotective Activities. *Planta Med.* **2009**, *76*, 294–297. [CrossRef]

68. Rom, S.; Zuluaga-Ramirez, V.; Reichenbach, N.L.; Erickson, M.A.; Winfield, M.; Gajghate, S.; Christofidou-Solomidou, M.; Jordan-Sciutto, K.L.; Persidsky, Y. Secoisolariciresinol diglucoside is a blood-brain barrier protective and anti-inflammatory agent: Implications for neuroinflammation. *J. Neuroinflamm.* **2018**, *15*, 25. [CrossRef]

69. Yamagata, K. Do Coffee Polyphenols Have a Preventive Action on Metabolic Syndrome Associated Endothelial Dysfunctions? An Assessment of the Current Evidence. *Antioxidants* **2018**, *7*, 26. [CrossRef]

70. Godos, J.; Vitale, M.; Micek, A.; Ray, S.; Martini, D.; Del Rio, D.; Riccardi, G.; Galvano, F.; Grosso, G. Dietary Polyphenol Intake, Blood Pressure, and Hypertension: A Systematic Review and Meta-Analysis of Observational Studies. *Antioxidants* **2019**, *8*, 152. [CrossRef]

71. Behl, M.; Bliwise, D.; Veledar, E.; Cunningham, L.; Vázquez, J.; Brigham, K.; Quyyumi, A. Vascular endothelial function and self-reported sleep. *Am. J. Med. Sci.* **2014**, *347*, 425–428. [CrossRef]

72. Cooper, D.C.; Ziegler, M.G.; Milic, M.S.; Ancoli-Israel, S.; Mills, P.J.; Loredo, J.S.; Von Känel, R.; Dimsdale, J.E. Endothelial function and sleep: Associations of flow-mediated dilation with perceived sleep quality and rapid eye movement (REM) sleep. *J. Sleep Res.* **2013**, *23*, 84–93. [CrossRef]

73. Thomas, S.J.; Calhoun, D. Sleep, insomnia, and hypertension: Current findings and future directions. *J. Am. Soc. Hypertens.* **2017**, *11*, 122–129. [CrossRef]

74. Lajous, M.; Rossignol, E.; Fagherazzi, G.; Perquier, F.; Scalbert, A.; Clavel-Chapelon, F.; Boutron-Ruault, M.-C. Flavonoid intake and incident hypertension in women. *Am. J. Clin. Nutr.* **2016**, *103*, 1091–1098. [CrossRef]

75. Grosso, G.; Stepaniak, U.; Micek, A.; Kozela, M.; Stefler, D.; Bobak, M.; Pajak, A. Dietary polyphenol intake and risk of hypertension in the Polish arm of the HAPIEE study. *Eur. J. Nutr.* **2017**, *57*, 1535–1544. [CrossRef]

76. Godos, J.; Sinatra, D.; Blanco, I.; Mulè, S.; La Verde, M.; Marranzano, M. Association between Dietary Phenolic Acids and Hypertension in a Mediterranean Cohort. *Nutrients* **2017**, *9*, 1069. [CrossRef]

77. Suzuki, A.; Nomura, T.; Jokura, H.; Kitamura, N.; Saiki, A.; Fujii, A. Chlorogenic acid-enriched green coffee bean extract affects arterial stiffness assessed by the cardio-ankle vascular index in healthy men: A pilot study. *Int. J. Food Sci. Nutr.* **2019**, *70*, 901–908. [CrossRef]

78. Wang, S.; Sarriá, B.; Mateos, R.; Goya, L.; Bravo-Clemente, L. TNF-α-induced oxidative stress and endothelial dysfunction in EA.hy926 cells is prevented by mate and green coffee extracts, 5-caffeoylquinic acid and its microbial metabolite, dihydrocaffeic acid. *Int. J. Food Sci. Nutr.* **2018**, *70*, 267–284. [CrossRef]

79. Gautier-Sauvigné, S.; Colas, D.; Parmantier, P.; Clement, P.; Gharib, A.; Sarda, N.; Cespuglio, R. Nitric oxide and sleep. *Sleep Med. Rev.* **2005**, *9*, 101–113. [CrossRef]

80. Salvucci, E. The human-microbiome superorganism and its modulation to restore health. *Int. J. Food Sci. Nutr.* **2019**, *70*, 781–795. [CrossRef]

81. Ceppa, F.A.; Mancini, A.; Tuohy, K. Current evidence linking diet to gut microbiota and brain development and function. *Int. J. Food Sci. Nutr.* **2018**, *70*, 1–19. [CrossRef]

82. Mörkl, S.; Wagner-Skacel, J.; Lahousen, T.; Lackner, S.; Holasek, S.J.; Bengesser, S.A.; Painold, A.; Holl, A.K.; Reininghaus, E.Z. The Role of Nutrition and the Gut-Brain Axis in Psychiatry: A Review of the Literature. *Neuropsychobiology* **2018**, *79*, 80–88. [CrossRef]

83. Caracciolo, B.; Xu, W.; Collins, S.; Fratiglioni, L. Cognitive decline, dietary factors and gut–brain interactions. *Mech. Ageing Dev.* **2014**, *136*, 59–69. [CrossRef]

84. Tomas-Barberan, F.; Selma, M.V.; Espín, J.C. Interactions of gut microbiota with dietary polyphenols and consequences to human health. *Curr. Opin. Clin. Nutr. Metab. Care* **2016**, *19*, 471–476. [CrossRef] [PubMed]

85. , .; Taleski, V. Association between the Gut Microbiota and Obesity. *Open Access Maced. J. Med. Sci.* **2019**, *7*, 2050–2056. [CrossRef]

86. Ozdal, T.; Sela, D.A.; Ulrih, N.P.; Boyacioglu, D.; Chen, F.; Capanoglu, E. The Reciprocal Interactions between Polyphenols and Gut Microbiota and Effects on Bioaccessibility. *Nutrients* **2016**, *8*, 78. [CrossRef] [PubMed]

87. Crispi, S.; Filosa, S.; Di Meo, F. Polyphenols-gut microbiota interplay and brain neuromodulation. *Neural Regen Res.* **2018**, *13*, 2055–2059. [CrossRef] [PubMed]

88. Espín, J.C.; González-Sarrías, A.; Tomas-Barberan, F. The gut microbiota: A key factor in the therapeutic effects of (poly)phenols. *Biochem. Pharmacol.* **2017**, *139*, 82–93. [CrossRef]

89. Zhi, C.; Huang, J.; Wang, J.; Cao, H.; Bai, Y.; Guo, J.; Su, Z. Connection between gut microbiome and the development of obesity. *Eur. J. Clin. Microbiol. Infect. Dis.* **2019**, *38*, 1987–1998. [CrossRef]

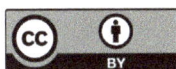

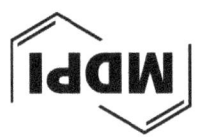

MDPI
St. Alban-Anlage 66
4052 Basel
Switzerland
Tel. +41 61 683 77 34
Fax +41 61 302 89 18
www.mdpi.com

Nutrients Editorial Office
E-mail: nutrients@mdpi.com
www.mdpi.com/journal/nutrients